Clinical Management of Infectious Diseases:

A Guide to Diagnosis and Therapy

Clinical Management of Infectious Diseases:

A Guide to Diagnosis and Therapy

Seymour I. Schlager, MD, PhD

Senior Medical Director
American Institute of Therapeutics
Lake Bluff, Illinois

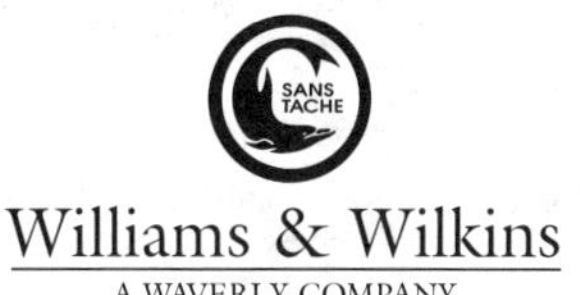

Williams & Wilkins

A WAVERLY COMPANY

BALTIMORE • PHILADELPHIA • LONDON • PARIS • BANGKOK
BUENOS AIRES • HONG KONG • MUNICH • SYDNEY • TOKYO • WROCLAW

Editor: Jonathan W. Pine, Jr.
Managing Editor: Molly L. Mullen
Marketing Manager: Peter Darcy
Project Editor: Ulita Lushnycky
Design Coordinator: Mario Fernandez

Copyright (©) 1998 Williams & Wilkins

351 West Camden Street
Baltimore, Maryland 21201-2436 USA

Rose Tree Corporate Center
1400 North Providence Road
Building II, Suite 5025
Media, Pennsylvania 19063-2043 USA

Accurate indications, adverse reactions and dosage schedules for drugs are provided in this book, but it is possible that they may change. The reader is urged to review the package information data of the manufacturers of the medications mentioned.

Printed in Canada

Library of Congress Cataloging-in-Publication Data
Schlager, Seymour I.
    Clinical management of infectious diseases : a guide to diagnosis and therapy / Seymour I. Schlager.
        p.   cm.
    Includes bibliographical references and index.
    ISBN 0-683-30568-9
    1. Communicable diseases—Handbooks, manuals, etc.   I. Title.
    [DNLM: 1. Communicable Diseases—diagnosis—handbooks.
2. Communicable Diseases—therapy—handbooks.   3. Diagnosis, Differential—handbooks.   WC 39 S338c 1998]
RC111.S367 1998
616.9—DC21
DNLM/DLC   97-50109
for Library of Congress   CIP

The publishers have made every effort to trace the copyright holders for borrowed material. If they have inadvertently overlooked any, they will be pleased to make the necessary arrangements at the first opportunity.

To purchase additional copies of this book, call our customer service department at **(800) 638-0672** or fax orders to **(800) 447-8438.** For other book services, including chapter reprints and large quantity sales, ask for the Special Sales department.

Canadian customers should call **(800) 665-1148**, or fax **(800) 665-0103.** For all other calls originating outside of the United States, please call **(410) 528-4223** or fax us at **(410) 528-8550.**

Visit Williams & Wilkins on the Internet: http://www.wwilkins.com or contact our customer service department at **custserv@wwilkins.com**. Williams & Wilkins customer service representatives are available from 8:30 am to 6:00 pm, EST, Monday through Friday, for telephone access.

98 99 00 01 02
1 2 3 4 5 6 7 8 9 10

Preface

Who among us has not faced the challenge of the patient with an infection the origin of which we could not discern? Or, once discovered, the infection whose treatment defied our best efforts? Most physicians are exposed sometime during their training to the art and science of the diagnosis and treatment of infectious diseases, but today the challenge is to do so as quickly, as effectively, and as cost-efficiently as possible. It is the challenge posed simultaneously by patients who expect their care givers to be familiar with the most cutting edge treatment, and by third-party payers who require physicians to exercise frugality.

This text was designed to aid the practicing physician in achieving a balance between carrying out a comprehensive diagnostic workup of infectious diseases and executing the appropriate treatment, while also pursuing a cost-effective, fiscally responsible management plan. In contrast to the didactic and comprehensive coverage of standard textbooks, this book provides concise and highly focused information in a practical and easy-to-use format. In adopting a telegraphic style of presentation, the clinical data are meant to be highly accessible to and user-friendly for the clinician. Grounded in an algorithmic style, the format of the material is designed to enable the reader to enter the flow of logic at any point. The user who is certain of his or her patient's diagnosis may use this text to review treatment options and the relative costs of treatment. The care giver who suspects a diagnosis may review a list of differential diagnostic options to broaden the area of consideration, even to ailments outside of infectious diseases. Perhaps, most importantly, the practitioner may use this book to move through the complete diagnostic and therapeutic algorithm to fully "work up" a patient. In that case the user may start with the patient's presenting complaints, proceed through the creation of a list of possible diagnoses, construct a reasonable plan of diagnostic tests, arrive at the most probable definitive diagnosis, and finally, select a workable and affordable treatment and follow-up plan.

In all cases, diagnostic suggestions are given in the most cost-effective order, i.e., to give the diagnostician the most likely chance to arrive at a correct diagnosis using the least expensive and least invasive tests. Similarly, differential diagnoses are presented in the order of most likely to least likely, giving the patient's presenting signs and symptoms appropriate weight. In all cases, a variety of therapeutic options is presented for each diagnostic entity. Information is available that allows the user to compare the treatment options for their relative cost and potential for causing adverse events and drug interactions.

The material is presented in 15 chapters, a Drug Index, and a comprehensive Bibliography. The first eight chapters are organized by organ system and include infectious processes that are primarily organ-specific. Chapter 9 deals with a large body of specialized infectious organisms that affect multiple organ systems, the rickettsiae, spirochetes, and a variety of parasites. Chapter 10 details the specialized problems associated with the multitude of infectious processes that are encountered in immuno-compromised hosts. Chapters 11 and 12 consider systemic microbial processes and the more serious problems of sepsis and nosocomial infections. Finally, the last three chapters provide practical information regarding immunizations, prophylactic antibiotic usage, and travel medicine; these are areas that are encountered commonly in everyday practice, but for which information is not readily available to the medical practitioner.

Within each chapter, topics are subdivided in a logical format that allows the user to find needed information quickly and easily. In some cases, material may be repeated in a somewhat different format (e.g., the discussion of pneumonias in Chapter 4: Lower Respiratory Tract; and Chapter 10: Immuno-compromised Hosts [including AIDS and malignancies]; or bacterial endocarditis in Chapter 5: Cardiac Infections and Chapter 14: Prophylaxis). The design is strictly to aid the clinician in his or her search for information.

The Drug Index contains a wealth of information. Each drug recommended in the text is characterized according to cost (by generic form and trade name), adverse reactions, drug interactions, dosage adjustments in patients with renal or hepatic impairment, and use in pregnancy.

This text is intended for a broad audience. Any medical care giver who is responsible for diagnosing and treating infectious diseases, for administering vaccinations, or for dispensing advice regarding travel to foreign lands will find this text helpful. Primary care physicians, specialists in medical or surgical disciplines, emergency medicine physicians, house staff officers, and medical students should find a friend here. Based on authoritative, up-to-date sources, yet sensitive to cost containment, this manual is designed as a practical and dependable guide for the management of infectious diseases, both common and unusual.

This manual is intended to aid in patient care in the hospital, emergency settings, the intensive care unit, and the physician's office. It can also be used as a teaching tool to help medical students organize their own logic and algorithmic thinking in the management of infectious diseases.

In this age in which the physician is simultaneously expected to be an expert in medicine and economics, this is an attempt to provide guidance in both areas.

Seymour I. Schlager, MD, PhD
Princeton, New Jersey
November 1997

Acknowledgments

This has been a labor of love and renewal. As such, there are many to thank.

To Dr. John Somberg for providing me with the atmosphere that made this work possible.

To Drs. Walid Khayr, Thomas Merigan, and John Phair for providing me with excellent critical reviews of the work.

To O. W. for believing in me and trusting me.

And to my Melinda for sharing my labor and love.

S.I.S.

Contents

Contents

- *Chlamydia* pneumonia (TWAR)
- Empyema and pleural effusion
- Lung abscess
- Cystic fibrosis
- Aspergillosis (aspergilloma of the lung)
- Blastomycosis
- Mycobacterium tuberculosis

- Infective endocarditis
- Suppurative thrombophlebitis
- Prosthetic valve endocarditis (PVE)
- Vascular graft infections
- Myocarditis
- Pericarditis
- Mediastinitis

- Esophagitis
- Peptic ulcer disease (*Helicobacter pylori* infection)
- Pseudomembranous colitis
- Inflammatory enteritides and acute diarrhea
- Enteric fever (typhoid fever)
- Foodborne infections
- Tropical sprue
- Whipple's disease
- Acute viral hepatitis
- Chronic hepatitis
- Peritonitis
- Intraperitoneal abscess
- Subphrenic abscess
- Pancreatic abscess
- Hepatic abscess

Contents

Skin and Soft Tissues

1

INFECTIONS COVERED

ABSCESSES

Presenting Symptoms:

SUBJECTIVE	OBJECTIVE
Pain	Fluctuant soft tissue
Redness	swelling surrounded
History of minor skin	by erythema
trauma	Regional
Fever may be present	lymphadenopathy
	Drainage of pus

Differential Diagnosis:

Cellulitis
Necrotizing subcutaneous infection
Furunculosis

Suggested Workup:

- Diagnosis generally made based on appearance of lesion
- Culture and Gram stain of surgical drainage: *Staphylococcus aureus* or other, depending on site

Definitive Diagnosis:

Abscess, unspecified skin site   ICD-9-CM 682.9

Suggested Treatment:

- Incision, irrigation, and drainage of the fluctuant area, followed by local heat and elevation
- Antibiotic treatment should be reserved for patients with suspected systemic infection, immunocompromised patients, or those with facial abscesses in the area drained by the cavernous sinus:
  - Dicloxacillin 500 mg orally every 6 hours for 14 days
- Penicillin allergy:
  - Erythromycin 250 to 500 mg orally every 6 hours, or

- Clindamycin 150 to 300 mg orally every 8 hours, or
- Cephalexin 250 to 500 mg orally every 6 hours for 14 days
- For more serious infections:
  - Cefuroxime 1.5 g intravenously (IV)/ intramuscularly every 8 hours for 7 days, or
  - Cefazolin 1 g IV every 8 hours for 7 days, or
  - Nafcillin 1 g IV every 6 hours for 7 days, or
  - Vancomycin 1 g IV every 12 hours for 7 days, then switch to oral therapy as above

Follow-Up:

- Standard monitoring following incision, irrigation, and drainage
- **Watch for:** signs and symptoms of
  - Reaccumulation of pus
  - Loculation
  - Systemic infection
  - Lymphangitic spread of infection

ACNE ROSACEA

Presenting Symptoms:

SUBJECTIVE	OBJECTIVE
Skin flush around nose, forehead, and cheeks	Erythema around affected areas
	Blood vessels prominent in affected area—collapse under pressure
	Acneiform lesions forming papules, pustules, and nodules

Telangiectasis
Rhinophyma
(occasionally)
NO comedones

Differential Diagnosis:

Drug eruptions
Granulomatous lesions
Cutaneous lupus erythematosus
Carcinoid syndrome
Fungal infection
Acne vulgaris
Seborrheic dermatitis

Suggested Workup:

- Diagnosis typically made on the basis of appearance
- Skin biopsy rarely indicated

Definitive Diagnosis:

Rosacea   ICD-9-CM 695.3

Suggested Treatment:

Doxycycline 100 mg orally every 12 hours during exacerbations, and
Metronidazole 0.75% gel applied topically 2 times a day, or
Erythromycin 2% gel applied topically 2 times a day, or
Clindamycin 1% solution applied topically 2 times a day

Follow-Up:

- Periodic monitoring, especially during exacerbations
- **Watch for:** signs and symptoms of
    - Rhinophyma (especially in men)
    - Conjunctivitis
    - Blepharitis
    - Keratitis

ACNE VULGARIS

Presenting Symptoms:

SUBJECTIVE	OBJECTIVE
"Pimples" on face, shoulders, chest, and/or back	Closed comedones (whiteheads)
	Open comedones (blackheads)
	Nodules or papules
	Pustules, with or without erythema
	Oiliness and thickening of the affected skin

Differential Diagnosis:

Folliculitis
Contact dermatitis
Acne rosacea
Steroid acne

Suggested Workup:

Diagnosis is made on the basis of history and physical examination

Definitive Diagnosis:

Acne vulgaris   ICD-9-CM 706.1

Suggested Treatment:

Tetracycline 250 mg orally 4 times a day for 7 to 10 days, followed by a taper to the lowest effective dose, or

Erythromycin 250 mg orally 4 times a day for 7 to 10 days, followed by a taper to the lowest effective dose,

and/or

Metronidazole 0.75% gel applied topically every 12 hours, or

Erythromycin 1% gel applied topically every 12 hours, or

Clindamycin 1% solution applied topically every
day (the topical antibiotics are most effective
against cystic lesions and can be used as
required on a rotating basis to reduce the
likelihood of development of resistance)

Follow-Up:

- Follow monthly until adequate clinical
  response is observed
- **Watch for:** signs and symptoms of
    - Acne conglobata (severe
      confluent inflammatory acne
      with systemic symptoms)
    - Facial scarring
    - Psychosocial problems

CELLULITIS

Presenting Symptoms:

SUBJECTIVE	OBJECTIVE
Involved area is red, hot, and swollen	Area of swelling, heat, and erythema
Malaise	Borders not elevated or demarcated
Fever and chills	demarcated
Itching (facial cellulitis)	Regional lymphadenopathy
Foul-smelling drainage from site (dissecting cellulitis of scalp)	

Differential Diagnosis:

Acute gout or pseudogout
Fasciitis or myositis
Mycotic infection
Ruptured Baker's cyst
Physical trauma
Impetigo
Thrombophlebitis

Osteomyelitis
Herpetic whitlow
Cutaneous diphtheria
Erysipelas

Suggested Workup:

- Physical examination
  - Raised and demarcated border of erythema?
    - ____Y: consider impetigo
    - ____N: consider cellulitis
  - Bullae?
    - ____Y: consider pemphigus/pemphigoid or erysipelas
    - ____N: consider cellulitis
  - Crusting?
    - ____Y: consider erysipelas or impetigo
    - ____N: consider cellulitis
  - Vesicles?
    - ____Y: consider erysipelas, impetigo, or herpes infection
    - ____N: consider cellulitis
- Aspirate point of maximum inflammation for Gram stain and culture (45% positive culture rate):
  - *S. aureus*
  - Group A *Streptococcus*
  - *Haemophilus influenzae*
- Skin biopsy for difficult cases: Dermal eosinophilia with inflammatory changes (will rule out mycotic or viral infection)
- Plain radiograph: soft tissue changes with bubbles (gas-forming cellulitis only)

Definitive Diagnosis:

Cellulitis   ICD-9-CM 682.9 (code may change if an anatomical site is specified)

Suggested Treatment:

- Mild, early infection (suspected *Streptococcus* etiology or no clues to etiology):
  - Dicloxacillin 500 mg orally every 6 hours for 14 days
  - Penicillin allergy: Erythromycin 500 mg orally every 6 hours for 14 days
- Severe infection:
  - Nafcillin 1 to 1.5 g IV every 4 hours for 10 to 14 days
  - Penicillin allergy: Vancomycin 1 g IV every 12 hours for 10 to 14 days
- Gram-negative infections:
  - Gentamicin 3 to 5 mg/kg/day IV given every 8 hours for 10 to 14 days, plus
  - Nafcillin 1 g IV every 6 hours for 10 to 14 days
  - Penicillin allergy: Erythromycin 1 g IV every 6 hours for 10 to 14 days (in place of nafcillin)
- Rapidly progressing cellulitis (especially after a fresh water injury):
  - Nafcillin or erythromycin plus gentamicin as above
- Cellulitis following a human bite:
  - Amoxicillin-clavulanic acid 500/125 mg orally every 8 hours for 10 to 14 days
  - Penicillin allergy: Erythromycin 500 mg orally every 8 hours for 10 to 14 days, or Doxycycline 100 mg orally every 12 hours for 10 to 14 days
- Cellulitis following an animal bite:
  - Nafcillin 1 g IV every 4 hours for 7 days, then
  - Nafcillin 500 mg orally every 6 hours for 10 to 14 days

- Penicillin allergy: Cefoxitin 1 g IV every 4 hours for 7 days, then Erythromycin 500 mg orally every 8 hours for 10 to 14 days
- Facial cellulitis (*H. influenzae* etiology suspected or confirmed):
  - Cefotaxime 1 to 2 g IV every 6 hours for 7 days, then
  - Ampicillin 500 mg orally every 6 hours for 10 to 14 days, or
  - Penicillin allergy: Erythromycin 500 mg orally every 8 hours for 10 to 14 days
- Gas-forming cellulitis:
  - PCN G 5 million units (U) IV every 6 hours for 10 to 14 days, then
  - PCN V 500 mg orally every 6 hours for 14 to 21 days, or
  - Penicillin allergy: Metronidazole 500 mg IV every 6 hours, plus
    Clindamycin 600 mg IV every 8 hours for 10 to 14 days, then
    Clindamycin 300 to 600 mg orally every 8 hours, or
    Erythromycin 500 mg orally every 8 hours for 14 to 21 days
- Cellulitis in a diabetic patient:
  - Mild-moderate:
    Cefoxitin 1 to 2 g IV every 6 hours for 10 to 14 days, or
    Ampicillin + sulbactam 1 to 2 g IV every 6 hours for 10 to 14 days
  - Toxic-appearing:
    Clindamycin 600 mg IV every 8 hours, plus
    Gentamicin 3 to 5 mg/kg/day given every 8 hours for 10 to 14 days
- Cellulitis in an intravenous drug abuser:
  - Vancomycin 0.5 to 1.0 g IV every 12 hours, plus

- Gentamicin 3 to 5 mg/kg/day IV given every 8 hours for 10 to 14 days
- Cellulitis in an immunocompromised host:
  - Clindamycin 300 mg IV every 8 hours, plus
  - Gentamicin 3 to 5 mg/kg/day IV given every 8 hours for 14 to 21 days
- Cellulitis in a burn patient:
  - Vancomycin 0.5 to 1.0 g IV every 12 hours, plus Gentamicin 3 to 5 mg/kg/day IV given every 8 hours for 10 to 14 days

Follow-Up:

- Blood culture at the end of treatment to ensure cure
- Repeat needle aspirate for culture
- **Watch for:** signs and symptoms of
  - Recurrent cellulitis
  - Bacteremia and sepsis/shock
  - Meningitis (especially in children with facial cellulitis)
  - Local abscess formation
  - Superinfection with Gram-negative organisms
  - Lymphangitis
  - Thrombophlebitis of lower extremities (especially in older patients)
  - Gas formation and gangrene
  - Glomerulonephritis (after Group A *Streptococcus*)

FOLLICULITIS

Presenting Symptoms:

SUBJECTIVE	OBJECTIVE
Painful, red ''bumps'' around hairs,	Yellow or gray pustules surrounded

growing in any part of the body

Most common on face, limbs, or scalp

No systemic symptoms or fever

Pruritus (occasionally)

by erythema and pierced by a hair

Lesions are commonly grouped

Differential Diagnosis:

Pseudofolliculitis barbae
Keratosis pilaris
Contact dermatitis
Tinea
Acne
Pustular miliaria
Flat warts
Molluscum contagiosum

Suggested Workup:

- History and physical examination usually reveal pathognomonic findings
- Scraping of area for Gram stain and culture: Gram-positive cocci
- Potassium hydroxide (KOH) preparation to rule out mycotic infection
- Biopsy in resistant cases or if diagnosis is in doubt

Definitive Diagnosis:

Folliculitis   ICD-9-CM 704.8

Suggested Treatment:

- Inflammation without infection:
    - Cleanse with antibacterial soap
    - Apply moist heat to affected area 2 to 3 times a day as needed
    - Avoid exposure to causative factors
- Inflammation with suspected infection of unknown etiology:

- • Mupirocin 2% ointment topically 3 times a day for 10 days
- *S. aureus* infection suspected or confirmed:
  - • Dicloxacillin 250 mg orally every 6 hours for 10 days
  - • Penicillin allergy: Erythromycin 250 mg orally every 6 hours for 10 days
- *Pseudomonas aeruginosa* infection suspected or confirmed:
  - • Ciprofloxacin 500 mg orally 2 times a day for 10 days, or
  - • Ofloxacin 400 mg orally 2 times a day for 10 days

Follow-Up:

- Recheck in 2 weeks for clinical improvement
- Resistant cases should be followed every 2 weeks until cleared
- **Watch for:** signs and symptoms of
  - • Furunculosis
  - • Carbuncle formation with subcutaneous suppuration
  - • Superficial abscess
  - • Mycotic infection
  - • Underlying immunodeficiency or diabetes (in severe or resistant cases)

FURUNCULOSIS/CARBUNCLES

Presenting Symptoms:

SUBJECTIVE	OBJECTIVE
Painful red nodules	Erythematous,
Central pustule	perifollicular
Located in hirsute	swelling
areas only	Papules or nodules:
No systemic symptoms	1 to 5 cm

No fever

Pustular discharge from necrotic plug

Differential Diagnosis:

Folliculitis
Pseudofolliculitis
Carbuncles
Ruptured epidermal cyst
Hidradenitis suppurativa

Suggested Workup:

- Physical examination is often pathognomonic: 1 to 5 cm nodules on the neck, breasts, face, buttocks, later becoming pustules 5 to 30 mm in diameter, with central necrosis and discharging a core of necrotic tissue and sanguineous purulent exudate. Especially suspicious in areas prone to minor friction (underneath belt; on anterior thighs)
- History is helpful: most common in teenagers and young adults; uncommon in children
- Collect exudate for Gram stain and culture: *S. aureus*

Definitive Diagnosis:

Furunculosis/carbuncle   ICD-9-CM 680.9

Suggested Treatment:

- Local, topical care:
  - Moist, warm compresses for 30 minutes 4 times a day
  - Incise and drain large, fluctuant or pointing lesions
- Systemic antibiotics usually reserved for:
  - Furuncles in the nose or central facial area,
  - Fever, or
  - Extensive surrounding cellulitis

- Treat with:
    Dicloxacillin 250 mg orally 4 times a day
      for 14 days
    Penicillin allergy: Erythromycin 250 to
      500 mg orally 3 times a day for
      14 days
- Recurrent/persistent infections:
  - As with systemic antibiotics above for 1 to
    3 months
  - May add rifampin 600 mg orally once daily
    for 10 days
  - Culture nares, skin, axilla, perineum to
    detect pathogenic strain of *S. aureus:* treat
    on the basis of antibiotic sensitivity testing
    after culture

Follow-Up:

- Acute infections are self-limiting and should
  resolve with compresses alone
- Recurrent infections need to be cultured
- Patient education regarding self-care and
  sanitary practices
- **Watch for:** signs and symptoms of
  - Scarring
  - Bacteremia
  - Seeding of remote sites (e.g.,
    prosthetic or defective heart
    valves, arthritic or artificial
    joints)

IMPETIGO

Presenting Symptoms:

SUBJECTIVE	OBJECTIVE
Red, tender nodule on arms, legs, or face	Superficial, vesiculopustular
Rapid spread	eruption that may

Weeping shallow red ulcer
Honey-colored crusts
Blistering, especially on buttocks, trunk, and face
Concentrated around mouth
include lesions at different stages of the infection:
—Erythematous tender papule
—Bullae or vesicles
—Honey-colored crusts

Differential Diagnosis:

Nonbullous eruption
—Chickenpox
—Herpes
—Folliculitis
—Erysipelas
—Insect bite
—Eczematous dermatitis
—Scabies
—Tinea corporis
Bullous eruption
—Burn
—Pemphigus vulgaris
—Bullous pemphigoid
—Stevens-Johnson syndrome

Suggested Workup:

- Diagnosis is usually based on clinical findings (as above)
- History is also very revealing: especially prevalent in 2- to 5-year-olds, living in a warm, humid environment, with poor hygiene, and after minor trauma to skin or insect bite
- Collect exudate from weeping ulcer or unroof crust to sample base of lesion for Gram stain and culture: coagulase-positive *Staphylococcus;* Beta-hemolytic *Streptococcus*

Definitive Diagnosis:

Impetigo   ICD-9-CM 684

Suggested Treatment:

- For most infections without bullous eruption: Mupirocin 2% ointment topically 3 times a day for 7 to 10 days
- For more serious infections (especially with bullous disease) and patients showing no response to mupirocin after 3 to 5 days of treatment:
  - Amoxicillin/clavulanate
    - —Adult: 250 mg orally 3 times a day for 10 days
    - —Pediatric: 20 to 40 mg/kg/day of amoxicillin orally given every 8 hours for 10 days, or
  - Cephalexin
    - —Adult: 250 mg orally 4 times a day for 10 days
    - —Pediatric: 25 to 50 mg/kg/day orally given every 6 hours for 10 days, or
  - Cefaclor
    - —Adult: 250 mg orally 3 times a day for 10 days
    - —Pediatric: 20 to 40 mg/kg/day orally given every 8 hours for 10 days, or
  - Cephradine
    - —Adult: 500 mg orally 2 times a day for 10 days
    - —Pediatric: 25 to 50 mg/kg/day orally given every 6 to 12 hours for 10 days
  - Penicillin allergy: Should be treated with cephalexin as above, NOT erythromycin (up to 40% of coagulase-positive *Staphylococcus* are resistant to erythromycin)

Follow-Up:

- Follow carefully for 7 to 10 days; if not clinically clear, culture the lesions
- Provide patient education regarding good family and personal hygiene, especially hand washing
- **Watch for:** signs and symptoms of
    - Ecthyma (ulcerative impetigo)
    - Erysipelas
    - Post-streptococcal acute glomerulonephritis (may occur even with appropriate antibiotic treatment)
    - Deep cellulitis
    - Bacteremia

ERYSIPELAS

Presenting Symptoms:

SUBJECTIVE	OBJECTIVE
Prodrome of malaise, fever, and chills	Patchy erythema with a raised, sharply demarcated border
Headache	Desquamation
Vomiting	Vesicle formation
Arthralgias	Fever
Pruritus	Facial redness
Fever	

Differential Diagnosis:

Erysipeloid
Contact dermatitis
Angioneurotic edema
Scarlet fever
Herpes zoster
Lupus
Polychondritis of the ear
Dermatophytid
Tuberculoid leprosy

Suggested Workup:

- Physical examination
  - Erythema with raised, sharply demarcated border?
    - ____Y: erysipelas
    - ____N: cellulitis, impetigo, furunculosis all possible
- Fever?
  - ____Y: erysipelas
  - ____N: consider mild cellulitis, impetigo, contact dermatitis, angioneurotic edema
- Antinuclear antibody (ANA)-positive?
  - ____Y: consider lupus
  - ____N: consider erysipelas
- Antistreptolysin-positive?
  - ____Y: erysipelas likely
  - ____N: erysipelas unlikely
- Dermatomal distribution?
  - ____Y: herpes zoster likely (confirm with Tzanck test)
  - ____N: erysipelas likely
- Blood culture: Group A beta-hemolytic *Streptococcus* → erysipelas
- Collect exudate from vesicle for Gram stain and culture: Group A beta-hemolytic *Streptococcus* → erysipelas

Definitive Diagnosis:

Erysipelas   ICD-9-CM 035

Suggested Treatment:

- Typical cases:
  - PCN VK
    - —Adult: 250 to 500 mg orally every 6 hours for 10 to 14 days
    - —Pediatric: 25 to 50 mg/kg/day orally given every 6 hours for 10 to 14 days

- Penicillin allergy:
  - —Adult: Erythromycin 250 mg orally every 6 hours for 10 to 14 days
  - —Pediatric: Erythromycin 30 to 40 mg/kg/day orally given every 6 hours for 10 to 14 days
- Severe or complicated cases:
  - PCN G
    - —Adult: 1.2 mill U IV every 6 hours for 3 to 4 days, then PCN VK orally as above
    - —Pediatric: PCN G 40,000 U/kg/day IV given every 6 hours for 3 to 4 days, then PCN VK orally as above
  - Penicillin allergy:
    - —Adult: Erythromycin 1 g IV every 6 hours for 3 to 4 days, then 500 mg orally every 8 hours for 10 to 14 days
    - —Pediatric: Erythromycin 15 to 20 mg/kg/day IV given every 6 hours, then 30 to 40 mg/kg/day orally given every 6 hours for 10 to 14 days

Follow-Up:

- Patients should be treated and followed until all symptoms and skin manifestations have resolved
- If infection is recurrent, work up other possible sources of *Streptococcus* infection:
  - Tonsils
  - Sinuses
  - Teeth
- **Watch for:** signs and symptoms of
  - Bacteremia/sepsis
  - Scarlet fever
  - Pneumonia
  - Abscess
  - Embolism

- Gangrene
- Meningitis
- Post–streptococcal glomerulonephritis

HUMAN OR ANIMAL BITES

Presenting Symptoms:

SUBJECTIVE	OBJECTIVE
History of human or animal bite	Bite wound with erythema and other indicia of inflammation
Pain and redness at bite site	
Fever and chills	Regional lymphadenopathy
Malaise	
Headache	

Differential Diagnosis:

History makes differential diagnosis unnecessary

Suggested Workup:

- History and appearance are pathognomonic
- Blood culture:
  - *S. aureus* and *Eikenella* → human bite
  - *S. aureus, Pasteurella multocida, Capnocytophaga canimorsus*, anaerobes → cat/dog bite
  - *Streptococcus moniliformis, Spirillum minus* → rat bite

Definitive Diagnosis:

Wound, open, unspecified site, bite	ICD-9-CM 879.8
As above, with complications	ICD-9-CM 879.9

Suggested Treatment:

- Amoxicillin-clavulanate 500 mg orally every 8 hours for 14 days, or PCN V 1 to 2 g/day orally given every 6 hours for 14 days

- Penicillin allergy: Tetracycline 500 mg orally every 6 hours for 14 days, or Cephalexin 500 mg orally every 6 hours for 14 days
- For animal bites, add:
  - Rabies prophylaxis with anti-rabies vaccine and rabies immune globulin (RIG):
  - Postexposure rabies vaccine should be given as 1.0 mL of reconstituted vaccine intramuscularly in deltoid muscle on days 0, 3, 7, 14, 30, and 90.
  - RIG given as 20 international units (IU)/kg intramuscularly at the wound site and/or in gluteal region, concomitantly with first vaccine dose; it may be repeated through the seventh day of vaccine treatment.
  - **NOTE: Vaccine and RIG should be given at *separate sites***
- For all bites, add:
  - Tetanus prophylaxis with tetanus toxoid and tetanus immune globulin (TIG):
  - A single injection of 0.5 mL tetanus toxoid is given intramuscularly in deltoid muscle or the anterolateral aspect of upper thigh, only in patients who have not received a tetanus booster in the past 10 years.
  - TIG is unnecessary in patients who have sustained clean, minor wounds. It may be given to patients with more serious wounds and/or patients with uncertain tetanus toxoid immunization histories or who have received less than three previous tetanus immunizations.
  - TIG 250 U is given by deep intramuscular injection into the deltoid muscle or the anterolateral aspect of the upper thigh.
  - **NOTE: Tetanus toxoid and TIG should be given at *separate sites*, and NOT in the**

gluteal region for fear of damage to the sciatic nerve

Follow-Up:

- Patients should be followed closely until wound healing occurs and all immunizations are completed
- **Watch for:** signs and symptoms of
    - Bacteremia and sepsis
    - Wound superinfections with Gram-negative bacteria or mycotic infections
    - Tetanus
    - Rabies

CAT-SCRATCH DISEASE

Presenting Symptoms:

SUBJECTIVE	OBJECTIVE
Papule or pimple at the site of a cat scratch	Erythematous, crusted papule or pustule, 2 to 6 mm
Fever	Regional lymphadenopathy
Malaise	Lymph nodes may be firm, or fluctuant with drainage
Headache	Parinaud's oculoglandular syndrome (a unilateral granulomatous conjunctivitis associated with a visibly enlarged and tender ipsilateral preauricular or
Anorexia	

submandibular
lymph node)

Differential Diagnosis:

Cellulitis
Mycotic infection (especially sporotrichosis)
Erysipelas

Suggested Workup:

- History of cat contact and physical examination findings as above are highly suggestive
- Cat-scratch skin test: if positive, confirms diagnosis
- Biopsy skin site or lymph node in difficult cases:
    - Granuloma formation?
        ____Y: cat scratch likely
        ____N: cat scratch less likely
    - Presence of *Rickettsia, Rochalimaea, Bartonella henselae, Bartonella quintana?*
        ____Y: cat-scratch confirmed
        ____N: look for other etiologies

Definitive Diagnosis:

Cat-scratch disease   ICD-9-CM 078.3

Suggested Treatment:

- Most patients with mild disease:
    - Local warm compresses and analgesics
    - No antibiotics warranted
- For persistent disease, there is anecdotal, but not universally accepted, evidence for the use of:
    - Ciprofloxacin 500 mg orally 2 times a day for 10 to 14 days, or
    - Doxycycline 100 mg orally every 12 hours for 10 to 14 days

- Fluctuant lymph node: Incision and drainage
- Disseminated or life-threatening illness:
  - Gentamicin 5 mg/kg/day IV given every 8 hours for 10 to 14 days, or
  - Cefoxitin 1 g IV every 4 hours for 10 to 14 days

Follow-Up:

- Most cases resolve completely without recurrence, especially where antibiotics are used
- Close monitoring required only where infection is resistant or recurrent, and lymph node pain and sinus drainage are present
- **Watch for:** signs and symptoms of
  - Systemic disease and sepsis
  - Parinaud's granulomatous conjunctivitis
  - Lymph node sinus or abscess formation

BURNS

Presenting Symptoms:

SUBJECTIVE	OBJECTIVE
History	First-Degree:
	—Erythema of involved tissue
	—Skin blanches with pressure
	—Skin may be tender
	—Partial thickness: only superficial layers of epidermis involved
	—Full thickness does not occur

Second-Degree:
—Skin is red and
  blistered
—Skin is very tender
—Partial thickness:
  involves varying
  degrees of epidermis
  and part of dermis
Third-Degree:
—Burned skin is tough
  and leathery
—Skin is not tender
—Partial thickness
  does not occur
—Full thickness:
  destruction of all
  skin elements with
  coagulation of
  subdermal plexus

Differential Diagnosis:

Toxic epidermal necrolysis
Scalded skin syndrome

Suggested Workup:

- Careful physical examination to determine degree and thickness of burn as per criteria above
- Electrolytes, blood urea nitrogen (BUN), hematocrit (HCT), type and cross, blood glucose
- Arterial blood gas for carboxyhemoglobin if smoke inhalation is suspected (xenon scan may be necessary to confirm)
- Chest radiograph
- Electrocardiogram (ECG), urine myoglobin, creatine kinase (CK) isoenzymes if electric burn is suspected

- Accurate estimate of percent of body surface area (BSA) involved:
  - Each upper extremity = 9% (adult and child)
  - Each lower extremity = 18% (adult) or 14% (child)
  - Anterior trunk = 18% (adult and child)
  - Posterior trunk = 18% (adult and child)
  - Head and neck = 10% (adult) or 18% (child)
  - For smaller burns, surface area of patient's hand represents approximately 1% of his or her BSA

Definitive Diagnosis:

Burn, otherwise unspecified	ICD-9-CM 949.0
—First-degree	ICD-9-CM 949.1
—Second-degree	ICD-9-CM 949.2
—Third-degree	ICD-9-CM 949.3
Burn, extent to be specified:	
—less than 10% BSA	ICD-9-CM 948.0
—10% to 19%	ICD-9-CM 948.1
—20% to 29%	ICD-9-CM 948.2
—30% to 39%	ICD-9-CM 948.3
—40% to 49%	ICD-9-CM 948.4
—50% to 59%	ICD-9-CM 948.5
—60% to 69%	ICD-9-CM 948.6
—70% to 79%	ICD-9-CM 948.7
—80% to 89%	ICD-9-CM 948.8
—more than 90% BSA	ICD-9-CM 948.9

Suggested Treatment:

- Hospitalization in a burn center is required for:
  - Second-degree burns over 10% BSA, or
  - Any third-degree burn, or
  - Burns of hands, feet, face, or perineum, or
  - Electrical or lightning burns, or

- Inhalation injury, or
- Chemical burns, or
- Circumferential burns
- General measures:
  - Remove all jewelry from affected extremities to prevent tourniquet effect
  - Flush areas of chemical burns for approximately 2 hours
  - Twice daily dressing changes
  - Surgical debridement with or without hydrotherapy
- Mild to moderate burns in nonhospitalized patients:
  - Apply 1% silver sulfadiazine cream topically twice a day and as needed, or
  - Mafenide acetate cream topically 2 times a day and as needed to keep burn covered, and
  - Dicloxacillin 500 mg orally every 6 hours for 10 to 14 days
  - Penicillin allergy: Clindamycin 150 to 300 mg orally every 8 hours for 10 to 14 days, and
  - Tetanus toxoid 0.5 mL intramuscularly in deltoid muscle or in anterolateral aspect of upper thigh
- Severe to serious burns in hospitalized patients:
  - Oxygen (100%)
  - Consider early intubation
  - Foley catheter
  - Nasogastric tube
  - Pain relief (intravenous ℞meperidine [™Demerol] or morphine)
  - Fluid resuscitation: generally, 2 to 4 mL Ringer's lactate × body weight (kg) × % BSA of burn, half given over the first 8 hours, and the rest over the next 16 hours

- Whirlpool hydrotherapy
- Apply 1% silver sulfadiazine cream topically twice a day, or mafenide acetate cream topically 2 times a day after hydrotherapy
- Other surgical therapy as needed (e.g., escharotomy and/or skin grafts)
- If suspect *Pseudomonas* superinfection:
  - —Ticarcillin-clavulanate 3 g IV every 6 hours, or
  - —Piperacillin + tazobactam 3 g piperacillin IV every 6 hours, or
  - —Ceftazidime 3 to 6 g/day IV given every 8 hours, or
  - —Imipenem 1 to 4 g/day IV given every 6 hours, or
  - —Vancomycin 1 to 2 g IV every 12 hours, and
  - —Gentamicin 3 to 5 mg/kg/day IV given every 8 hours, all for 10 to 14 days, or
  - —Aztreonam 2 g IV every 8 hours for 10 to 14 days
- Tetanus toxoid as above

Follow-Up:

- According to extent of burn and treatment:
  - First-degree: expect complete resolution with little or no complications
  - Second-degree: follow carefully until re-epithelialization occurs or skin grafts are viable
  - Third-degree: no potential for re-epithelialization; skin graft will be required, as well as intensive care unit (ICU) care depending on extent of burn, smoke inhalation, and age
- **Watch for:** signs and symptoms of
  - Gastroduodenal ulceration (Curling's ulcer)

- Squamous cell carcinoma in old burn site (Marjolin's ulcer)
- Gram negative sepsis
- Pneumonia
- Flexion contractures (preventable with early mobilization)
- Malnutrition (preventable with nasogastric feedings or total parenteral nutrition [TPN] as needed)

ANAEROBIC AND NECROTIZING INFECTIONS

Presenting Symptoms:

SUBJECTIVE	OBJECTIVE
Local pain	Involvement of subcutaneous soft tissues and superficial or deep fascia
Swelling	
Bluish, greenish, or black discoloration of skin	
	Acute, rapidly progressive process
Fever	
Rapid pulse	Involvement is usually of the extremities, but can occur anywhere on the body (especially abdominal wall, perianal and groin areas, and postoperative wounds)
Malaise	
Malodorous discharge from affected site	
	History of trauma (laceration, abrasion, burn, insect bite) or

surgical procedure
with or without a
penetrated viscus
Affected area is
initially:
—Erythematous,
changing to red-
purple and
eventually to
blue-gray
—Swollen without
sharp margins
—Hot
—Shiny
—Exquisitely tender
Over 3 to 5 days,
affected area:
—Develops frank skin
breakdown with
fluid-filled bullae
—Cutaneous gangrene
appears
—No longer
painful—anesthesia
develops because of
nerve destruction
Subcutaneous gas is
often present, seen
as a superficial or
deep fluctuance or
crepitance
Blunt probing of the
lesion allows easy
passage of the
instrument along
fascial planes
(pathognomonic)

Fever and systemic
toxicity are typical
Marked regional
lymphangitis

Differential Diagnosis:

Gas gangrene
Postoperative clostridial infection of muscle and
soft tissues
Clostridial myonecrosis
Clostridial myositis
Anaerobic streptococcal infection of muscle and
soft tissues
Necrotizing cellulitis
Hemolytic streptococcal gangrene
Acute, infectious staphylococcal gangrene
Anaerobic cellulitis
Crepitant phlegmon
Clostridial cellulitis
Necrotizing fasciitis
Anaerobic cutaneous gangrene
Synergistic necrotizing cellulitis
Fournier's gangrene
Perineal phlegmon
Clostridial contamination of a wound (traumatic
or surgical)
Pneumogranuloma (especially common after
industrial accidents)
Infected vascular gangrene

Suggested Workup:

- Collection of exudate/discharge from lesions
  for Gram stain and culture and antibiotic
  sensitivity; presence of these organisms
  suggests anaerobic/necrotizing infections
  rather than a simple cellulitis:
  - Gram-positive cocci = *Peptostreptococcus*
    (anaerobic *Streptococcus*), *Streptococcus*

> *pyogenes*, Group A beta-hemolytic *Streptococcus*
> - Gram-positive bacilli = *Clostridia*, especially *C. perfringens*
> - Gram-negative aerobic bacilli = *Escherichia coli, Klebsiella pneumoniae, Enterobacter, Proteus*
> - Gram-negative anaerobic bacilli = *Bacteroides fragilis*

- Blood cultures (aerobic and anaerobic)
- Plain radiographs of affected areas: gas in tissues
- Magnetic resonance imaging (MRI): edema and subcutaneous gas
- Surgical exploration of skin, fascia, and muscles: look for necrotic tissue—confirms diagnosis

CRITERIA FOR ESTABLISHING DIAGNOSIS AMONG CONDITIONS INCLUDED IN THE DIFFERENTIAL DIAGNOSIS ABOVE

- **Clostridial cellulitis:**
  - Occurs after local trauma or surgery
  - Incubation usually longer than 3 days
  - Gradual onset
  - Mild pain with moderate swelling
  - Minimal discoloration of skin
  - Thin, dark, foul exudate
  - Gas + + + +
  - Minimal systemic toxicity
  - No muscle involvement
- **Nonclostridial anaerobic cellulitis:**
  - Occurs in diabetics and after localized infection
  - Incubation over several days
  - Gradual or rapid onset
  - Mild pain with moderate swelling
  - Minimal discoloration of skin

- Dark, foul pus exudate
- Gas $++++$
- Moderate systemic toxicity
- No muscle involvement
- **Gas gangrene:**
  - Occurs after local trauma or surgery
  - Incubation over 1 to 2 days
  - Acute onset
  - Marked pain and swelling
  - Skin is yellow-bronze with dark bullae and green-black patches of necrosis
  - Serosanguinous exudate that may be foul or sweet
  - Gas $++$
  - Marked systemic toxicity
  - Muscle involvement $++++$
- **Streptococcal myositis:**
  - Occurs after local trauma
  - Incubation over 3 to 4 days
  - Acute onset
  - Marked pain with moderate swelling
  - Erythematous skin
  - Abundant seropurulent exudate with a slightly sour odor
  - Gas $\pm$
  - Systemic toxicity late in course of infection
  - Muscle involvement $+++$
- **Necrotizing fasciitis:**
  - Occurs after abdominal surgery, perineal infections in diabetics and obese patients (Fournier's gangrene)
  - Incubation over 1 to 4 days
  - Acute onset
  - Moderate/severe pain with marked swelling
  - Erythematous cellulitis with areas of skin necrosis

- • Seropurulent, foul exudate
- • Gas + +
- • Moderate/marked systemic toxicity
- • No muscle involvement
- **Infected vascular gangrene:**
  - • Occurs in patients with peripheral arterial insufficiency
  - • Incubation over more than 5 days
  - • Gradual onset
  - • Variable amount of pain with moderate/ marked swelling
  - • Skin discolored or black
  - • No exudate
  - • Gas + + +
  - • Minimal systemic toxicity
  - • Muscle involvement severe: dead muscle
- **Synergistic necrotizing cellulitis:**
  - • Occurs in diabetics, patients with cardiorenal disease, obesity, and/or perirectal infections
  - • Incubation over 3 to 14 days
  - • Acute onset
  - • Severe pain with moderate/marked swelling
  - • Scattered areas of skin necrosis
  - • Dishwater-appearing pus with foul odor
  - • Marked systemic toxicity
  - • Muscle involvement + +

Definitive Diagnosis:

Gangrene (unspecified site)	ICD-9-CM 785.4
Gas gangrene (unspecified site)	ICD-9-CM 040.0
Phlegmon (cellulitis and abscess at unspecified site)	ICD-9-CM 682.9
Necrotizing fasciitis	ICD-9-CM 608.83

Suggested Treatment:

- Surgical exploration:
  - Debridement of necrotic tissue or radical excision depending on degree of involvement
  - Drainage of pus
  - Exploration to determine extent of tissue and muscle involvement
- Mixed aerobic/anaerobic infection (90% of cases):
  - Ceftriaxone 2 to 4 g/day IV given every 24 hours, and
  - Clindamycin 900 mg IV every 8 hours for 14 to 21 days
- Gram-positive cocci or bacteria:
  - Select the best agent on the basis of antibiotic sensitivity testing:
  - PCN G 3 to 5 million U IV every 6 hours for 14 to 21 days, or
  - Clindamycin 600 mg IV every 8 hours for 14 to 21 days, or
  - Metronidazole 500 mg IV every 6 hours for 14 to 21 days, or
  - Cefazolin 1 g IV every 8 hours for 14 days
- Gram-negative bacilli (*Bacteroides*):
  - Select the best agent on the basis of antibiotic sensitivity testing:
  - Clindamycin 600 mg IV every 8 hours for 14 to 21 days, or
  - Metronidazole 500 mg IV every 6 hours for 14 to 21 days, or
  - Cefoxitin 1 g IV every 4 hours for 14 to 21 days (be careful, as many *B. fragilis* are resistant), or
  - Ticarcillin 1 to 2 g IV every 4 hours for 14 to 21 days, or

- Mezlocillin 1 to 2 g IV every 4 hours for 14 to 21 days
- Gram-negative coliforms:
  - Select the best agent on the basis of antibiotic sensitivity testing:
  - Gentamicin 3 to 5 mg/kg/day IV given every 8 hours for 10 to 14 days, or
  - Tobramycin 3 to 5 mg/kg/day IV given every 8 hours for 10 to 14 days, or
  - Amikacin 15 mg/kg/day IV given every 8 to 12 hours for 10 to 14 days
  - Ampicillin 1 g IV every 6 hours for 14 to 21 days, or
  - Cefamandole 1 g IV every 6 hours for 10 to 14 days, or
  - Cefoxitin 1 g IV every 4 hours for 10 to 14 days, or
  - Ceftazidime 1 to 2 g IV every 8 hours for 10 to 14 days, or
  - Imipenem 1 to 4 g/day IV given every 6 hours

Follow-Up:

- Monitor in ICU for clinical response to treatment and:
  - Blood levels of antibiotics
  - Electrolytes
  - Nutritional status
  - CK levels
- Surgical consult
- **Watch for:** signs and symptoms of
  - Progression of gangrene
  - Bacteremia and sepsis
  - Disulfiram reactions caused by antibiotics

- Underlying illnesses:
  —Immune deficiency
  —Diabetes mellitus
  —Peripheral vascular disease
  —Malignancy

DIABETIC WOUND INFECTIONS

Presenting Symptoms:

SUBJECTIVE

History of diabetes mellitus

Nonhealing ulcer or wound, typically on lower extremities or feet

Few systemic complaints early in course of infection; little pain noted

Fever (occasionally)

OBJECTIVE

Acute or subacute ulcerated lesion, typically on lower extremity

History of diabetes mellitus with complications of peripheral neuropathy and/or vascular insufficiency

Few systemic symptoms early in course of infection

Differential Diagnosis:

Venous stasis ulcer
Decubitus ulcer
Mycotic infection
Squamous cell carcinoma
Deep vein thrombosis
Infectious thrombi from remote source

Suggested Workup:

- Tests for diabetes mellitus if diagnosis not already established: most revealing is two to three fasting blood sugar measurements

several days apart; may consider oral glucose tolerance testing
- Sample exudate or tissue from wound edge for Gram stain and culture: diabetics typically will have mixed cultures of aerobes and anaerobes, *S. aureus,* and Group A *Streptococcus; Clostridia* spp. may be present
- Consider punch biopsy: evidence of necrotic tissue with disruption of underlying vascular supply
- Plain radiograph/bone scan of affected area to evaluate for osteomyelitis

Definitive Diagnosis:

Diabetes with skin ulcer   ICD-9-CM 250.8

Suggested Treatment:

- Surgical debridement as needed
- Early infection, or no systemic symptoms:
  - Amoxicillin + clavulanate 500 mg orally every 8 hours, or
  - Ciprofloxacin 500 to 750 mg orally every 12 hours, and
  - Clindamycin 300 mg orally every 8 hours, all for 14 to 21 days
- Advanced infection, or presence of systemic symptoms:
  - Ampicillin + sulbactam 1 to 2 g IV every 6 hours, or
  - Ciprofloxacin 400 to 800 mg/day IV given every 8 hours, and
  - Clindamycin 1.8 to 2.7 g/day IV given every 6 to 8 hours for 10 to 14 days, then change to oral antibiotics as above

Follow-Up:

- Careful evaluation is required on a regular basis until healing is assured

- Re-evaluate glycemic control; monitor blood glucose levels daily
- **Watch for:** signs and symptoms of
    - Bacteremia and sepsis
    - Superinfection with fungi or Gram-negative bacteria
    - Sinus formation
    - Worsening vascular insufficiency

HERPES SIMPLEX (ORAL AND CUTANEOUS)

Presenting Symptoms:

SUBJECTIVE	OBJECTIVE
Multiple vesicles occurring as clusters around mouth or on finger	Erythematous based, clustered, umbilicated vesicles with vermilion border
Intense itching and pain	Occur around lips (**herpes labialis**— herpes simplex virus 1 [HSV-1]) or localized on a finger (**herpetic whitlow**)
Malaise	
Fever	May present as diffuse, pox-like eruption complicating atopic dermatitis (**eczema herpeticum**), accompanied by high fever and local edema
	May present as vesicular eruption on pharyngeal and oral

mucosa, palate,
tongue, and floor of
mouth (**herpetic
gingivostomatitis**)
Elicit precipitating
events (trauma,
stress, intense sun
exposure, menses,
fever)
Elicit history of
prodrome of pain,
burning, or itching 6
to 48 hours prior to
appearance of
vesicles
Vesicles may ulcerate
and crust within 48
to 72 hours of
appearance
Local lymphadenopathy

Differential Diagnosis:

Impetigo
Herpes zoster
Syphilitic chancre
Stevens-Johnson syndrome
Herpangina (rare on lips; usually found in
  oropharynx)
Kaposi's varicelliform eruption (varicella or
  Coxsackievirus A 16)
Molluscum contagiosum

Suggested Workup:

- History and physical appearance usually
  reveal pathognomonic findings
- Collect scraping from base of vesicular lesion
  for Tzanck test: multinucleated giant cells are
  diagnostic for herpes

- Anti-herpes antibody:
  - High titer is diagnostic, but will not reliably distinguish between HSV-1 and HSV-2
  - May be difficult to distinguish between acute infection and previous exposure
- HSV culture usually not indicated, except for persistent or frequently recurring cases (requires 2 to 6 days)

Definitive Diagnosis:

Herpes labialis   ICD-9-CM 054.9
Eczema herpeticum   ICD-9-CM 054.0
Herpetic gingivostomatitis   ICD-9-CM 054.2
Herpetic whitlow   ICD-9-CM 054.6

Suggested Treatment:

- General measures:
  - Intermittent cool, moist dressings with Domeboro or Burow's solution
  - Analgesics
- Immunocompetent patients:
  - Generally accepted principle is that acyclovir is not indicated, but anecdotal reports claim a benefit in reducing severity and duration of infection, decrease in recurrent infections, and lowering transmission/viral shedding:
  - Acyclovir 200 mg orally 5 times a day for 5 to 7 days

Follow-Up:

- Observe closely for disappearance of lesions (10 to 14 days for herpes labialis and herpetic gingivostomatitis and 2 to 3 weeks for herpetic whitlow and eczema herpeticum)

- Educate patient regarding expected recurrences
- **Watch for:** signs and symptoms of
  - Herpes pneumonia
  - Aseptic meningitis
  - Herpes encephalitis
  - Herpes septicemia

HERPES SIMPLEX (GENITAL)

Presenting Symptoms:

SUBJECTIVE

Sixty to 70% are asymptomatic

Thirty to 40% complain of:
—Fever
—Headache
—Malaise
—Myalgia
—Burning genital pain
—Dysuria (females)
—Dyspareunia
—Vesicular eruption in genital or perirectal areas

OBJECTIVE

Sixty to 70% show no objective findings

Thirty to 40% display clinical findings:

Umbilicated vesicles on an edematous, erythematous base

May ulcerate and crust over

Elicit history of prodrome of burning, numbness, tingling, and paresthesias of genitals

Distribution:
—Female: labia, inner thighs, vaginal mucosa, cervix, perianal skin
—Male: glans penis, penile shaft, urethra

Primary lesions are typically bilateral and diffuse

Recurrent lesions are
usually unilateral
and localized
Elicit history of sexual
activity within 1 to
45 days (usually 6
days) of appearance
of lesions
Inguinal
lymphadenopathy
Sacral paresthesia

Differential Diagnosis:

Primary syphilis
Chancroid
Lymphogranuloma venereum
Atypical genital warts
Scabies
Molluscum contagiosum
Allergic contact dermatitis
Trauma
Candidiasis
Herpes zoster
Behçet's syndrome
Stevens-Johnson syndrome
Inflammatory bowel disease
Granuloma inguinale

Suggested Workup:

- History and physical examination findings are
  usually typical
- Collect scraping from base of vesicular lesion
  for Tzanck test: multinucleated giant cells are
  diagnostic for herpes
- Anti-herpes antibody: high titer is diagnostic,
  but will not reliably distinguish between
  HSV-1 and HSV-2

- Herpes simplex viral culture is usually not indicated, except for persistent or frequently recurring cases (requires 2 to 6 days)

Definitive Diagnosis:

Herpes genitalis   ICD-9-CM 054.10

Suggested Treatment:

- General measures:
  - Burow's solution topically 4 to 6 times a day
  - Ice packs to perineum
  - Sitz baths
  - Lidocaine topically
- Primary or first episode:
  - Acyclovir 200 mg orally 5 times a day for 7 to 10 days
- Recurrent episodes (occur in more than 50% of patients with variable frequency):
  - Acyclovir 200 mg orally 5 times a day for 5 days, or
  - Acyclovir 400 mg orally 3 times a day for 5 days, or
  - Acyclovir 800 mg orally 2 times a day for 5 days
- Chronic suppression for patients with frequent (at least 6 times a year) or disabling recurrences:
  - Acyclovir 400 mg orally 2 times a day chronically, or
  - Acyclovir 200 mg orally 3 to 5 times a day chronically
  - (These dosages appear to be safe and efficacious for at least 6 years)
- Severe, disabling local or disseminated disease:
  - Acyclovir 5 mg/kg IV every 8 hours for 7 days

Follow-Up:

- Patient with an acute, primary episode can be followed as an outpatient on an as-needed basis; symptoms will typically resolve spontaneously and completely within 21 days
- Female patients with latent, recurrent infections should receive annual Pap smears and have careful prenatal care
- All patients with latent, recurrent infections should be counseled regarding:
  - Avoiding intercourse in the presence of symptomatic genital lesions
  - Use of condoms and spermicide in all sexual activity
  - Avoiding multiple sexual partners, and
  - Avoiding stress
- **Watch for:** signs and symptoms of
  - Secondary bacterial infection
  - Urinary retention
  - Aseptic meningitis
  - Neonatal transmission
  - Increased risk for human immunodeficiency virus (HIV) infection

HERPES ZOSTER (SHINGLES)

Presenting Symptoms:

SUBJECTIVE	OBJECTIVE
Red papules or grouped vesicles on face or trunk	Elicit history of prodrome: tingling, itching, or sharp pain
Fatigue	Acute phase:
Headache	erythematous,
Low grade fever	maculopapular rash
Weakness	

Malaise
Pain at rash site
Constitutional
 symptoms

in a dermatomal
distribution,
evolving to grouped
vesicles
Vesicles become
pustular and/or
hemorrhagic within
3 to 5 days
Vesicles crust by 14 to
21 days
Rash is almost always
unilateral
Elicit history of having
had chicken pox
(varicella) in
childhood
One to 5% of patients
may present with
motor nerve
weakness in the
distribution of the
rash (herpes zoster
motoricus), resulting
in facial nerve
weakness or spinal
motor radiculopathy

Differential Diagnosis:

Herpes simplex virus
Coxsackievirus dermatitis
Superficial pyoderma
Pain may mimic:
—Cholecystitis
—Pleuritis
—Myocardial infarction
—Trigeminal neuralgia
—Facial nerve palsy

Suggested Workup:

- History and physical appearance typically reveal pathognomonic findings (as above)
- Unroof vesicle and obtain smear for Tzanck test: multinucleated giant cells with typical inclusions does not distinguish from herpes simplex

Definitive Diagnosis:

Herpes zoster (shingles)   ICD-9-CM 053.9
(not site-specific)

Suggested Treatment:

- General measures:
    - Wet dressings of Burow's solution applied topically for 30 to 60 minutes 4 to 6 times a day
    - Silver sulfadiazine cream 1% topically twice a day for secondarily infected rash
    - Analgesia as needed (avoid aspirin-containing products to minimize subsequent development of Guillain-Barré syndrome)
- Antiviral (should be initiated within 48 hours of appearance of rash):
    - Acyclovir 800 mg orally every 4 hours (5 doses/day) for 7 to 10 days, or
    - Valacyclovir 1 g orally 3 times a day for 7 days, or
    - Famciclovir 500 mg orally every 8 hours for 7 days
- Serious infection and/or ophthalmic involvement: Acyclovir 10 mg/kg IV every 8 hours for 7 to 10 days
- Varicella vaccines: not indicated; they do not protect against herpes zoster

Follow-Up:

- Most patients have resolution of rash within 14 to 21 days without complication
- Educate patient regarding transmission of virus causing chickenpox (varicella) to susceptible persons until rash has crusted entirely
- **Watch for:** signs and symptoms of
    - Postherpetic neuralgia (50% in patients over age 80 years, but less than 10% in patients younger than 50)
    - Ocular involvement (especially with facial zoster)
    - Meningoencephalitis
    - Cutaneous dissemination
    - Bacterial superinfection of dermal lesions
    - Hepatitis
    - Pneumonitis
    - Peripheral motor weakness
    - Segmental myelitis
    - Cranial nerve involvement, especially ophthalmic and facial (Ramsay Hunt's syndrome)
    - Corneal ulceration
    - Guillain-Barré syndrome

MOLLUSCUM CONTAGIOSUM

Presenting Symptoms:

SUBJECTIVE	OBJECTIVE
Flesh colored or pearly white papules	Discrete, flesh-colored to pearly white, umbilicated papules,
In children, on face, trunk, and	2 to 6 mm diameter

extremities	Erythematous base
In adults, in groin area or genitalia	Grouped in one or two areas
Lesions are pruritic and/or tender	Beneath umbilicated center is white curd-like core
	Adults: elicit history of sexual contact 2 to 8 weeks previously
	Children: elicit history of swimming pool contact 2 to 8 weeks previously

Differential Diagnosis:

Basal cell carcinoma
Furunculosis
Keratoacanthomas
Warts
Pyodermas (folliculitis, furunculosis)
Pyogenic granuloma
Mycotic infection

Suggested Workup:

- History and physical appearance strongly suggestive; white, curd-like core easily expressed from beneath umbilication
- Biopsy: Poxvirus (cannot be cultured) with other pathognomonic histologic changes (intracytoplasmic inclusion bodies with hypertrophied and hyperplastic dermis)

Definitive Diagnosis:

Molluscum contagiosum   ICD-9-CM 078.0

Suggested Treatment:

- Curettage is treatment of choice
- Alternatives to curettage: topical treatment (these have been reported to be effective, but

no clinical trials exist in which safety and efficacy were tested):

- Podophyllin 25% applied topically for 1 to 4 hours weekly until lesions are healed, or
- Silver nitrate 10% ointment or solution applied topically weekly until lesions are healed, or
- Tretinoin 0.025% gel or cream applied topically daily until lesions are healed

Follow-Up:

- Treat weekly until lesions have healed (usually requires 2 to 4 treatments)
- Recheck 2 to 4 weeks after treatment for development of new lesions; recurrences are uncommon
- Educate adult patients as to safe sex practices
- **Watch for:** signs and symptoms of
    - Extension of infection
    - Underlying immune deficiency

FUNGAL INFECTIONS—DERMATOPHYTES

Presenting Symptoms:

SUBJECTIVE	OBJECTIVE
	Tinea corporis
Red, ring-like rash on body	Pink to red papulosquamous annular lesions with raised borders and scaly appearance
Intense itching	
Few other systemic symptoms	Lesions expand peripherally with time and clear centrally
	Lesions may occur singly or in groups of three or four

Each plaque is smaller
than 5 cm in
diameter

Tinea pedis

Itchy, scaly, inflamed
areas in the spaces
between the toes
May also involve the
sides of the foot or
the toenails

Macerated lesions with
scaling borders in
the toe-web spaces
that can involve the
plantar surface of the
foot in a "moccasin"
distribution, and the
arch of the foot
Vesicles may form in
acute flare-ups
Pruritus common

Tinea unguium

Thickened, dull
toenails or
fingernails
Nail separation from
nailbed

Thickened and
lusterless toenails or
fingernails
Separated nail-plate
with nail destruction

Tinea capitis

Round patches of scale
or bald areas on
scalp
Stumps of broken hairs
in scaly areas
"Ringworm"

Round patches of
scaly, erythematous
lesions and alopecia
on scalp
Characteristic "black
dot" pattern may
develop where hair
breaks off
Extreme inflammation
may result in **kerion**
(exudative pustular
nodulation leading
to granuloma
formation)

Tinea cruris

Itchy, red rash of groin area	Well-marginated, erythematous half-moon shaped plaques in crural folds of the groin May spread to the upper thighs Advancing border may show scaling and/or vesicles Usually bilateral, involving scrotum, penis, buttocks, and gluteal cleft areas

Tinea versicolor

Multiple white or brown patches on skin of chest, shoulders, or back Not itchy Periodic recurrences	Sharply marginated, 3 to 4 mm diameter patches, ranging from white on sun-exposed areas to brown or red-brown on covered areas Usually on chest, shoulders, or back, but may occur in any sebum-rich area There may be fine scales, visible only with scraping More prominent in summer Periodic recurrence

Differential Diagnosis:

Pityriasis rosea
Eczema
Drug eruption
Erythema multiforme
Contact dermatitis
Psoriasis
Secondary syphilis
Subacute lupus erythematosus
Intertrigo
Hyperkeratosis
Nummular eczema
Elastosis perforans serpiginosa
Erythema annulare
Erythrasma
Seborrhea dermatitis
Alopecia areata
Pyoderma
Gyrate erythemas
Candidiasis
Vitiligo
Hyperhidrosis

Suggested Workup:

- Pathognomonic appearance helps suggest diagnosis
- Confirm fungal etiology with skin/hair scraping for KOH preparation
  - Branching hyphae with septa establishes fungal cause of infection (most likely *Trichophyton* if on body, feet, nails, or groin)
  - Short, stubby hyphae or Y-shaped hyphae with spore clusters on hyphae establishes *Pityrosporon orbiculare* (**tinea versicolor**)
  - Scalp hair with spore sheath surrounding hair shaft confirms *Trichophyton* infection (**tinea capitis**)

- Examine skin or scalp under Wood's light
  - Fluorescence to a bright green establishes *Microsporum* infection (**tinea capitis**) (*Trichophyton* does not fluoresce under Wood's light)
  - Fluorescence to golden yellow establishes *Pityrosporon* infection (**tinea versicolor**)
- Fungal culture is usually not necessary, but may be performed on Sabouraud's dextrose agar (reserved for cases where patient has been partially treated or has confounding conditions [e.g., psoriasis, seborrheic dermatitis])

Definitive Diagnosis:

Tinea capitis   ICD-9-CM 110.0
Tinea corporis   ICD-9-CM 110.5
Tinea cruris   ICD-9-CM 110.3
Tinea pedis   ICD-9-CM 110.4
Tinea unguium   ICD-9-CM 110.1
Tinea versicolor   ICD-9-CM 111.0

Suggested Treatment:

- Tinea capitis:
  - Griseofulvin microsized 10 mg/kg/day orally given 2 times a day or once a day for 6 weeks, or
  - Itraconazole 200 mg orally once daily for 6 weeks, or daily for 1 week each month for 3 to 4 months
- Tinea corporis:
  - For mild infection:
    - Miconazole 2% cream topically 2 times a day for 2 weeks, or
    - Clotrimazole 1% cream topically 2 times a day for 2 weeks, or
    - Ketoconazole 2% cream topically once daily for 2 weeks, or
    - Econazole 1% cream topically once daily for 2 weeks

May use longer if infection persists; use
for 1 week after infection resolves
- For resistant, extensive, and/or invasive
infections:
  Griseofulvin ultramicrosized orally for 4
  weeks: 375 mg/day in adults; 7 mg/kg/
  day in children older than 2 years, or
  Itraconazole 200 mg daily for 4 weeks, or
  daily for 1 week each month for 3
  to 4 months
- Tinea cruris:
  - Clotrimazole 1% cream topically 2 times a
    day for 2 to 4 weeks, or
  - Ciclopirox 1% cream topically 2 times a
    day for 2 to 4 weeks, or
  - Econazole 1% cream topically 2 times a day
    for 2 to 4 weeks, or
  - Miconazole 2% cream topically 2 times a
    day for 2 to 4 weeks, or
  - Tolnaftate 1% cream or solution topically 2
    times a day for 2 to 4 weeks, or
  - Terbinafine 1% cream topically 2 times a
    day for 1 to 4 weeks
  - If these topical agents are unsuccessful:
    Ketoconazole 2% cream topically daily for
    14 days
  - All therapy must be continued for 10 days
    after symptoms have resolved
- Tinea unguium:
  - Ciclopirox 1% cream topically once daily
    for 6 to 12 months, or
  - Itraconazole 200 mg orally once a day for 3
    months
- Tinea pedis:
  - Acute vesicular stage:
    Burow's wet dressings topically, then
    Clotrimazole 1% cream topically 2 times
    a day for 4 weeks

- Subacute macerated, scaling stage:
    Clotrimazole 1% cream or solution 2
      times a day for 4 weeks, and
    Tolnaftate 1% powder in the shoes
- Chronic infection:
    Initially, same treatment as for subacute
      stage; if this fails—Griseofulvin
      ultramicrosized 375 mg orally 2 times
      a day for 4 to 8 weeks (if toenail is
      involved, may need to treat for 6
      months)
- Tinea versicolor:
  - Selenium sulfide shampoo applied topically
    and allowed to dry for 40 minutes on body
    before showering daily for 1 week, or
    allowed to dry on body for 12 to 24 hours
    before showering once a week for 4 weeks, or
  - Clotrimazole 1% cream topically 2 times a
    day for 3 to 4 weeks, or
  - Miconazole 2% cream/solution topically 2
    times a day for 3 to 4 weeks, or
  - Ketoconazole 2% cream topically 2 times a
    day for 3 to 4 weeks
  - If strongly resistant to topical therapy, may
    use ketoconazole 400 mg orally once daily
    for 2 days

Follow-Up:

- Recheck after 2 and 6 weeks of therapy to
  document clinical improvement or cure
- Recheck periodically to monitor recurrence
- Liver function testing before therapy and at
  regular intervals for patients taking oral
  ketoconazole
- Regular monitoring of complete blood count
  (CBC), and renal and hepatic function for
  patients taking oral griseofulvin

- Patient education:
  - Tinea capitis
    —Good personal hygiene
    —Do not share headwear
  - Tinea unguium
    —Wearing gloves to wash dishes
    —Keeping hands clean and dry
  - Tinea pedis
    —Wearing rubber sandals in community showers or bathing facilities
    —Careful drying between toes after bathing
    —Applying drying/dusting powder to feet
    —Changing socks frequently
- **Watch for:** signs and symptoms of
  - Permanent hair loss and scarring (tinea capitis)
  - Secondary bacterial superinfection (all dermatophyte infections)
  - Generalized, invasive dermatophyte infection (tinea corporis)
  - Development of paronychia or onychia (tinea unguium)
  - Eczematoid changes (tinea pedis)
  - Frequent recurrences (all dermatophyte infections)

FUNGAL INFECTIONS— MUCOCUTANEOUS CANDIDIASIS

Presenting Symptoms:

SUBJECTIVE	OBJECTIVE
Interdigital Candidiasis	
Small, erosive, scaly lesion in space between fingers	Round to ovoid erosion, surrounded by a delicate

No itching or bleeding

No systemic symptoms

cigarette–paper-like scaling collar that follows the borders of the lesions

No regional lymphadenopathy

Intertrigo

Unilateral, eczema-like lesions in groin area or where there are two apposing folds of skin

Mild/moderate itching

No systemic symptoms

Nonindurated, sharp, but irregularly demarcated erythematous area with cigarette–paper-like scaling collar that follows the borders of the lesions

Occurs mainly in groin area or where there are two apposing folds of skin (e.g., submammary regions, axillae, and skin folds secondary to obesity)

Usually presents as a main lesion with satellite lesions

Skin around lesions may be pustular, macerated, and/or raw and denuded

No regional lymphadenopathy

Vulvovaginitis

Red rash on vulva, vagina and/or perineum

Meaty red erythema of vulva, vaginal skin, and mucus

Thin, watery to thick, cheesy vaginal discharge

May be asymptomatic or intensely pruritic with burning sensation

membrane, and/or perineum

Vaginal discharge may range from thin to thick, creamy-white, curdy

There may be satellite pustules on skin

May elicit history of use of antibiotics, oral contraceptives, or steroids (oral or inhaled), or of pregnancy

Regional lymphadenopathy uncommon

Balanitis

Erosive, scaling lesions of glans penis

Slight edema of preputium and glans

Mild to moderate pain

No urethral discharge

No systemic symptoms

Linear erosions with slight edema and erythema on preputium

Delicate cigarette–paper-like scaling associated with lesions

Erosive areas on glans penis

No history of high-risk sexual intercourse

Strong possibility of underlying diabetes mellitus

Oral candidiasis

White, raised, painless patches in mouth

Thrush: Confluent white or cream-

Red, raw, deep fissures at the corners of the mouth causing distortion of the angles of the mouth, and pain

Few systemic symptoms

colored pustules on the palate, tongue, buccal mucus membranes, or gums

Lesions are easily scraped away, leaving an erythematous, raw, bleeding base

Angular cheilitis/ perlèche: Red, scaly, raw fissures at the corners of the mouth

Elicit history of ill-fitting dentures

Differential Diagnosis:

Leukoplakia
Lichen planus
Seborrheic dermatitis
Reiter's syndrome
Contact dermatitis
Lichen sclerosis et atrophicus
Syphilis
Hyperhidrosis
Psoriasis
Diaper dermatitis
Balanitis xerotica obliterans
Cheilosis

Suggested Workup:

- History, physical appearance, and location of lesions are very suggestive
- Cigarette–paper-like scaling collar is a pathognomonic feature of *Candida* infections
- Obtain a sample that is coating the infected area, ulcer, or vaginal discharge for KOH

preparation: yeast forms and pseudohyphae seen under the microscope confirm *Candida*
- Obtain a sample that is coating the infected area, ulcer, or vaginal discharge for Gram stain: Gram-positive yeast forms and pseudohyphae seen under the microscope confirm *Candida*
- Fungal cultures on blood or Sabouraud's agar reserved for difficult cases or infections resistant to antifungal medication

Definitive Diagnosis:

Candidiasis of mouth	ICD-9-CM 112.0
Vulvovaginal candidiasis	ICD-9-CM 112.1
Candidal balanitis	ICD-9-CM 112.2
Intertrigo	ICD-9-CM 695.89
Candidiasis, unspecified site	ICD-9-CM 112.9

Suggested Treatment:

- Interdigital candidiasis:
    - Nystatin (100,000 U/g) ointment, topically 2 times a day for 1 to 3 months, or
    - Miconazole 2% cream topically 2 times a day for 1 to 3 months, or
    - Clotrimazole 1% cream topically 2 times a day for 1 to 3 months, or
    - Ketoconazole 2% cream topically once daily for 1 to 3 months, or
    - Ciclopirox 1% cream topically once daily for 1 to 3 months
- Intertrigo:
    - As with interdigital candidiasis above; if not effective, may use ketoconazole 200 to 400 mg orally once daily for 10 to 14 days
- Vulvovaginitis:
    - Miconazole 2% cream, 1 applicator intravaginally each night at bedtime for 7 days, or

- Miconazole 200 mg intravaginal suppositories, 1 suppository each night at bedtime for 3 days, or
- Clotrimazole 500 mg intravaginal suppositories, 1 suppository each night at bedtime for 5 days, or
- Nystatin (100,000 U/intravaginal tablet) 1 tablet 2 times a day for 7 days, or
- Terconazole 0.8% cream, 1 applicator intravaginally each night at bedtime for 3 days (or 0.4% cream can be used each night at bedtime for 7 days), or
- Terconazole 80 mg intravaginal suppositories, 1 suppository each night at bedtime for 3 days, or
- Fluconazole 150 mg orally for 1 dose
- Balanitis:
  - As with intertrigo above
  - If bacterial superinfection is suspected, Bacitracin ointment (500 U/g) topically 4 times a day for 10 to 14 days, or Neosporin ointment topically 4 times a day for 10 to 14 days, or Trimethoprim-sulfamethoxazole (TMP-SMX) DS 1 tablet orally 2 times a day for 7 to 10 days
- Oral candidiasis:
  - Nystatin oral suspension 100,000 U/mL, 5 to 10 mL swish and swallow 4 to 5 times a day for 14 to 21 days, or
  - Nystatin pastilles 500,000 U, 1 to 2 pastilles orally 4 to 5 times a day for 14 to 21 days, or
  - Clotrimazole 10 mg troche, 1 troche slowly dissolved in mouth five times a day for 7 to 14 days
  - (The three medications listed above should be given for at least 48 hours after the disappearance of thrush), or

- Ketoconazole 200 to 400 mg orally once daily for 14 to 21 days, or
- Fluconazole 50 to 200 mg orally once daily for 14 to 21 days
- Angular cheilitis/perlèche:
  - Clotrimazole 1%-betamethasone 0.05% cream topically 2 times a day for 2 to 4 weeks, or
  - Nystatin 100,000 U/g + triamcinolone 0.1% cream topically 2 times a day for 2 to 4 weeks

Follow-Up:

- For immunocompetent individuals, a benign course and excellent prognosis is the norm, but close monitoring of patients on long-term (1 to 3 months) therapy is prudent to evaluate clinical response
- Liver function testing before therapy and at regular intervals for patients taking long-term oral fluconazole
- May be necessary to evaluate recurrences (especially oral and vulvovaginal candidiasis) by routine visual inspections or KOH preparations during physical examinations
- Patient education regarding avoidance of antibiotics, oral contraceptives, and douching
- Patient education regarding use of loose cotton underwear
- Patient education about keeping hands clean and dry
- Patient education regarding proper denture fitting and good oral hygiene
- Low threshold to work up other predisposing factors for candidiasis: diabetes mellitus, Cushing's disease, immunosuppression, uremia, malignancy

- **Watch for:** signs and symptoms of
  - Chronic/recurrent candidiasis
  - Hematogenously disseminated candidiasis and/or candidemia (rare in immunocompetent patients)
  - Esophagitis (rare in immunocompetent patients)

PARONYCHIA

Presenting Symptoms:

SUBJECTIVE	OBJECTIVE
Pain and inflammation of the skin around a fingernail or toenail	Erythematous swelling of skin around a nail plate
May have followed trauma to nail or history of frequent immersion of hands into water	Purulent discharge may be present
	Regional lymphangitis is occasional finding
Appearance may be acute or chronic	

Differential Diagnosis:

Herpetic whitlow
Felon (infection of pulp space of finger pad following minor trauma, prick, or splinter)

Suggested Workup:

- History and physical appearance are pathognomonic
- Collect exudate or swab nail bed for Gram stain, culture and sensitivity, and KOH preparation to determine likely organisms:
  - *S. aureus*
  - *Streptococcus*

- *Pseudomonas*
- *Candida albicans*

Definitive Diagnosis:

Paronychia of finger   ICD-9-CM 681.02
Paronychia of toe   ICD-9-CM 681.11
Candidal paronychia   ICD-9-CM 112.3

Suggested Treatment:

- For mild cases in nondiabetic patients:
  - Warm compresses or soaks
  - Elevation
  - Drying agents as needed (e.g., Castellani paint 1.5%)
- For more severe cases, suppuration, and/or in diabetic patients:
  - Dicloxacillin 250 to 500 mg orally every 6 hours for 7 to 10 days, or
  - Penicillin allergy: Erythromycin 500 mg orally every 6 hours for 7 to 10 days, or Cephalexin 250 mg orally every 6 hours for 7 to 10 days
- For chronic cases with positive KOH preparation:
  - Nystatin cream topically 2 times a day until infection is cleared, or
  - Itraconazole 200 mg orally once daily for 3 months, or
  - Ketoconazole 200 mg orally once daily for 3 months
- Where abscess is present:
  - Incision and drainage
  - If abscess is subungual, or ingrown nail is present, partial or complete removal of nail may be necessary

Follow-Up:

- Routine monitoring until healed
- Patient education regarding keeping hands and feet dry and clean
- For diabetic patients, re-educate regarding careful foot and hand care and good glycemic control
- **Watch for:** signs and symptoms of
    - Subungual abscess
    - Secondary damage and/or loss of nail

Central Nervous System and Eye 2

BACTERIAL MENINGITIS

Presenting Symptoms:

<u>SUBJECTIVE</u>

Prodromal upper respiratory tract symptoms
Stiff neck
Fever
Headache
Vomiting
Lethargy
Photophobia
Profuse sweats
Rigors
Weakness
Seizures (20% to 30% of cases)

<u>OBJECTIVE</u>

Meningismus with positive Kernig and/or Brudzinski signs
Nuchal rigidity
Signs of cerebral dysfunction
Altered mental status
Focal neurologic deficits (50% of patients)
Confusion (especially in the elderly)
There may be rash associated with meningococcemia: initially, erythematous, macular lesions, becoming petechial or purpuric
Palsy of cranial nerve (CN) III, VI, VII, VIII (10% to 20% of cases)

Differential Diagnosis:

Bacteremia
Sepsis
Brain abscess
Seizure disorder
Aseptic meningitis
Skull fracture

Suggested Workup:

- Lumbar puncture: pathognomonic findings (Table 2.1)
- Blood cultures
- Computed tomography (CT) scan of head if there is concern for increased intracranial pressure or intracranial abscess
- Sinus/skull radiographs if there is concern for cranial osteomyelitis, paranasal sinusitis, or skull fracture
- Guidelines for evaluation of cerebrospinal fluid (CSF):
  - Normal findings:
    - —Opening pressure = 5 to 15 mm water
    - —White blood cells (WBCs) = fewer than 10 cells/mm^3 (5 to 10 cells/mm^3 is suspect of an infection)
    - —Protein = 15 to 45 mg/dL
    - —Glucose = 40 to 80 mg/100 mL (or CSF/blood glucose ratio greater than 0.6)
  - Abnormal CSF without infection: (Table 2.2)

Definitive Diagnosis:

Bacterial meningitis   ICD-9-CM 320

Suggested Treatment:

- Should begin **immediately** following lumbar puncture, even before admission to hospital
- Empiric therapy until culture results are available:
  - Age younger than 1 month (requires 14 to 21 days of treatment):
    Ampicillin 300 to 400 mg/kg/day intravenously (IV) given every 4 to 6 hours, and
    Cefotaxime 200 mg/kg/day IV given every 4 to 6 hours, or

Table 2.1.

Lumbar Puncture—Typical Findings for Bacterial Meningitis

	Adult	Pediatric
CSF opening pressure (mm)	>180	>180
CSF clarity	Turbid	Turbid
WBCs in CSF (no./mm^3)	>1,000 (with ↑ polys)	>5–10
CSF protein (mg/dL)	>1500	>500 (>1500 in neonates)
CSF glucose (mg/dL)	<40	<50
CSF: blood glucose ratio	<0.4	<0.6
Gram stain of CSF	Gram+ cocci and/or Gram− bacilli	
Culture of CSF	*Streptococcus pneumoniae, Neisseria meningitides, Escherichia coli, Listeria monocytogenes, Haemophilus influenzae*	

CSF = Cerebrospinal fluid; **WBCs** = white blood cells; **polys** = polymorphonuclear leukocytes; **Gram+** = Gram-positive; **Gram−** = Gram-negative.

Table 2.2.
Abnormal Cerebrospinal Fluid Without Infection

Cause of Abnormality	WBC	RBC	Protein	Glucose
Traumatic tap	Incr.	Incr.	Incr.	NL
Chemical meningitis	Incr. LNC	NL	Incr.	NL
Cerebral contusion or hemorrhage	Incr. PMN	Incr.	Incr.	Decr.
Vasculitis	Incr.	NL	Incr.	NL
Postictal	Incr.	Incr.	NL	NL
CNS tumors	Incr. PMN	NL	Incr.	Decr.
Postneurosurgical	Incr. Monos.	Incr.	Incr.	NL
CNS sarcoidosis	Incr. Monos.	NL	Incr.	NL/Decr.

WBC = white blood cells; RBC = red blood cells; Incr. = increased; Decr. = decreased; NL = normal; LNC = lymphocytes; PMN = polymorphonuclear leukocytes; Monos. = monocytes.

Ceftriaxone 100 mg/kg/day IV given
every 12 to 24 hours,
OR
Ampicillin 300 to 400 mg/kg/day IV
given every 4 to 6 hours, and
Tobramycin 7.5 mg/kg/day IV given
every 6 to 8 hours
Penicillin allergic patients may substitute
for ampicillin: Vancomycin 15 to
20 mg/kg/day IV given every 6 to
8 hours
- Age 1 to 3 months (requires 10 days of
treatment):
Ampicillin + third-generation
cephalosporin or
Tobramycin as above
Penicillin allergic patients may substitute
for ampicillin: Vancomycin 40 mg/kg/
day IV given every 6 to 8 hours
- Age 3 months to 18 years (10 days of
treatment):
Cefotaxime 200 mg/kg/day IV given
every 4 to 6 hours (adult dose is 2 g IV
every 4 hours), or
Ceftriaxone 100 mg/kg/day IV given
every 12 to 24 hours (adult dose is 2 g
IV every 12 hours), or
Ampicillin 300 to 400 mg/kg/day IV
given every 4 to 6 hours (adult dose is
2 g IV every 4 to 6 hours), and
Chloramphenicol 50 to 100 mg/kg/day
IV given every 6 hours
- Age 18 to 50 years (10 days of treatment):
PCN G 18 to 24 million units (U)/day IV
given every 4 to 6 hours, or
Ampicillin 2 g IV every 4 to 6 hours, and
Cefotaxime 2 g IV every 4 hours, or

> Ceftriaxone 2 g IV every 12 hours
> Penicillin allergy: may substitute for PCN G or Ampicillin: Vancomycin 1 g IV every 12 hours

- Age older than 50 years (14 to 21 days treatment):
  > Ampicillin 2 g IV every 4 to 6 hours, and Cefotaxime or Ceftriaxone as above
  > Penicillin allergy: may use vancomycin as above

- Corticosteroid use (these agents may decrease sensorineural hearing loss and mortality, and thus are recommended for all patients more than 1 month old or younger than 50 years old): Dexamethasone 0.15 mg/kg IV every 6 hours for 4 days (infusion should be started 15 to 20 minutes before antibiotics)

Follow-Up:

- Average case fatality rate is 14% and as high as 26% with *Streptococcus pneumoniae;* inpatient care with admission to intensive care unit (ICU) if needed
- Vigorous supportive care, especially in presence of seizure activity and to prevent hypothermia and dehydration
- Brainstem auditory evoked response (BAER) testing should be done with infants before hospital discharge
- **Watch for:** signs and symptoms of
  - Seizure activity
  - Coma
  - Sensorineural hearing loss in children
  - Neurodevelopmental sequelae (e.g., learning deficits can occur in 30% of cases)

- Cranial nerve palsies (usually self-limiting and reversible with appropriate antibiotic treatment)
- Obstructive hydrocephalus
- Subdural effusions
- CSF fistula (especially in patients with recurrent bacterial meningitis)

ASEPTIC (VIRAL) MENINGITIS

Presenting Symptoms:

SUBJECTIVE	OBJECTIVE
Fever	Fever and malaise without meningeal signs, **OR**
Severe headache	
Stiff neck	
Nausea and vomiting	Fever, headache, malaise with stiff neck and back, **OR**
Photophobia	
Generalized aches and pains	All of the above, plus signs of encephalitis and cerebral dysfunction:
	—Altered mental state
	—Personality change
	—Seizure activity
	—Focal neurological signs
	—Cranial nerve abnormalities

Differential Diagnosis:

Bacterial meningitis
Encephalitis
Acute encephalopathy
Postinfectious encephalomyelitis

Parameningeal infections (e.g., subdural
  empyema)
Carcinomatous meningitis
Parasitic infection
Meningeal leukemia
Migraine headache
Viral syndrome
Chemical meningitis
Brain abscess
Tuberculosis (CNS)
Syphilis
Leptospirosis

Suggested Workup:

- Lumbar puncture: pathognomonic findings:
  (Table 2.3)
- Blood cultures
- CT scan or magnetic resonance imaging (MRI)
  of brain, or electroencephalogram (EEG)
  usually reserved for those cases where
  encephalitis is a consideration, or results of
  lumbar puncture are equivocal, or to rule out
  brain abscess

Definitive Diagnosis:

Aseptic (viral) meningitis   ICD-9-CM 047.9

Suggested Treatment:

- Antibiotics or antiviral agents are generally
  NOT indicated for the treatment of **confirmed**
  aseptic (viral) meningitis, but may be initiated
  until a viral etiology is firmly established
- Antibiotic therapy until bacterial etiology is
  ruled out:
  - Ampicillin 2 g IV every 4 to 6 hours
  - Penicillin allergy: Vancomycin 1 g IV every
    12 hours, and
  - Cefotaxime 2 g IV every 4 hours, or
  - Ceftriaxone 2 g IV given every 12 hours

Table 2.3.

Lumbar Puncture—Typical Findings for Meningitis

	Aseptic Meningitis*	Bacterial Meningitis
CSF opening pressure	Normal to slightly elevated	Markedly elevated
CSF clarity	Clear to slightly turbid	Turbid
WBCs in CSF (no./mm^3)	50–200	>1,000
Nature of WBCs	Lymphocytes	Polys
CSF protein (mg/dL)	Elevated, but <1500	Elevated, usually 1500–4000
CSF glucose (mg/dL)	Normal (50–100)[†]	Decreased to <40
Gram stain of CSF	Negative	Positive
Bacterial culture of CSF	Negative	Positive
Latex agglutination for bacteria with CSF	Negative	Positive
Antiviral antibody in CSF	Positive	Negative
CBC (blood)	Normal	Elevated WBCs

CSF = Cerebrospinal fluid; WBCs = white blood cells; CBC = complete blood count.

*Patients pretreated with antibiotics prior to lumbar puncture may result in a "partially treated" bacterial meningitis, which may mimic aseptic (viral) meningitis with respect to CSF findings.

[†]CSF glucose may be decreased in meningitis caused by herpes or mumps viruses. CSF glucose may be artificially increased in patients with diabetes mellitus

- Analgesia, antipyretics, and antiemetics as needed

Follow-Up:

- Severity of symptoms dictates need for hospitalization
- Complete recovery is usual
- May check on persons coming in contact with patient, but transmission is low probability
- Once acute illness begins to resolve, follow at least daily for 7 to 10 days (repeat lumbar puncture usually not necessary unless clinical course is atypical)
- **Watch for:** signs and symptoms of
  - Deafness
  - Muscle weakness
  - Seizure activity (rare)

VIRAL ENCEPHALITIS

Presenting Symptoms:

SUBJECTIVE	OBJECTIVE
Prodrome of malaise, fever, and upper respiratory tract symptoms (e.g., rhinorrhea)	Meningeal signs with nuchal rigidity
Stiff neck	Lethargy may progress to coma
Headache	May elicit history of prodromal viral infection 2 to 12 days prior to onset of present symptoms
Photophobia	Progression variable (rapid or indolent)
Lethargy	Seizure activity may be present, especially involving frontal or temporal lobes
Seizure activity	

Differential Diagnosis:

Bacterial meningitis
Brain abscess
Tuberculosis (CNS)
Cat-scratch disease
Rocky Mountain spotted fever
Ehrlichiosis
Syphilis
Lyme disease
Leptospirosis
Toxoplasmosis
Intracranial hemorrhage
Intracranial tumor
Trauma
Thromboembolism
Systemic lupus erythematosus
Ingestion of toxin
Ingestion of drug
Hypoglycemia
Subdural hematoma

Suggested Workup:

- Lumbar puncture: abnormal, but not pathognomonic findings:
  - CSF WBCs:
    - Normal or increased to 10 to 2000/mm^3
    - Neutrophils predominate early, then shift to lymphocytes
  - CSF protein: normal to slightly elevated
  - CSF glucose: normal to slightly decreased
  - CSF red blood cells: normal to elevated (in herpes infection)
- EEG: pathognomonic findings:
  - Slowing or epileptiform activity
  - Temporal lobe abnormalities, especially periodic slow-wave complexes (PLEDS) (indicative of herpes virus encephalitis)

- CT or MRI of brain can be used to:
  - Exclude brain abscess, tumor, subdural empyema, subdural hematoma, sagittal sinus thrombosis
  - Detect temporal lobe inflammation
- CSF antibody index: pathognomonic for infectious agent:
  - CSF and serum are tested for albumin content and presence of immunoglobulin (Ig)G antibody to the common encephalitis-producing viruses:
    —Herpes simplex types 1 and 2
    —Epstein-Barr
    —Varicella-zoster
    —Adenovirus
    —Rabies
    —Dengue
    —Benign lymphocytic choriomeningitis V
    —California
    —Japanese B encephalitis
    —Russian spring-summer encephalitis
    —Murray Valley
    —Arboviruses (St. Louis, eastern equine, western equine, Venezuelan equine)
    —Enteroviruses (Coxsackie B, mumps, influenza, human T-cell lymphotropic virus type III [HTLV-III])
  - CSF antibody/albumin greater than serum antibody/albumin suggests infection caused by the viral specificity of the antibody
- Viral culture from CSF is usually not indicated because of low yields, except for enteroviruses (60% recovery rate)
- Brain biopsy can establish the diagnosis definitively, but its utility must be balanced against its significant morbidity (usually

reserved for patients with undiagnosed lesion on CT or MRI and a poor clinical response to empiric intravenous acyclovir)

Definitive Diagnosis:

Viral meningitis   ICD-9-CM 047.9

Suggested Treatment:

- Antiherpes therapy can be given empirically until another etiology is **definitively confirmed:**
  - Adult: Acyclovir 30 mg/kg/day IV given every 8 hours (infusion should be given over 1 hour)
  - Pediatric: Acyclovir 1500 mg/m^2/day IV given every 8 hours (infusion should be given over 1 hour)
  - Treatment should be continued for 10 to 14 days
  - No other specific antiviral therapy is recommended for other etiologies
- Supportive measures:
  - Fluid balance is critical, especially during treatment with acyclovir
  - Anticonvulsants as needed

Follow-Up:

- Hospitalization and possible ICU care required
- Adequate respiratory and circulatory support critical and likely to require close monitoring
- May need to monitor intracranial pressure in severe cases
- Prognosis varies with etiologic agent
- **Watch for:** signs and symptoms of
  - Seizures
  - Coma
  - Cerebral edema

- Syndrome of inappropriate secretion of antidiuretic hormone (SIADH)
- Neurologic impairment

BRAIN ABSCESS

Presenting Symptoms:

SUBJECTIVE

Gradual onset of headache, becoming progressively severe

Personality change

Nausea and vomiting

Low-grade fever

Mental changes

Neck stiffness

Seizures

OBJECTIVE

Altered mental status, progressing from lethargy to stupor and coma, developing over several days to weeks

Papilledema

Focal neurological findings (nature varies with location of abscess)

Meningeal signs

Differential Diagnosis:

Brain tumor

Stroke

Intracranial hemorrhage

Subdural empyema

Extradural abscess

Encephalitis

Bacterial or aseptic meningitis

Degenerative diseases

Suggested Workup:

- History of rapidly developing symptoms favors abscess over tumor

- CT or MRI of head usually provides findings pathognomonic of abscess
- Blood cultures
- Radionuclide imaging with indium (^{117}ln)-labeled leukocytes can distinguish abscess from tumor if CT or MRI is equivocal
- Lumbar puncture is **relatively contraindicated** for fear of transtentorial herniation
- Surgical burr hole with aspiration of abscess under CT stereotaxic guidance to make a specific bacteriologic diagnosis is reserved for cases where empiric antibiotic therapy is ineffective
- If a remote primary source of infection is suspected (e.g., lung, sinuses), appropriate workup should be conducted (i.e., chest radiograph, sinus radiographs)
- If degenerative disease is suspected, appropriate workup should be conducted:
  - Chemistry panel and complete blood count (CBC)
  - Thyroid function tests
  - Folate and B$_{12}$ levels
  - VDRL (Venereal Disease Research Laboratories) test
  - Electrocardiogram (ECG)/Holter monitoring to rule out atrial fibrillation
  - Human immunodeficiency virus (HIV) antibody testing
  - Visual evoked responses to rule out multiple sclerosis

Definitive Diagnosis:

Intracranial abscess   ICD-9-CM 324.0

Suggested Treatment:

- Empiric antibiotic therapy:
  - PCN G 24 million U IV/day given as every 4 hours

- Penicillin allergy: Vancomycin 1 g IV every 12 hours, or

    Ceftriaxone 1 to 2 g IV every 24 hours, and

    Metronidazole 3 g/day IV given as every 6 hours
- After cranial trauma, neurosurgery, or where endocarditis is suspected as primary infection, *Staphylococcus aureus* may be present and requires an additional antibiotic:
  - Nafcillin 3 g IV every 6 hours is **added** to the regimen above
  - Penicillin allergy: Vancomycin 1 g IV given every 12 hours
- If Gram-negative organisms (e.g., *Enterobacteriaceae*) are suspected (as where there are otic, genitourinary [GU], or gastrointestinal [GI] sources of primary infection), an additional antibiotic must be added:
  - Ceftizoxime 1.5 g IV every 6 hours, or
  - Ceftriaxone 1 to 2 g IV every 24 hours, or
  - Ceftazidime 1 g IV every 8 hours is **added** to the regimen for empiric antibody treatment above
- All the antibiotics in the regimens above are to be given for 6 to 8 weeks
- In patients who are HIV-positive (HIV+), the abscess is assumed to be caused by *Toxoplasma gondii*:
  - Pyrimethamine 50 to 75 mg orally once daily, and
  - Sulfadiazine 1 to 4 g/day orally given every 8 hours
  - These agents are given for 3 weeks, the patient's clinical response and tolerance of therapy is assessed, and the dosage is then modified for an additional 4 to 5 weeks

- Therapy may be life-long in patients with acquired immunodeficiency syndrome (AIDS)
- Anticonvulsant for patients with seizure activity:
  - Phenytoin (dosage should be adjusted to maintain blood levels of 10 to 20 μg/mL) usual starting dose is 100 mg orally 3 times a day in patients with no prior anticonvulsant therapy; dose is then adjusted based on blood levels
  - If intravenous/intramuscular usage is required, phenytoin **SHOULD NOT** be added to an intravenous infusion because of the lack of solubility and resultant precipitation. May give 100 to 200 mg intramuscularly every 4 hours and follow blood levels, or loading dose of 10 to 15 mg/kg intravenous push (not exceeding 50 mg/min), followed by 100 mg IV every 6 to 8 hours and follow blood levels
- Cerebral edema:
  - Dexamethasone 10 mg intravenous bolus, followed by 4 mg IV/intramuscularly every 6 hours until symptoms of cerebral edema subside, usually within 12 to 24 hours; dosage may then be reduced after 2 to 4 days and tapered off over a period of 5 to 7 days

Follow-Up:

- Inpatient care with serial CT or MRI to monitor resolution of abscess
- Adequate treatment of primary infection (e.g., otitis media, mastoiditis, dental abscess)
- **Watch for:** signs and symptoms of
    - Cerebral edema and transtentorial herniation
    - Permanent neurological deficits

- Surgical complications
- Multifocal or recurrent abscesses
- Seizures

SUBDURAL EMPYEMA

Presenting Symptoms:

SUBJECTIVE
Headache
Lethargy
Seizure activity
Fever (usually low-
  grade)
Nausea and vomiting

OBJECTIVE
Elicit history of
  prodromal sinus
  infection (especially
  frontal and ethmoid),
  ear infection, cranial
  trauma or surgery,
  or pulmonary
  infection
In children under 5
  years old, may
  follow bacterial
  meningitis
Focal neurologic
  deficits
Seizures
Lethargy progressing
  to coma
Meningeal signs may
  or may not be
  present

Differential Diagnosis:

Brain tumor
Stroke
Intracranial hemorrhage
Brain abscess
Extradural abscess
Encephalitis
Bacterial or aseptic meningitis

Suggested Workup:

- History of rapidly developing symptoms over several days or weeks favors empyema over tumor
- CT or MRI of head usually yields pathognomonic findings: a collection of pus between the dura and the arachnoid membranes
- Blood cultures
- Lumbar puncture is **relatively contraindicated** for fear of transtentorial herniation
- Subdural tap may be diagnostic only in infants: culture for anaerobes
- Surgical burr hole with aspiration of the empyema under CT stereotaxic guidance may be necessary for significant collections of pus and/or where the patient's response to empiric antibiotic therapy is unsatisfactory

Definitive Diagnosis:

Subdural empyema   ICD-9-CM 324.9

Suggested Treatment:

- Surgical drainage of the empyema is indicated where there is elevated intracranial pressure and/or cerebral edema, extension of the empyema into the underlying sinus, recurrent empyemas, or lack of clinical response to empiric antibiotics
- Empiric antibiotic therapy:
  - PCN G 24 million U IV/day given every 4 hours
  - Penicillin allergy: Vancomycin 1 g IV every 12 hours, and
  - Metronidazole 3 g/day IV given every 6 hours, or
  - Chloramphenicol 1 g IV every 6 hours

- After cranial trauma or neurosurgery, *S. aureus* may be present and requires an additional antibiotic:
  - Nafcillin 3 g IV every 6 hours is **added** to the regimen above
  - Penicillin allergy: Vancomycin 1 g IV every 12 hours
- If Gram-negative organisms (e.g., *Enterobacteriaceae*) are suspected (as where there are otic sources of primary infection), an additional antibiotic must be added:
  - Ceftizoxime 1.5 g IV every 6 hours, or
  - Ceftriaxone 1 to 2 g IV every 24 hours, or
  - Ceftazidime 1 g IV every 8 hours is **added** to the regimen for empiric antibiotic treatment above
- All the antibiotics in the regimens above are to be given for **6 to 8 weeks**
- In HIV+ patients, the empyema is likely to be caused by *T. gondii:*
  - Pyrimethamine 50 to 75 mg orally once daily, **and**
  - Sulfadiazine 1 to 4 g/day orally given every 8 hours
  - These agents are given for 3 weeks, the patient's clinical response and tolerance of therapy is assessed, and the dosage is then modified for an additional 4 to 5 weeks
  - Therapy may be life-long in AIDS patients
- Anticonvulsant for patients with seizure activity:
  - Phenytoin (dosage should be adjusted to maintain blood levels of 10 to 20 μg/mL); usual starting dose is 100 mg orally 4 times a day in patients with no prior anticonvulsant therapy; dose is then adjusted based on blood levels
  - If intravenous/intramuscular usage is required, phenytoin **SHOULD NOT** be

> added to an intravenous infusion because of the lack of solubility and resultant precipitation. May give 100 to 200 mg intramuscularly every 4 hours and follow blood levels, or a loading dose of 10 to 15 mg/kg intravenous push (not exceeding 50 mg/min), followed by 100 mg IV every 6 to 8 hours and follow blood levels

- Cerebral edema:
  - Dexamethasone 10 mg intravenous bolus, followed by 4 mg IV/intramuscularly every 6 hours until symptoms of cerebral edema subside, usually within 12 to 24 hours; dosage may then be reduced after 2 to 4 days and tapered off over a period of 5 to 7 days

Follow-Up:

- Inpatient care with serial CT or MRI to monitor the resolution of the empyema
- Adequate treatment of accompanying meningitis, otic, or sinus infections
- **Watch for:** signs and symptoms of
  - Cerebral edema and transtentorial herniation
  - Permanent neurological deficits (less likely than with intracranial abscess)
  - Surgical complications
  - Seizures

EPIDURAL ABSCESS

Presenting Symptoms:

SUBJECTIVE	OBJECTIVE
	Intracranial
Headache	Elicit history of
May or may not be	prodromal otitis/
alteration of mental	sinusitis

state
Facial pain may be
present
Prodrome of symptoms
of sinusitis or otitis
Lethargy leading to
weakness
Fever

Local pain at abscess
site
Change in mental
status
Focal neurologic signs
Focal or generalized
seizure activity
Papilledema (late
symptom)
Gradenigo syndrome
(unilateral facial
pain, lateral rectus
weakness, and
deficits in CN V and
VI where the abscess
is near the petrous
bone)
Edema or cellulitis of
the face may be
present

Spinal

Mid or lower back
pain
Headache
Stiff neck
Radicular symptoms

Focal vertebral pain
Focal tenderness to
percussion
Deficits of sensory,
motor, or sphincter
function leading to
paralysis
Nuchal rigidity
Impaired respiratory
function (cervical
cord involvement)
There may be recent
history of back
surgery, lumbar
puncture, epidural

anesthesia, penetrating injury to back, or decubitus ulcers

Differential Diagnosis:

Brain tumor
Intracranial abscess
Subdural empyema
Intracranial hemorrhage
Subdural hematoma
Extradural abscess
Encephalitis
Bacterial or aseptic meningitis
Vertebral osteomyelitis
Noninfectious radiculopathy
Sciatica
Spinal cord compression
Vertebral disc herniation
Spinal cord tumor
Intramedullary spinal cord lesions
Vertebral joint space infections

Recommended Workup:

- **Intracranial:**
  - CT or MRI of head usually show pathognomonic findings: superficial, circumscribed density between the outermost layer of meninges and the overlying skull or vertebral column
  - Lumbar puncture typically reveals nonspecific results and is **relatively contraindicated** because of the fear of tonsillar herniation
  - Blood cultures
  - Skull radiographs may reveal concomitant sinusitis or otitis
  - Neurosurgical drainage of intracranial epidural abscess may provide material for

microbiologic diagnosis as well as prevent formation of subdural empyema
- **Spinal:**
  - Blood cultures
  - MRI of spinal cord and vertebral column reveals pathognomonic findings: circumscribed area of diminished attenuation in epidural space, usually bulging into the spinal canal and possibly compressing the spinal cord
  - CT (with contrast) of spinal cord and vertebral column can be used to differentiate subdural from epidural infection, or in identifying vertebral osteomylelitis
  - Myelography can also be used to demonstrate spinal cord compression
  - Radiographs of the spine may show evidence of osteomyelitis

Definitive Diagnosis:

Epidural abscess, intracranial   ICD-9-CM 324.9
Epidural abscess, spinal cord   ICD-9-CM 324.1

Suggested Treatment:

- Neurosurgical drainage of all **intracranial** epidural abscesses to prevent development of subdural empyema
- Laminectomy and drainage of spinal epidural abscesses
- Empiric antibiotic treatment (may be modified after culture results are available):
  - Nafcillin 1.5 g IV every 4 hours
  - Penicillin allergy: Vancomycin 1 g IV every 12 hours, and
      Metronidazole 1 g intravenous load, then 500 mg IV every 6 hours, or
      Chloramphenicol 1 g IV every 6 hours for 4 to 6 weeks

- If Gram-negative infection is suspected (concomitant otitis or mastoiditis, or vertebral osteomyelitis), **add:** Ceftizoxime 1.5 g IV every 6 hours for 6 to 8 weeks

Follow-Up:

- Patients should be followed closely in hospital with serial CT or MRI scans to monitor resolution of abscess
- **Watch for:** signs and symptoms of
    - Spinal cord compression
    - Development of subdural empyema or intracranial abscess
    - Permanent neurological deficits
    - Surgical complications

SLOW INFECTIONS (PRION-RELATED) OF THE CENTRAL NERVOUS SYSTEM

Presenting Symptoms:

SUBJECTIVE	OBJECTIVE
	Kuru
Prodromal phase of long period of headaches and arthralgias	Cerebellar ataxia
	Action tremor
	Choreoathetosis
	Myoclonic jerks
Sudden onset of ataxia, tremor, and "jerky" involuntary movements	Coarse fasciculations
	Progressive dementia
	NO cranial nerve findings, motor weakness, or sensory loss (except in a few cases in the terminal stages of the disease)
Progressive dementia	
	Typically, onset of symptoms to death is 2 years

Creutzfeldt-Jakob Disease (CJD)

History of corneal transplantation, dural graft, use of contaminated neurosurgical instruments, or stereotactic depth electrodes

History of receiving human cadaveric growth hormone for treatment of pituitary disease

History of receiving human cadaveric pituitary gonadotropin for infertility

Rapidly progressive dementia with associated myoclonus

Visual disturbances (visual field cuts, cortical blindness, visual agnosia)

Cerebellar ataxia

Rapidly progressive mental deterioration

Exuberant myoclonus, induced or aggravated by a startle

Nystagmus

Hypokinesia and rigidity

Hyperreflexia and spasticity

Extensor plantar responses

NO/RARE cranial nerve or peripheral nervous system involvement

RARE seizure activity

Typically, onset of symptoms to death is 7 to 9 months

Subacute Sclerosing Panencephalitis (SSPE)

Age under 20 years

History of measles

Early complaints: diminished performance in school, forgetfulness, temper outbursts, distractibility,

Altered mental status

Grand mal seizure activity

Myoclonus

Athetosis, chorea, and ballistic movements

Dystonic movements

Paroxysmal

insomnia, and hallucinations

Later complaints: seizures, involuntary "jerky" movements, intellectual decline, changes in speech, difficulty in swallowing, visual disturbances, hyperthermia, diaphoresis

opisthotonos

Cortical blindness with optical atrophy

Focal chorioretinitis on funduscopic examination

Hypothalamic abnormalities including abnormalities of pulse and blood pressure

Focal neurologic deficits may occur

Typically, onset of symptoms to death is 1 to 3 years

Differential Diagnosis:

Oculomotor disorders
Wernicke's disease
Multiple sclerosis
Spinal chord or brain tumor
Vascular occlusion (basilar artery or its branches)
Encephalitis
Brain abscess
Cranial trauma
Hypoxic encephalopathy
Hepatic encephalopathy
Hypoparathyroidism
Tabes dorsalis
Friedreich's ataxia
Myxedema
Senile dementia
Drug/alcohol intoxication
Cerebrovascular disease
Meningitis

Thyrotoxicosis
Electrolyte disorders ($\downarrow$ Na$^+$, $\uparrow$ Ca^{2+}, $\downarrow$ K$^+$)
Subdural or epidural hematoma
Korsakoff's psychosis
Myoclonic epilepsy
Normal-pressure hydrocephalus
Pellagra
Cushing's disease
Schilder's disease
Huntington's chorea
Wilson's disease
Lipid storage diseases (e.g., Tay-Sachs, Niemann-
  Pick)
Mucopolysaccharidoses
Parkinson's disease
Tardive dyskinesia
Pheochromocytoma
Carcinoid syndrome
Lesch-Nyhan disease
Sydenham's chorea
Lupus erythematosus
Polycythemia vera
Senile chorea
Thalamic infarct or hemorrhage
Amyotrophic lateral sclerosis

Recommended Workup:

- **Kuru:** Laboratory tests are rarely helpful in
  making the diagnosis but can be used to
  exclude other diagnostic possibilities
  - CBC, differential, erythrocyte sedimentation
    rate (ESR) are all normal
  - CSF profile is unremarkable
  - EEG usually shows no gross abnormalities
  - CT/MRI typically show nonspecific
    findings
  - Molecular genetic studies may be helpful in
    some cases (patients with kuru may show a

higher than expected incidence of
homozygosity at codon 129 of the PrP gene)
- **Creutzfeldt-Jakob Disease:** Laboratory tests
  are rarely helpful in making the diagnosis but
  can be used to exclude other diagnostic
  possibilities
  - CBC, differential, ESR are all normal
  - Liver function tests (LFTs) may be slightly
    elevated
  - CSF is acellular with normal glucose and
    mildly elevated protein (pleocytosis or
    hypoglycorrhachia should prompt
    consideration of other diagnostic
    possibilities)
  - CSF enolase, creatine kinase-BB fraction
    (CK-BB), and ubiquitin are typically
    elevated
  - PrPc has been detected in CSF, but
    this test is not readily available in most
    diagnostic labs
  - CT of the brain may show nonspecific
    abnormalities
  - Profound and rapidly progressive dementia
    associated with CT findings of no significant
    cortical atrophy should suggest CJD
  - MRI of the brain may be more sensitive
    and show abnormally increased T2 signals
    in the striatum and thalamus or in the
    peripheral cortex
  - Positron emission tomography (PET) scans
    of the brain have been reported to show
    diagnostically useful patterns
  - EEG may be diagnostic in up to 90% of
    patients: pathognomonic slow background
    interrupted by generalized bilaterally
    synchronous bi- or triphasic periodic sharp
    wave complexes (PSWCs)

- Lack of PSWCs in a patient whose symptoms have persisted for longer than 4 months casts doubts on the diagnosis of CJD
- Brain biopsy will provide definitive diagnosis: typical neuropathological features of neuronal loss, reactive gliosis, and neuronal vacuolation with no inflammatory response
- Western immunoblotting of brain biopsy material with monoclonal and polyclonal anti-prion protein antibodies is both specific and sensitive for PrPsc gene product, a distinct CJD neuroprotein
- Molecular genetic studies of PrP gene mutations in codons 200 and 178, if available, may be used to confirm the diagnosis of CJD

- **Subacute Sclerosing Panencephalitis:** Diagnosis should be considered in a child or adolescent who shows progressive mental deterioration and myoclonic jerks or seizures; diagnosis can be confirmed by:
  - EEG: shows characteristic findings of paroxysmal synchronous bursts of high-voltage diphasic waves
  - CSF: has normal total protein content, but shows elevated gamma-globulin content constituting up to 60% of total CSF protein
  - Abnormally high titer of antimeasles antibody in blood and CSF is typical
  - CT of brain: shows dilatation of lateral ventricles and atrophy of cerebral cortex, brainstem, and cerebellum

Definitive Diagnosis:

Kuru	ICD-9-CM 046.0
Creutzfeldt-Jakob Disease	ICD-9-CM 046.1

CJD with dementia   ICD-9-CM 290.10
Subacute sclerosing   ICD-9-CM 046.2
   panencephalitis

Suggested Treatment:

- Kuru, CJD, and SSPE appear to be invariably fatal with no hope of recovery and for which no antimicrobial agent has been helpful; only symptomatic treatment, anticonvulsants, and supportive measures can be offered
- Treatments that have been tried and failed:
  - ℞ Idoxuridine (™Herplex)
  - ℞ Acyclovir (™Zovirax)
  - Interferons
  - Polyanions
  - ℞ Amphotericin B (™Amphocin, ™Fungizone)
- Anecdotal reports of stabilization or improvement have been noted with:
  - Amantadine
  - Vidarabine
  - Methisoprinol
  - **NOTE:** These results have NOT been confirmed, or represent anecdotal reports; these are not approved indications for these drugs

Follow-Up:

- Frequent follow-up with supportive measures and evaluation of disease progression are recommended
- Universal secretion precautions are prudent, although person-to-person spread of these diseases does not appear to occur without direct inoculation, implantation, or transplantation of infectious material
- Gloves should be worn when handling blood, urine, feces, CSF, and material soiled by these fluids

- Known prion-containing material should be sterilized either by steam autoclaving (1 hour at 132°C according to American Neurological Association (ANA) Guidelines, or 4.5 hours at 121°C at 15 psi according to published reports), or immersion into 1 N NaOH (1 hour or 30 minutes for 3 treatments, at room temperature)
- Ultraviolet (UV) light, alcohol, phenol, bleach, or formalin do not reliably reduce prion infectivity
- **Watch for:** signs and symptoms of disease progression as outlined above, culminating in patient's death

CONJUNCTIVITIS

Presenting Symptoms:

SUBJECTIVE

Redness and burning
  of eyes
Excess tearing
Modest to profuse
  exudate
Swelling of periorbital
  tissues
Fever and myalgia
  (viral)
Photosensitivity
Decreased visual acuity
  (occasionally)
Foreign body sensation
Rash (viral)

OBJECTIVE

In General:
Conjunctival
  hyperemia
Pruritus and tearing
Foreign body sensation
Exudation and matting
Chemosis
Pseudoptosis
Mild ocular pain
Usually normal visual
  acuity
Photosensitivity
Pruritus
Bacterial:
Minimal pruritus
Profuse, purulent
  exudate with
  moderate tearing

Usually unilateral (at
least initially)
Chemosis
Small tarsal plate
papillae
Rare lymphadenopathy
Viral:
Minimal pruritus
Minimal, clear exudate
with profuse tearing
Usually bilateral
Subconjunctival
hemorrhage
Tarsal plate lymphoid
follicles
Viral systemic
symptoms (fever,
myalgia, etc.)
Chemosis rare
Associated pharyngitis
common
Associated rash (e.g.,
measles or herpes)
Painfully enlarged
preauricular
lymphadenopathy
Chlamydial:
Minimal pruritus
Variable amounts of
exudate and tearing
Often bilateral
Associated
genitourinary
symptoms

Differential Diagnosis:

Uveitis (iritis, iridocyclitis, choroiditis)
Acute glaucoma
Allergic conjunctivitis

Chemical or irritative conjunctivitis
Corneal disease
Foreign body
Canalicular obstruction (canaliculitis,
  dacryocystitis)
Scleritis
Episcleritis
Kawasaki disease
Syphilis
Rickettsial, parasitic, or fungal infection
Thyroid disease
Stevens-Johnson syndrome
Reiter's syndrome
Sjögren's syndrome
Wegener's granulomatosis
Sarcoidosis
Carcinoid syndrome
Psoriasis
Trachoma
Trauma

Recommended Workup:

- Physical examination may be revealing in
  differentiating etiology of conjunctivitis:
  (Table 2.4)
- Conjunctival smear or smear of exudate for
  Gram stain and culture:
  - Gram-positive cocci: *S. aureus,*
    S. pneumoniae
  - Gram-negative cocci: *Neisseria* spp.,
    Branhamella spp.
  - Gram-positive bacteria: *Haemophilus*
    influenzae; rarely, *Pseudomonas,* coliforms,
    Klebsiella, Proteus spp.
- Conjunctival smear or smear of exudate for:
  - Bovin fixation and stain for herpes simplex
  - Viral culture
  - Giemsa stain:

Table 2.4.

Differentiating Etiology of Conjunctivitis

	Bacterial	Viral	Allergy	Iritis	Glaucoma
Lid swelling	Mod	Min	Sev	Min	Min
Pruritus	Min	Min	Sev	No	No
Lymphadenopathy	Min	Sev	Min	No	No
Eye pain	Min	Min	Min	Mod	Sev
Visual acuity diminished	No	No	No	Mod	Sev
Intraocular pressure elevated	No	No	No	No	Sev
Cornea	NL	NL	NL	PPT	Cloudy
Iris	NL	NL	NL	Dull & swollen	Congested & bulging
Pupil	NL	NL	NL	Small & irreg	Mid-dilated/unreactive
Pupil response to light	NL	NL	NL	Min	Min

Min = minimal; Mod = moderate; Sev = severe; No = none; NL = normal; PPT = precipitate; Irreg = irregular.

  —Polymorphonuclear leukocytes (PMNs) in
    bacterial conjunctivitis
  —Lymphocytes and mononuclear cells in
    viral conjunctivitis
  —PMNs, plasma cells, lymphoblastic cells
    with inclusion bodies in chlamydial
    conjunctivitis
- Fluorescein staining and examination under
  UV light used to rule out retained foreign
  body and corneal abrasion or ulcer

Definitive Diagnosis:

Acute bacterial conjunctivitis   ICD-9-CM 372.30
Acute viral conjunctivitis   ICD-9-CM 077.99
Acute herpetic conjunctivitis   ICD-9-CM 054.43
Acute chlamydial   ICD-9-CM 077.98
  conjunctivitis

Suggested Treatment:

- Bacterial conjunctivitis:
  - Tobramycin 0.3%, as ophthalmic drops:
    1 to 2 drops every 4 hours, or as
    ophthalmic ointment: ½-inch strip of
    ointment to lower conjunctival sac 4 times
    a day, for 5 to 7 days
    [**NOTE**: NOT for streptococcal infections], or
  - 10% sodium sulfacetamide, as ophthalmic
    drops: 1 to 2 drops every 4 hours, or as
    ophthalmic ointment: ½-inch strip of
    ointment to lower conjunctival sac 4 times
    a day and each night at bedtime for 5 to 7
    days, or
  - Erythromycin ophthalmic ointment (5 mg/g)
    4 times a day for 5 to 7 days
- If *Neisseria* spp. are involved or suspected, **add**
  to regimen above:
  - Cefixime 200 mg orally twice a day for 7 to
    10 days, or

- Ciprofloxacin 500 mg orally every 12 hours for 7 to 10 days, or
- Ceftriaxone 1 g intramuscularly for 1 dose; saline lavage of infected eye once
- For serious *Neisseria* infection:
  - Cefotaxime 1 g IV given every 6 hours, or
  - Ceftriaxone 2 g IV given every 12 hours for 7 to 10 days
- Viral conjunctivitis: Trifluridine 1% ophthalmic drops: 1 drop every 2 hours, up to 9 drops/day for 5 to 7 days
- Herpes conjunctivitis (for serious disease involving herpes simplex or zoster), **add** to regimen for viral conjunctivitis: Acyclovir 800 mg orally 5 times a day for 7 to 10 days
- Chlamydial conjunctivitis:
  - Doxycycline 100 mg orally 2 times a day for 3 weeks, or
  - Erythromycin 500 mg orally 4 times a day for 2 to 3 weeks
- Corticosteroids should **NOT** be used until a causative pathogen is **definitively excluded** and allergic conjunctivitis is established (use of topical corticosteroids in the presence of herpes or bacterial conjunctivitis can lead to spread of the infection to the cornea with subsequent ulceration and/or perforation

Follow-Up:

- Careful monitoring of clinical response, especially for first 24 hours
- Ophthalmologic consult recommended if severe infection or if clinical response is poor
- **Watch for:** signs and symptoms of
  - Chronic marginal blepharitis
  - Conjunctival scar
  - Corneal ulcer or perforation (especially with bacterial and herpes conjunctivitis)

- Hypopyon
- Lid scars and entropion (especially with varicella-zoster)
- Bacterial superinfection in viral and chlamydial conjunctivitis
- Clinical trachoma
- Bacteremia (especially with meningococcal conjunctivitis)
- Chronic conjunctivitis

KERATITIS

Presenting Symptoms:

SUBJECTIVE

Moderate to severe
  eye pain
Foreign body sensation
  in the eye
Excessive tearing
Photophobia
Blepharospasm
Decreased vision
  (variable, but more
  common than in
  conjunctivitis)
Corneal anesthesia
No discharge

OBJECTIVE

Loss of corneal
  transparency (early
  sign)
Focal epithelial defect
  ranging to frank
  corneal ulceration
  under ultraviolet
  (UV)/fluorescein
  examination
Suppurative corneal
  inflammation of
  stroma
Keratolysis
Corneal leukoma (late
  sign)
Vesicular blepharitis
  (herpes keratitis)
Corneal edema
Discharge typically
  absent, unless there
  is purulent bacterial
  keratitis (main

difference from
conjunctivitis)

Differential Diagnosis:

Bacterial or viral conjunctivitis
Keratoconjunctivitis
Uveitis
Allergic conjunctivitis
Chemical or irritative keratoconjunctivitis
Foreign body
Scleritis
Episcleritis
Kawasaki disease
Syphilis
Rickettsial, parasitic, or fungal infection
Thyroid disease
Stevens-Johnson syndrome
Reiter's syndrome
Sjögren's syndrome
Wegener's granulomatosis
Sarcoidosis
Trachoma
Hypersensitivity reaction
Diabetes mellitus-associated corneal ulcerations
Tuberculosis interstitial keratitis
Cogan syndrome
Corneal trauma/abrasion
—Sicca
—Improperly cared-for contact lenses
—Trichiasis
—Entropion
—Neurogenic corneal anesthesia
—Immunodeficiency state

Recommended Workup:

- Physical examination will yield evidence of
  corneal suppuration and/or ulceration
  distinctive of keratitis

- To distinguish infectious from noninfectious keratitis, and to identify the specific infection (bacterial, viral, or fungal) involved:
  - Local anesthetic without antiseptic properties (e.g., proparacaine HCl 0.5%) is applied to affected eye
  - Multiple samples from each area of suppuration, inflammation, and/or ulceration are obtained with
    —Kimura blunt platinum spatula,
    —Sterile surgical blade, or
    —Calcium alginate swab
  - Corneal scrapings are transferred to clean glass slide for:
    —Gram stain
    —Giemsa stain
    —Acid-fast stain
    —Calcofluor white stain
    —Methenamine silver stain
  - Corneal scrapings are used to inoculate:
    —Blood agar
    —Chocolate agar
    —Thioglycolate broth
    —Saboraud's agar
    —Anaerobic blood agar
    —Middlebrook agar or Bactec medium (if mycobacterial infection is suspected)
  - Samples from the unaffected eye are also collected to ascertain the patient's normal eye flora for comparison to the results from the affected eye
  - The microbiological profile generated will verify a microbial etiology and identify the pathogen
- Slit-lamp examination: pathognomonic findings consistent with keratitis

- Gram stain and culture of aqueous/vitreous humors are usually of little help because they remain sterile in most microbial keratitis until a late stage when infective endophthalmitis may occur

Definitive Diagnosis:

Keratitis (nonspecific)	ICD-9-CM 370.9
Keratitis with ulceration	ICD-9-CM 370.00
Herpes keratitis	ICD-9-CM 054.43
Purulent/suppurative keratitis	ICD-9-CM 370.8
Syphilitic keratitis	ICD-9-CM 090.3

Suggested Treatment:

- Most infections will respond to **topical therapy,** applied every hour during the day and every 2 hours at night for 5 days, then less frequently (3 to 4 times a day) for 5 days; this is identified below as "top"
- Resistant or difficult-to-treat infections may require **subconjunctival injections:** 1 dose is given daily for 4 days (the first dose may be repeated after 12 hours in severe cases); this is identified below as "subconj" and may be followed by top therapy for 5 to 7 days
- Severe, suppurative, or contiguously spreading infections (e.g., sclerokeratitis), or those threatening impending perforation may require **oral or intravenous** treatment for 7 to 14 days
- Bacterial keratitis:
  - Gram-positive:
    Cefazolin 50 mg/mL top or 100 mg/ 0.5 mL subconj or 15 mg/kg/day IV given every 6 hours, or
    PCN G 100,000 U/mL top or 1 million U

subconj or 2 million U IV every 4 to
6 hours, or
Penicillin allergy/penicillin-resistant:
Vancomycin 50 mg/mL top or 25 mg/
0.5 mL subconj, or
Erythromycin 1 g orally, then 500 mg
orally every 6 hours

- Gram-negative:
Gentamicin 10 to 20 mg/mL top or
20 mg/0.5 mL subconj or 3 to 5 mg/
kg/day IV given every 8 hours, or
Tobramycin 10 to 20 mg/mL top or
20 mg/0.5 mL subconj or 3 to 5 mg/
kg/day IV given every 8 hours, or
Ticarcillin 4 mg/mL top or 125 mg/
0.5 mL subconj or 1 to 2 g IV every
6 hours
Penicillin allergy: Ciprofloxacin 0.3%
ophthalmic solution top or 500 to
750 mg orally every 12 hours, or
400 mg IV every 12 hours

- *Pseudomonas*:
Ciprofloxacin 0.3% or ofloxacin 0.3% or
norfloxacin 0.3% ophthalmic solution
top, or
Gentamicin or tobramycin 10 to 20 mg/mL
top or 20 mg/0.5 mL subconj or 3 to
5 mg/kg/day IV given every 8 hours, or
Polymyxin B 1 to 2 mg/mL top or
10 mg/0.5 mL subconj, or
Ticarcillin or Piperacillin 1 g IV every
4 hours

- *Nocardia*:
Sodium sulfacetamide 10% to 30%
ophthalmic ointment or solution top, or
Amikacin 50 to 100 mg/mL top or
25 mg/0.5 mL subconj or 10 to 15 mg/
kg/day IV given every 8 hours

- *Chlamydia*:
    Doxycycline 100 mg orally every
        12 hours, or
    Erythromycin 5 mg/g ophthalmic
        ointment top or 500 mg orally every
        6 hours
- Fungal keratitis:
    - Natamycin 5% suspension top or
      amphotericin B 1.5 to 3 mg/mL top or
    - Miconazole 1% solution or 2% ointment
      top, or
    - Miconazole 5 to 10 mg/0.5 to 1.0 mL
      subconj or amphotericin B 0.5 to 1.0 mg
      subconj, or
    - Ketoconazole 200 mg orally once daily or
      Itraconazole 200 mg orally once daily , or
    - Fluconazole 200 mg orally once, then
      100 mg orally once daily or 100 to 200 mg/
      day continuous intravenous infusion (may
      be required in cases of *Candida* keratitis)
- Parasitic keratitis (most commonly,
  Acanthamoeba):
    - Neomycin 20 mg/mL top plus
      propamidine solution 0.1 mg/mL or
      ointment 0.15% top, or
    - Paromomycin 10 mg/mL top plus
      propamadine solution 0.1 mg/mL or
      ointment 0.15% top, or
    - Ketoconazole 200 mg orally every 12 hours
      for severe cases
- Viral keratitis (primarily herpes simplex):
    - Trifluridine 1% ophthalmic solution top, or
    - Vidarabine 3% ophthalmic ointment top, or
    - Idoxuridine 0.1% ophthalmic solution top, or
    - Acyclovir 400 to 800 mg orally 5 times a
      day (**only** for patients with severe herpetic
      keratitis, particularly in atopic individuals

who are susceptible to aggressive ocular and dermal herpetic disease)
- Atropine 1% ophthalmic drops, 1 to 2 drops 3 times a day may be added in patients with accompanying herpetic uveitis
- **NOTE:** concurrent prophylactic antibacterial antibiotics are relatively contraindicated because of the increased risk for drug toxicity; they should be used only where there is significant danger of bacterial superinfection
- Empiric antibacterial therapy (no organism identified, but lesion suggestive of bacterial infection):
  - Cefazolin 50 mg/mL top or 100 mg/0.5 mL subconj or 15 mg/kg/day IV given every 6 hours, plus gentamicin 10 to 20 mg/mL top or 20 mg/0.5 mL subconj or 3 to 5 mg/ kg/day IV given every 8 hours, or
  - Tobramycin 10 to 20 mg/mL top or 20 mg/0.5 mL subconj, plus bacitracin 10,000 units/mL top, or
  - Polymyxin B 1 to 2 mg/mL top or 10 mg/ 0.5 mL subconj, plus vancomycin 50 mg/ mL top or 25 mg/0.5 mL subconj
- Empiric antifungal therapy (no organisms identified, but lesion suggestive of fungal infection):
  - Natamycin 5% suspension top, or
  - Amphotericin B 1.5 to 3 mg/mL top or 0.5 to 1.0 mg subconj (rarely necessary)
- Use of corticosteroids:
  - **Controversial:** risk-benefit ratio not settled
  - May minimize inflammatory sequelae of bacterial keratitis
  - May be used *cautiously* after antifungal therapy has been well underway to

     minimize corneal destruction from the host immune response to the fungi
- Contraindicated in herpetic epithelial keratitis
- Very useful in herpetic stromal keratitis and/or concurrent scleritis
- Agents that may be used include:
  —Dexamethasone sodium phosphate 0.05% ophthalmic ointment, thin coating to affected eye 3 to 4 times a day, or 0.1% ophthalmic solution, 1 to 2 drops 3 to 4 times a day, or
  —™Cortisporin ophthalmic ointment (polymyxin B 5000U, bacitracin 400U, neomycin 3.5 mg, and hydrocortisone 10 mg per g ointment) 3 to 4 times a day, or
  —™NeoDecadron ophthalmic ointment (neomycin 3.5 mg and dexamethasone 0.5 mg per g ointment) 3 to 4 times a day, or
  —™TobraDex ophthalmic ointment or suspension (tobramycin 0.3% and dexamethasone 0.5%) 3 to 4 times a day, or
  —™Blephamide ophthalmic suspension (sulfacetamide 10% and prednisolone 0.2%) 3 to 4 times a day

NOTE: In areas where natamycin is not available, may substitute amphotericin B 0.5% top or 1 to 2 mg subconj

- For treatment failures or patients unresponsive to conventional therapy, consider:
  - "Fortified" topical solutions at very high frequency (every 15 minutes to 1 hour), composed of formulations of parenteral antibiotics added to commercially available ocular lubricants

- Continuous lavage of cornea with antibiotic solutions
- Soft hydrophilic contact lenses with frequent topical administration of antibiotics for enhanced drug delivery
- Collagen corneal shields soaked with antibiotic solutions for enhanced antibiotic penetration*[†]
- Polymer inserts soaked with antibiotics
- Liposomal delivery systems or reformulations of topical antibiotics
- Transcorneal iontophoresis of antibiotics*
- Placement of temporary punctal occlusion plugs*
- Parenteral (intravenous/intramuscular) antibiotics, especially for severe suppurative keratitis or sclerokeratitis

Follow-Up:

- Usually hospitalize patients for treatment to prevent corneal perforation
- Frequent slit lamp examinations until there is clinical improvement
- Patients with fungal keratitis usually require corneal transplant
- **Watch for:** signs and symptoms of
    - Corneal ulceration and/or perforation
    - Endophthalmitis
    - Central corneal scarring
    - Spread of infection to sclera (sclerokeratitis)
    - Visual loss

*Requires consulting ophthalmologist
[†]Experimental technique with only anecdotal data

- Decreased corneal sensation (may lead to increased chance for corneal trauma)
- Medullary infarction
- Indications for corneal transplant

ENDOPHTHALMITIS

Presenting Symptoms:

SUBJECTIVE

Severe pain on movement of eye
Redness of sclera and vitreous
Photophobia
Profound blurring of vision
Commonly, history of penetrating eye injury or intraocular surgery, with inflammatory symptoms occurring rapidly within 24 to 48 hours (bacterial) or slowly after several weeks (fungal)
Common in intravenous drug users and diabetics (hematogenous spread from distant locus)

OBJECTIVE

Inflammation of ocular cavity and adjacent structures
Difficulty or lack of visualization of fundus from inflammation of anterior chamber and vitreous
Exaggerated conjunctival hyperemia
Chemosis
Lid edema
Specific findings of vitreal abscess on slit lamp examination (see below)
Chorioretinitis
Hypopyon

Differential Diagnosis:

Bacterial or viral conjunctivitis
Keratoconjunctivitis
Uveitis
Allergic conjunctivitis
Chemical or irritative keratoconjunctivitis
Foreign body
Scleritis
Episcleritis
Hypersensitivity reaction
Eye trauma
Retained lens material following cataract surgery
Neoplasm
Syphilis
Retinal vasculitis
Periarteritis
Chorioretinitis
Papillitis
Whipple's disease

Recommended Workup:

- History may be helpful in revealing the etiologic agent of endophthalmitis:
  - Intraocular surgery and cataract extraction: bacterial
  - Sudden onset in unoperated, nontraumatized eye: bacterial hematogenous spread from distant focus (especially prevalent in intravenous drug user)
  - Previous fungal keratitis with extension: fungal
  - Use of contaminated ophthalmic irrigation solution: fungal
  - Delayed onset of signs and symptoms for several weeks following ocular trauma or intraocular surgery: fungal

- - Indwelling catheter-acquired candidemia: fungal
  - Immunocompromised patient: fungal
  - Penetrating nonsurgical trauma: bacterial very rare
- Slit lamp examination by an experienced ophthalmologist will yield pathognomonic findings of endophthalmitis and may distinguish bacterial, viral, fungal, and parasitic etiologies
- Blood cultures (especially if hematogenous spread is suspected)
- Aspiration of 0.5 to 1.0 mL of vitreous under local anesthesia through a pars plana sclerotomy using a 23G needle; aspirate is examined to identify organisms:
  - Gram stain
  - Giemsa stain
  - Periodic acid-Schiff (PAS) stain
  - Gomori methenamine silver stain
  - Calcofluor white stain (fungi)
  - Fluorochrome stain (mycobacteria)
  - Inoculation for culture and antimicrobial susceptibility testing onto:
    —Blood agar
    —Chocolate agar
    —Thioglycolate broth
    —Saboraud's agar
  - Cytology
  - Enzyme-linked immunosorbent assay (ELISA) testing (best used for specimen of aqueous humor material) for specific antibodies (especially useful for diagnosis of *Toxocara* infection)
- Ultrasound, or CT/MRI, if unable to visualize retina

Definitive Diagnosis:

Infective unspecified endophthalmitis	ICD-9-CM 360.00
Panophthalmitis	ICD-9-CM 360.02
Vitreous abscess	ICD-9-CM 360.04
Parasitic endophthalmitis	ICD-9-CM 360.13

Suggested Treatment:

- Endophthalmitis is a true ophthalmologic emergency, requiring:
  - Early diagnostic aspirates,
  - **Immediate** empiric broad-spectrum antimicrobial coverage,
  - Anti-inflammatory therapy to reduce the host immune response,
  - Modification of the antimicrobial therapy based on the results of microbial identification and susceptibility testing, and
  - Possible vitrectomy
- Bacterial endophthalmitis:
  - Empiric:
    Vancomycin 1 mg/0.1 mL plus amikacin 0.4 mg/0.1 mL by intravitreal injection, and
    Ceftazidime 1 to 2 g IV every 8 hours or Vancomycin 1 g IV every 12 hours
  - Post-traumatic (*Bacillus cereus*):
    Clindamycin 1 mg/0.1 mL by intravitreal injection plus 600 to 900 mg IV every 8 hours
  - Post-surgical (*S. aureus, Pseudomonas, Staphylococcus epidermidis, Propionibacterium acnes*):
    —Cefazolin 2.25 mg/0.1 mL by intravitreal injection, and PCN G 2 million U IV every 4 to 6 hours, or
    —Penicillin allergy: Vancomycin 1 g IV every 12 hours, and

—Pars plana vitrectomy and removal of all residual lens material and capsule
- Hematogenous:
  Vancomycin 1 mg/0.1 mL by intravitreal injection, and
  Ceftazidime 1 to 2 g IV every 8 hours
- Fungal endophthalmitis:
  - Post-surgical (*Neurospora, Candida, Scedosporium, Paecilomyces*):
    —Amphotericin B 0.3 to 1.0 mg/kg/day IV given as a slow infusion over 4 to 8 hours, plus
    —Natamycin 5% suspension top, plus
    —Vitrectomy
  - Hematogenous spread (*Candida, Aspergillus*):
    —Amphotericin B 0.3 to 1.0 mg/kg/day IV given as a slow continuous infusion over 4 to 8 hours, plus
      Flucytosine 50 to 150 mg/kg/day orally given every 6 hours, plus
    —Vitrectomy
    —Itraconazole 200 to 400 mg/day orally given every 12 hours may be given after the infection has become more indolent or toxicity from amphotericin B becomes life-threatening
  - *Cryptococcus* and *Coccidioides:*
    Amphotericin B 0.3 to 1.0 mg/kg/day IV given as a slow continuous infusion over 4 to 8 hours and 0.01 mg given as an intravitreal injection
    NOTE: This treatment is based on several **anecdotal reports** where a positive response was seen in 20% to 50% of a limited number of patients treated

- *Histoplasma:*
  - —Prednisone 60 mg orally daily; gradual taper over 10 to 14 days, and
  - —Photocoagulation or cryopexy of macular lesions not involving the fovea
- Viral endophthalmitis:
  - Herpes simplex:
    - Atropine 1% ophthalmic drops, 1 to 2 drops 3 times a day, and
    - Dexamethasone phosphate 0.05% ophthalmic ointment or 0.1% suspension, thin coating or 1 to 2 drops to affected eye 3 to 4 times a day
  - Varicella-zoster: Acyclovir 800 mg orally 5 times a day
  - Cytomegalovirus:
    - —Ganciclovir 5 mg/kg IV twice a day during induction therapy; 5 mg/kg/day IV for maintenance, plus
    - —Address underlying immunodeficiency (e.g., reduce or discontinue immunosuppressive therapy; treat HIV infection, etc.)
- Parasitic endophthalmitis:
  - *Toxoplasma:*
    - Pyrimethamine 200 mg orally once, then 50 to 75 mg orally once daily, plus
    - Sulfadiazine 1 to 1.5 g orally every 6 hours or
    - Sulfa allergy: Clindamycin 600 mg orally every 6 hours, plus
      - Folinic acid (leucovorin) 10 to 20 mg orally once daily, plus
      - Dexamethasone phosphate 0.05% ophthalmic ointment or 0.1%

> suspension 3 to 4 times a
> day, plus
> Prednisone 60 mg orally daily; gradual
> taper over 14 to 21 days

- *Toxocara:*
  > Methylprednisolone acetate 1 to 2 mg
  > as a periocular depot administered
  > daily, or
  > Prednisone 60 mg orally once a day;
  > gradual taper over 10 to 14 days

- Corticosteroid use:
  - Even where not specifically mentioned above, intraocular instillation of corticosteroids is highly recommended in all cases of infectious endophthalmitis to prevent the visually destructive secondary processes that can occur from host immune and inflammatory responses to the causative organism; if vision is to be retained, control of these secondary processes MUST accompany effective antimicrobial therapy:
    - —Hydrocortisone ophthalmic ointment 0.5%
    - —Prednisolone acetate suspension 0.125% and 1%
    - —Prednisolone sodium phosphate solution 0.125% and 1%
    - —Dexamethasone sodium phosphate suspension 0.1% and ointment 0.05%

Follow-Up:

- Hospitalization is typically necessary
- Frequent slit lamp examinations are used to follow the clinical course of the patient
- If hematogenous spread is suspected, a septic focus must be identified and treated, consider:

- Meningitis
- Abdominal infection
- Endocarditis
- Pneumonia
- Otitis media
- Breast abscess
- Paronychia
- Pharyngitis
- Lymphangitis

- Be prepared to arrange for emergency vitrectomy
- **Watch for:** signs and symptoms of:
    - Panophthalmitis
    - Blindness

PERIOCULAR INFECTIONS

Presenting Symptoms:

SUBJECTIVE	OBJECTIVE
	Eyelids
	Blepharitis
Foreign-body sensation	Inflammation of the lid
Itching, burning, redness of lid margins	margins, either at anterior of margin involving the lash follicles, or posteriorly involving the meibomian gland
Excessive tearing	
Conjunctival irritation	
Glue-like discharge from eyes during sleep	Staphylococcal ulcerative
Crusts or scales on the lid margins	blepharitis: tenacious adherent crusting lesions on the anterior lid margins with small pustules on the lash follicles

Herpetic ulcerative blepharitis: follicular conjunctivitis with ipsilateral preauricular lymphadenopathy

Hordeolum (Stye)

Pain, redness, tenderness of lid margin

Small, round, tender area of swelling at lid margin

Excessive tearing

Photophobia

Foreign body sensation

Small yellowish spot on lid

Drainage of pus from lid margin

Internal: diffuse lid swelling, erythema and tenderness

Small abscess of meibomian glands pointing to skin or conjunctival surface of the lid

External: Discrete, small, superficial, elevated, erythematous pustules on lid margin pointing toward the skin

Affects glands of Zeis (sebaceous glands connected to eyelash follicles) and glands of Moll (apocrine sweat glands near the lid margin)

Internal or External: collection of pus/ discharge may be present

Lacrimal Apparatus (Dacryocystitis)

Pain, redness, swelling around lacrimal sac

Epiphora

Erythema and edema around lacrimal sac

Conjunctivitis/

Conjunctivitis
Blepharitis
Fever
Pus may drain from
   lacrimal punctum

blepharitis
May elicit history of:
—Mucosal polyps
—Congenital
   dacryostenosis
—Nasal trauma
—Deviated septum
—Hypertorphic
   rhinitis
Pus may regurgitate
   through punctum

Orbit and Cavernous Sinus
Orbital Cellulitis

Extreme orbital pain
Lid swelling
Fever
Malaise
Rhinorrhea

Chemosis
Orbital edema
Exophthalmos and
   proptosis
Impaired ocular
   motion
Conjunctival
   hyperemia
Increased orbital
   pressure
Congestion of retinal
   veins
Chorioretinal striae
Leukocytosis
May elicit history of:
—Paranasal sinusitis
—Trauma to the eyelid
   (especially puncture
   wound)
—Retained foreign
   body in eye

Cavernous Sinus Thrombosis

Severe headache
Diminished level of

Exophthalmos
Papilledema

<table>
<tr><td>

consciousness
Seizure activity
High fever

</td><td>

Severe signs of
  cerebritis
Meningeal signs
Cranial nerve palsies
  (often bilateral
  trigeminal
  involvement)
Internal and external
  ophthalmoplegia
Paretic eye muscles
  (bilateral)
Diminished sensorium
Septic fever curve
May elicit history of:
—Orbital cellulitis
—Sphenoidal or
  ethmoidal sinusitis
—Otitis media or
  interna

</td></tr>
</table>

Differential Diagnosis:

Chalazion
Noninfectious dermatoblepharitis
Blepharitis
Eyelid neoplasms (usually basal cell carcinoma, but may be squamous cell or sebaceous cell carcinoma)
Allergies/hypersensitivities
Seborrheic blepharitis
Dacryoadenitis
Dacryostenosis (usually congenital)
Entropion
Ectropion
Xanthelasma
Conjunctivitis
Panendophthalmitis
Exophthalmos secondary to hyperthyroidism

Arteriovenous aneurysm of internal carotid artery
Carotid-cavernous fistula
Meningioma
Unilateral high myopia
Nasal or facial bone fracture
Canaliculitis
Meningitis
Encephalitis
Physical or chemical trauma to the eye

Recommended Workup:

- Blepharitis:
  - Physical examination of eye is usually sufficient to establish the diagnosis
  - May collect drainage or scrapings from lid margins for Gram stain and culture
  - Biopsy atypical cases or where carcinoma is suspected
- Hordeolum:
  - Physical examination of eye is usually sufficient to establish the diagnosis
  - May collect discharge or scrapings from lid margins for Gram stain and culture
  - Lacrimal duct irrigation should be attempted; successful irrigation rules out dacryocystitis
- Dacryocystitis:
  - Physical examination of eye is usually sufficient to establish the diagnosis
  - Jones tests may be used to evaluate the patency of the lacrimal drainage system:
    —Jones I test: 2% fluorescein dye is instilled into the conjunctival sac. Secretions are collected on nasal applicator beneath the inferior turbinate: if no dye is collected, proceed to
    —Jones II test: cannulate nasolacrimal sac and irrigate with sterile saline. If dye is

       collected from nasal secretions, there is nasolacrimal duct obstruction and dacryocystitis is strongly suggested

- Orbital cellulitis:
  - Collect samples for Gram stain, PAS stain, and culture from:
    —Conjunctiva
    —Skin
    —Blood
    —Oral mucosa
    —Nasal mucosa
    —Discharge/exudate
  - Culture evaluation should include inoculation of samples into:
    —Blood agar
    —Chocolate agar
    —Saboraud's agar
    —Thioglycollate broth
    —Anaerobic culture tubes
  - Ultrasound of orbit will detect possible abscess formation
  - Radiographs, CT, or MRI of orbit to evaluate sinus and bony abnormalities, abscess formation, and presence of foreign body
  - In children, a primary source of infection (in absence of obvious trauma or foreign body) should be investigated; consider:
    —Skin
    —Nasopharynx
    —Teeth
    —Oral cavity
- Cavernous sinus thrombosis:
  - MRI or CT with contrast of cavernous and air sinuses, orbit and brain to delineate extent of infection and possible abscess formation

- Carotid angiography may be attempted to investigate infarction of ocular arterial supply and retinal artery (**CAUTION:** this is a potentially dangerous test)
- Orbital venography to investigate extent of thrombosis of orbital veins
- Lumbar puncture is of little diagnostic value; nonspecific pleocytosis with typically negative cultures; it may be useful to rule out meningitis
- Nasal discharge and blood should be collected for culture
- If air sinus is drained, material should be sent for culture
- A primary source of infection should be investigated in all patients; consider:
  - —Face
  - —Nasal cavity
  - —Paranasal sinuses
  - —Ear
  - —Eye (orbital infection)
  - —Source of trauma

Definitive Diagnosis:

Blepharitis	ICD-9-CM 373.0
Hordeolum	ICD-9-CM 373.1
Dacryocystitis	ICD-9-CM 375.30
Orbital cellulitis	ICD-9-CM 376.01
Cavernous sinus thrombosis	ICD-9-CM 325

Suggested Treatment:

- Blepharitis:
  - Erythromycin 0.5% or sodium sulfacetamide 10% ophthalmic ointment topically 4 times a day for 7 to 10 days
  - Scrub eyelids with diluted shampoo applied to lid margins

- If infection is resistant or recurrent,
    Tetracycline 100 mg daily for 3 to 9 weeks
- Hordeolum:
  - Hot compresses applied topically for 10
    minutes 3 to 4 times a day are usually
    sufficient
  - If infection persists, can use erythromycin
    0.5% or sodium sulfacetamide 10%
    ophthalmic ointment topically 4 times a
    day for 7 to 10 days
  - On rare occasions that infection persists
    despite topical therapy, may use:
      Dicloxacillin 250 mg orally 4 times a day
        for 7 to 10 days, or
      Penicillin allergy: Erythromycin 250 mg
        orally 4 times a day for 7 to 10 days
  - Contents of hordeolum should be
    expressed as soon as suppuration is
    evidenced
- Dacryocystitis:
  - Mild cases: Cephalexin 500 mg orally every
    6 hours for 7 to 10 days
  - Severe cases: Cefazolin 1 g IV every 6
    hours for 10 to 14 days
  - This is empiric therapy that should be
    begun as soon as a diagnosis is made;
    antibiotics should be changed as results of
    culture and sensitivity testing become
    available
  - Hot compresses applied topically for 10
    minutes 4 times a day are helpful
  - Appearance of abscess requires incision
    and drainage with Gram stain and culture
    of collected material
  - If nasolacrimal duct obstruction is found on
    workup, patient should be instructed to
    massage lacrimal sac area 3 to 4 times a

day; if this is unsuccessful in relieving obstruction, probing of sac should be performed
- For resistant, recurrent, or chronic cases, may need:
  —Nasolacrimal intubation
  —Dacryocystorhinostomy
  —Removal of lacrimal sac
- Orbital cellulitis:
  - Empiric antibiotics should be started **immediately;** coverage may be changed once results of culture and antibiotic sensitivity testing are known
  - Mild disease: Cephalexin 500 mg orally every 6 hours for 14 days
  - Severe disease:
      Cefazolin 1 g IV every 6 hours for 7 days, or
      Nafcillin 1.5 g IV every 4 hours, or
      Penicillin allergy: Vancomycin 1 g IV every 12 hours
  - Resistance to antibiotics or lack of clinical response may be caused by abscess formation; incision and drainage will be necessary
- Cavernous sinus thrombosis:
  - Nafcillin 1.5 g IV every 4 hours for 10 to 14 days, or
      Penicillin allergy: Vancomycin 1 g IV every 12 hours for 10 to 14 days
  - Prednisone 40 mg orally daily with slow taper is recommended for its anti-inflammatory effects
  - If oral therapy is not feasible, may give Prednisolone sodium phosphate 40 to 60 mg IV/intramuscularly daily in divided doses every 4 to 8 hours with slow taper

- Anticoagulation with heparin subcutaneously has been used with some efficacy, but its role is still unclear [THIS IS STILL AN EXPERIMENTAL/UNTESTED ENTITY]
- Resistance to antibiotics or lack of clinical response may be caused by abscess formation; may need to drain infected air sinus

Follow-Up:

- Blepharitis and Hordeolum: patients should be seen several weeks after therapy to assess effectiveness of therapy
- Dacryocystitis: patients should be monitored closely, initially every second or third day, then weekly until clinical resolution; patients should be taught to massage the lacrimal sac area firmly several times daily
- Orbital cellulitis: patients are typically hospitalized for intravenous antibiotics and surgical consultation
- Cavernous sinus thrombosis: patients are typically hospitalized for intravenous antibiotics and surgical or neurosurgical consultation
- **Watch for:** signs and symptoms of
    - Blepharitis:
        - —Hordeolum scarring of eyelid margin
        - —Trichiasis
        - —Corneal infection/ulceration
    - Hordeolum: generalized cellulitis of eyelid
    - Orbital cellulitis:
        - —Scarring of eyelid
        - —Loss of vision

- —Optic neuritis
- —Thrombophlebitis of orbital
  veins
- —Cavernous sinus thrombosis
- —Panophthalmitis
- —Osteomyelitis
- —Strabismus
- —Afferent pupillary defect
- —Spread of infection to
  meninges and brain
- —Formation of orbital or
  subperiosteal abscess with
  rupture through orbital
  septum
- Cavernous sinus thrombosis:
  - —Mortality rate of 30% despite
    antibiotic therapy
  - —Spread of infection to
    meninges and brain

Upper Respiratory Tract, Trachea, and Bronchi

3

INFECTIONS COVERED

ACUTE SINUSITIS

Presenting Symptoms:

SUBJECTIVE	OBJECTIVE
Nasal congestion and discharge	For all of these signs: if Y, acute sinusitis is likely; if N, unlikely
Sinus pressure	
Malaise	Purulent nasal discharge?
Headache	
Fever	Periorbital edema?
Facial pain, ↑ with bending	Pain on percussion of sinus areas?
Cough	Fever?

Differential Diagnosis:

Rhinitis
Fungal infection
Cyst
Tumor
Foreign body
Wegener's granulomatosis

Suggested Workup:

- Transillumination of maxillary and frontal sinuses →dullness?
  ____Y: sinusitis likely
  ____N: sinusitis unlikely
- Sinus radiographs →cloudiness?
  - Air-fluid levels?
    ____Y: sinusitis likely;
    ____N: sinusitis unlikely
  - Opacity?
    ____Y: sinusitis likely;
    ____N: sinusitis unlikely
  - Thickened mucosa?
    ____Y: sinusitis likely;
    ____N: sinusitis unlikely

- Aspirate sinus/collect nasal discharge for Gram stain/culture: if *Haemophilus influenzae* and *Streptococcus pneumoniae:* think bacterial sinusitis

Definitive Diagnosis:

Acute sinusitis   ICD-9-CM 461.9

Suggested Treatment:

- Amoxicillin 500 mg orally every 8 hours for 14 to 21 days, or
  - Cefuroxime 250 mg orally every 12 hours for 14 to 21 days, or
  - Cefaclor 500 mg orally every 8 hours for 14 to 21 days
- Penicillin allergy: Trimethoprim-sulfamethoxazole (TMP-SMX) DS orally twice a day for 14 to 21 days, or
  - Clarithromycin 500 mg orally 3 times a day for 14 days, or
  - Azithromycin 250 mg orally once daily for 6 days
- Nasal decongestant may be used.

Follow-Up:

- Follow until clinically clear
- **Watch for:** signs and symptoms of
  - Meningitis
  - Abscess formation
  - Osteomyelitis
  - Orbital infection
  - Septic cavernous thrombosis

ORAL INFECTIONS AND STOMATITIS

Presenting Symptoms:

SUBJECTIVE	OBJECTIVE
Mouth and jaw pain	Intraoral ulcers may be:
Fever	—Lingual
Malaise	—Buccal

—Palatal
—Gingival
—Tonsillar
Gingival erythema
Gingival swelling

Differential Diagnosis:

Stomatitis
—Bacterial
—Viral (herpes)
—Fungal (thrush)
Vincent's angina
Gingivitis
Dental abscess
Tumor
Aphthous stomatitis
Behçet's syndrome

Suggested Workup:

- Detailed History and Physical:
  - Intense oral erythema?
    ____Y: stomatitis
    ____N: consider tumor; Behçet's syndrome
  - Necrotic ulceration of interdental papillae?
    ____Y: Vincent's angina
    ____N: stomatitis
  - White, curdy patches on tongue or palate?
    ____Y: thrush
    ____N: nonmycotic infection
  - Concomitant genital ulcers?
    ____Y: Behçet's syndrome
    ____N: primary oral infection
  - Collect scraping or exudate for Gram stain, Gomori's methenamine-silver (GMS) stain, and culture:
    —Candida/yeast forms?: thrush
    —Mix of anaerobes and *Streptococcus*: dental abscess

—Strict anaerobes: Vincent's angina
—Positive Tzanck test: herpes simplex

Definitive Diagnosis:

Stomatitis   ICD-9-CM 528.0
Herpes simplex   ICD-9-CM 054.2
Vincent's angina   ICD-9-CM 101
Behçet's syndrome   ICD-9-CM 136.1
Candida   ICD-9-CM 112.0

Suggested Treatment:

- Dental/periodontal infection/Vincent's angina:
  - Metronidazole 500 mg orally every 12 hours, plus
  - PCN V 250 mg orally every 6 hours, or
  - Clindamycin 300 mg orally every 8 hours (for Penicillin allergy) for 10 to 14 days
- Thrush:
  - Nystatin oral suspension (100,000 U/mL) 4 mL swish and swallow 4 times a day for 10 days, or
  - Clotrimazole 10 mg troches 4 times a day for 10 days, or
  - Ketoconazole 200 mg once daily for 7 to 14 days
- Herpes simplex:
  - Acyclovir 200 mg orally every 4 hours (5 times a day) for 10 days (generally not an indication, but anecdotal reports claim a benefit)

Follow-Up:

- Follow until clinically clear
- **Watch for:** signs and symptoms of
  - Abscess formation
  - Fungemia or viremia

- Pharyngeal/laryngeal spread of infection
- Pneumonia
- Meningitis

ACUTE OTITIS MEDIA

Presenting Symptoms:

SUBJECTIVE
Earache
Fever
Nasal discharge
Cough
Decreased hearing

OBJECTIVE
Erythematous, bulging
    tympanic membrane
Decreased eardrum
    mobility on
    pneumatic otoscopy
Decreased hearing

Differential Diagnosis:

Mandibular lesion
Dental problem

Suggested Workup:

- Good History and Physical reveals pathognomonic findings above
- Tympanocentesis only for treatment failures or for resistant *S. pneumoniae*

Definitive Diagnosis:

Acute otitis media   ICD-9-CM 382.0

Suggested Treatment:

- Adult: Amoxicillin 250 mg orally every 8 hours for 10 days
- Adult: Penicillin allergy: TMP-SMX DS twice a day for 10 days, or
  - Cefaclor 250 mg orally every 8 hours for 10 days
- Pediatric: Amoxicillin 40 mg/kg/day orally given every 8 hours for 10 days

- Pediatrics: Penicillin allergy: TMP 8 mg/kg/
  day + SMX 40 mg/kg/day orally given every
  12 hours for 10 days, or
    - Cefaclor 40 mg/kg/day orally given every
      8 hours for 10 days

Follow-Up:

- Otoscopic examination 2 to 4 weeks after
  diagnosis
- **Watch for:** signs and symptoms of
    - Perforation
    - Hearing loss
    - Acute mastoiditis
    - Facial nerve paralysis

OTITIS EXTERNA ("SWIMMER'S EAR")

Presenting Symptoms:

SUBJECTIVE	OBJECTIVE
Itching of ear	Erythematous/
Plugging of ear	edematous ear
Otalgia	canal
	Purulent discharge
	from canal
	Periauricular
	lymphadenitis
	Deficit of cranial nerve
	(CN) VII, IX–XII
	possible

Differential Diagnosis:

Cranial nerve palsy
Hearing loss
Nonspecific ear pain
Malignant external otitis
Eczema

Suggested Workup:

Thorough examination:
- Eczema present?
  - ____Y: eczematous (noninfectious) otitis
  - ____N: bacterial otitis externa likely
- Granulation tissue at external junction of osseus and cartilaginous portions of external ear?
  - ____Y: consider malignant otitis externa
  - ____N: bacterial otitis externa likely
- History of diabetes?
  - ____Y: consider malignant otitis externa
  - ____N: bacterial otitis externa likely
- Gram stain and GMS stain of purulent ear discharge:
  - *Aspergillus, Rhizopus,* yeast present?
    - ____Y: fungal otitis externa
    - ____N: bacterial otitis externa
- *Pseudomonas* and *Staphylococcus* present?: typical otitis externa

Definitive Diagnosis:

Infective otitis externa   ICD-9-CM 380.10
  (unspecified organism)

Suggested Treatment:

- Bacterial otitis externa:
  - 2% Acetic or boric acid topically 4 times a day for 10 days, or
    - Neomycin + polymyxin otic drops 3 times a day for 10 days, and
    - Hydrocortisone otic solution 3 times a day for 5 days
  - Be certain there is no otomycosis
- Fungal otitis externa:
  - Nystatin cream topically 2 times a day for 10 days, or

- 2% Acetic or boric acid topically 4 times a day for 10 days, or
- M-cresyl acetate otic drops 3 times a day for 10 days
- Necrotizing, malignant otitis externa
  - Ciprofloxacin 500 mg intravenously (IV) every 12 hours for 4 to 6 weeks, or
  - Tobramycin 3 to 5 mg/kg/day IV given every 8 hours for 4 to 6 weeks, or
  - Cefoperazone 2 g IV every 12 hours for 4 to 6 weeks, or
  - Ceftazidime 1 to 2 g IV every 8 hours for 4 to 6 weeks

Follow-Up:

- Follow until clinically clear: rapid for bacterial or fungal otitis externa; prolonged for malignant form
- **Watch for:** signs and symptoms of
  - Meningitis
  - Osteomyelitis
  - Abscess formation
  - Cranial nerve involvement

PERIMANDIBULAR INFECTIONS

Presenting Symptoms:

SUBJECTIVE	OBJECTIVE
Ear pain	Perimandibular,
Perimandibular mass	auricular, or cervical
Perimandibular	lymphadenitis
tenderness	Perimandibular mass
Oral pain	Enlarged parotid gland
Fever	Mandibular sinus or
	fistula with drainage
	(late in course)

Differential Diagnosis:

Cervicofacial actinomycosis
Parotitis
Anaerobic space infection
Acute cervical adenitis
Post-auricular cellulitis
Tumor

Suggested Workup:

- Surgical aspiration with Gram stain/culture of drainage/aspirate
    - *Actinomyces israeli:* "lumpy jaw" syndrome (perimandibular actinomycosis)
    - *S. aureus:* parotitis likely
    - Anaerobes: anaerobic space infection
    - *Streptococcus pyogenes, S. aureus,* and anaerobes: acute cervical adenitis
- Facial radiograph: perimandibular soft tissue mass with or without bone involvement

Definitive Diagnosis:

Cervicofacial actinomycosis   ICD-9-CM 039.3
Parotitis   ICD-9-CM 527.2
Anaerobic space infection   ICD-9-CM 041.84
Acute cervical adenitis   ICD-9-CM 289.3

Suggested Treatment:

- Actinomycosis:
    - PCN G 3 million U IV every 6 hours for 2 weeks, then
    - PCN V 1 g orally 4 times a day for 3 to 6 months
    - Penicillin allergy: Clindamycin 600 mg IV every 8 hours for 2 weeks, then
        Clindamycin 300 mg orally every 6 hours, or

> Tetracycline 500 mg orally every 6 hours, or
>
> Erythromycin 250 to 500 mg orally every 8 hours for 3 to 6 months

- Bacterial Parotitis:
  - Dicloxacillin 250 mg orally every 6 hours for 10 to 14 days
  - Penicillin allergy: Cephalexin 250 mg orally every 6 hours, or
    - Clindamycin 300 mg orally every 8 hours for 10 to 14 days
  - Surgery: Drainage procedure
  - Other: Sialogogues as needed
- Anaerobic space infection:
  - Clindamycin 600 mg IV every 8 hours, or
    - Cefoxitin 1 g IV or intramuscularly every 6 hours, or
    - PCN G 1 million U IV every 6 hours + Metronidazole 500 mg IV every 12 hours for 2 to 3 weeks
  - Surgery: Drainage procedure
- Acute cervical adenitis:
  - *S. pyogenes*
    - —PCN G 2 million U IV every 6 hours
    - —Penicillin allergy: Erythromycin 1 g IV every 6 hours
  - Anaerobes: Clindamycin 600 mg IV every 8 hours
  - *S. aureus:*
    - —Dicloxacillin 250 to 500 mg orally every 6 hours
    - —Penicillin allergy: Cephalexin 250 to 500 mg orally every 6 hours
  - All treatment given for 14 days, then re-evaluate clinically

Follow-Up:

- Follow until clinically clear
- Reassess clinically and microbiologically after 4 and 8 weeks of treatment
- **Watch for:** signs and symptoms of
    - Fungemia
    - Ocular involvement
    - Meningitis
    - Sepsis

ACUTE MASTOIDITIS

Presenting Symptoms:

SUBJECTIVE	OBJECTIVE
Otalgia	Bulging, erythematous tympanic membrane
Post-auricular tenderness	Post-auricular mass and erythema
Fever	Protrusion of auricle

Differential Diagnosis:

Otitis media
Abscess
Cholesteatoma
Cellulitis
Tumor
Aditus ad antrum

Suggested Workup:

- Plain skull radiograph →clouding of mastoid air cells?
    - ____Y: acute mastoiditis likely
    - ____N: acute mastoiditis unlikely
- CT of head→ clouding of mastoid air cells?
    - ____Y: acute mastoiditis likely
    - ____N: unlikely

- CT of head→ loss of bony septation in air cells?
  - ____Y: acute mastoiditis likely
  - ____N: unlikely
- If otorrhea present, collect discharge for Gram stain/culture:
  - Group A beta-hemolytic streptococci, *S. pneumoniae*, *H. influenzae*
    - ____Y: acute mastoiditis
    - ____N: unlikely

Definitive Diagnosis:

Acute mastoiditis   ICD-9-CM 383.00
Acute mastoiditis with   ICD-9-CM 383.01
   subperiosteal abscess

Suggested Treatment:

- Severe infection:
  - Ampicillin 1 to 2 g IV every 6 hours for 14 days
  - Penicillin allergy: Cefuroxime 750 mg IV every 8 hours for 14 days
- Moderate infection:
  - Amoxicillin + clavulanate 500/125 mg orally every 8 hours for 14 days
  - Penicillin allergy: Cefuroxime 500 mg orally every 12 hours for 14 days
- Ancillary procedures:
  - May require myringotomy with placement of pressure equalizing tube, and aspiration of subperiosteal abscess
  - Patients who do not respond to antibiotics within 72 hours or those with meningeal or intracranial complications may require mastoidectomy

Follow-Up:

- Follow closely for 2 to 4 weeks, with frequent cleaning of ear canal

- **Watch for:** signs and symptoms of
    - Subperiosteal abscess
    - CN VI palsy
    - Meningitis
    - Intracranial abscess

ACUTE PHARYNGITIS AND TONSILLITIS

Presenting Symptoms:

SUBJECTIVE	OBJECTIVE
Sore throat	Tonsillar enlargement with exudate
Fever	Pharyngeal erythema
Chills	Cervical lymphadenopathy
Malaise	Cough?
Headache	____Y: pharyngitis or tonsillitis unlikely
	____N: pharyngitis or tonsillitis possible

Differential Diagnosis:

Acute bacterial pharyngitis/tonsillitis
Acute viral pharyngitis/tonsillitis
Chronic allergic rhinitis
Chemical irritation
Viral laryngitis
Vincent's angina

Suggested Workup:

- Throat culture or spot screen: Group A streptococci?
    - ____Y: streptococcal pharyngitis/tonsillitis
    - ____N: viral infection more likely
- Monospot test:
    - ____Positive: Epstein-Barr virus infection

  _____Negative: Epstein-Barr virus infection
    less likely (repeat test in 7 to
    10 days)
- Rhinitis/cough?
  _____Y: viral infection more likely
  _____N: bacterial infection more likely
- Conjunctival injection?
  _____Y: consider allergy/viral infection
  _____N: bacterial infection more likely
- Palatal enanthem?
  _____Y: viral infection more likely
  _____N: bacterial infection more likely

Definitive Diagnosis:

Acute pharyngitis   ICD-9-CM 462
Acute tonsillitis   ICD-9-CM 463
Strep sore throat   ICD-9-CM 034.0

Suggested Treatment:

- Streptococcal pharyngitis/tonsillitis:
  - PCN VK 250 mg orally every 8 hours for
    10 days
      Penicillin allergy: Erythromycin 200 to
      400 mg orally 3 times a day for 10
      days, or
      Cephalexin 250 mg orally every 8 hours
      for 10 days
  - Treat presumptively until evidence is
    obtained that no bacterial infection is
    present
- Viral pharyngitis/tonsillitis
  - Salt water gargles
  - Acetaminophen as needed for pain
  - Dyclomine lozenges
  - Humidifier

Follow-Up:

- As needed
- **Watch for:** signs and symptoms of

- Rheumatic fever
- Post-streptococcal glomerulonephritis
- Peritonsillar abscess
- Sinusitis
- Pneumonia

EPIGLOTTITIS

Presenting Symptoms:

SUBJECTIVE
Acute onset without
  prodrome
Fever
Dysphagia, drooling
  (child)
Sore throat
Respiratory distress
Hoarseness
Minimal or no cough

OBJECTIVE
Edematous pharynx
Inspiratory stridor
Expiratory rhonchi
Diminished breath
  sounds
Respiratory distress
"Tripod" appearance
  with toxic
  appearance
Cervical
  lymphadenopathy
Inspiratory retractions

Differential Diagnosis:

Viral croup
Sepsis
Aspirated foreign body
Bacterial tracheitis
Peritonsillar or retropharyngeal abscess
Diphtheria

Recommended Workup:

- Toxic patients in imminent respiratory failure: INTUBATION
  - Post-intubation workup:
    - Indirect laryngoscopy to visualize inflammation of epiglottis, vallecula, and arytenoids

—Epiglottic swab for Gram stain and culture: *H. influenzae* and Group A streptococci?

____Y: epiglottitis likely

____N: epiglottitis unlikely, but not excluded

- Blood culture may be positive for *H. influenzae* and Group A streptococci in toxic patients
- Nontoxic patients not in imminent respiratory failure:
  - Lateral neck radiograph→ positive "thumb sign?"

    ____Y: epiglottitis confirmed

    ____N: unlikely, but not excluded

Definitive Diagnosis:

Acute epiglottitis without   ICD-9-CM 464.30
  obstruction

Acute epiglottitis with   ICD-9-CM 464.31
  obstruction

Suggested Treatment:

- Cefotaxime 100 mg/kg/day IV given every 6 hours, or
  Ceftriaxone 75 mg/kg/day IV given every 12 hours for 10 to 14 days
- Ensure patent airway: be prepared for:
  - Intubation, or
  - Needle cricothyroidotomy, or
  - Percutaneous tracheostomy if intubation is unsuccessful

Follow-Up:

- Laryngoscopy within 48 hours after extubation or clinical stabilization if not intubated
- **Watch for:** signs and symptoms of
  - Pneumonia
  - Meningitis

- Pericarditis
- Shock
- Pneumothorax

BACTERIAL TRACHEITIS

Presenting Symptoms:

SUBJECTIVE	OBJECTIVE
"Barking" cough	Inspiratory stridor
Fever	Respiratory distress
Gradual onset of upper airway symptoms	Subglottic edema
NO history of dysphagia or drooling	

Differential Diagnosis:

Epiglottitis
Foreign body aspiration
Retropharyngeal abscess
Pneumonia
Viral croup
Asthma
Viral laryngitis

Suggested Workup:

- Gram stain/culture tracheal secretions:
  - *S. aureus*
  - *H. influenzae*
  - *S. pneumoniae*
  - *Moraxella catarrhalis:* most common in bacterial tracheitis
- Direct laryngoscopy: Should visualize inflammation of subglottic epithelium $\pm$ membranous exudate
- Lateral neck radiograph: Subglottic narrowing? or Negative "thumb sign?"

____Y: tracheitis
____N: must rule out epiglottitis

Definitive Diagnosis:

Acute tracheitis   ICD-9-CM 464.1
Acute laryngotracheitis   ICD-9-CM 464.2

Suggested Treatment:

- Ampicillin + sulbactam 1 to 2 g ampicillin IV every 6 hours, or
- Nafcillin 0.5 to 1.0 g IV or intramuscularly every 6 hours, and
  - Cefuroxime 750 mg IV or intramuscularly every 8 hours, or
  - Cefotaxime 0.5 to 1.0 g IV or intramuscularly every 6 hours for 14 days
- Penicillin allergy: Clindamycin 600 mg IV every 8 hours, and
  - Chloramphenicol 1 g IV every 6 hours for 14 days

Follow-Up:

- Careful clinical evaluation, with intensive care unit (ICU) care if warranted
- **Watch for:** signs and symptoms of
  - Pneumonia
  - Toxic shock syndrome (*Staphylococcus*)
  - Endotoxin
  - Cardiopulmonary arrest

ACUTE LARYNGITIS

Presenting Symptoms:

SUBJECTIVE	OBJECTIVE
Hoarseness	Red, inflamed vocal chords
Abnormal sounding voice	Increased regional lymphadenopathy
Throat "tickling"	

Feeling of throat
  rawness
Fever
Malaise
Dysphagia
Cough

Aphonia
History of smoking or
  alcohol abuse

Differential Diagnosis:

Viral croup
Measles
Diphtheria
Vocal chord nodules
Laryngeal cancer

Suggested Workup:

- History and Physical usually provide diagnosis
- Direct laryngoscopy (rarely needed)
  - → Nodules? → vocal chord nodules
  - → Mass? → rule out malignancy
  - →Inflamed vocal chords with hemorrhage and/or exudate? → acute laryngitis likely
- Collect exudate noted on laryngoscopy for Gram stain and culture: beta-hemolytic streptococci?, *S. pneumoniae? M. catarrhalis?*: should treat with antibiotics

Definitive Diagnosis:

Acute laryngitis   ICD-9-CM 464.0

Suggested Treatment:

- If viral etiology is suspected, or Gram stain and culture are negative:
  - Analgesia
  - Inhalation of steam
  - Rest voice
- If bacterial etiology is suspected, or Gram stain is positive for beta-hemolytic

Streptococcus or *Pneumococcus:*
- PCN V 250 mg orally every 6 hours for 10 to 12 days
- Penicillin allergy: Erythromycin 250 mg orally every 6 hours for 10 to 12 days

Follow-Up:
- Usually not needed
- May consider influenza vaccine after infection is cleared
- **Watch for:** signs and symptoms of
    - Chronic laryngitis
    - Vocal chord fibrosis

ACUTE LARYNGOTRACHEOBRONCHITIS (CROUP)
Presenting Symptoms:

SUBJECTIVE	OBJECTIVE
Barking, spasmodic cough	Biphasic stridor
Fever	Hypoxia and cyanosis (80% of patients)
Upper respiratory infection prodrome	Inflamed subglottic region
Fatigue	NO involvement of supraglottic region
Increased respiratory rate	
NO hoarseness	
NO dysphagia or drooling	

Differential Diagnosis:
Epiglottitis
Foreign body aspiration
Subglottic stenosis
Bacterial tracheitis
Upper respiratory tract infection
Diphtheria

Suggested Workup:
- History and Physical usually provide diagnosis
- Fiberoptic laryngoscopy or bronchoscopy (rarely needed)

- $\rightarrow$ Inflammation of subglottic region, larynx, and trachea
  - $\rightarrow$ Inflammatory reaction of respiratory mucosa with thick mucoid secretions
- Rapid antigen test for virus panel may be positive for:
  - Parainfluenza 1
  - Paramyxovirus
  - Influenza virus type A
  - Respiratory syncytial virus (RSV)
  - Adenovirus
  - Rhinovirus
- Posterior to anterior (PA) and lateral neck radiograph: Funnel-shaped subglottic region with normal epiglottis

Definitive Diagnosis:

Acute laryngotracheobronchitis	ICD-9-CM 464.20
Acute laryngotracheobronchitis with obstruction	ICD-9-CM 464.21

Suggested Treatment:

- Dexamethasone 1 to 1.5 mg/kg every 8 to 12 hours (up to 8 times a day; no more than 20 mg/day)
- ℞Nebulized racemic epinephrine (™Vaponefrin) given as 0.2 to 0.5 mL of 2.25% racemic epinephrine in 2 to 3 mL of normal saline every 30 minutes
  - **SPECIAL WARNING:** ™Vaponefrin is known to cause the following adverse effects:
    —Reflex tachycardia
    —Rebound stridor with obstruction of airway

- Caution must be used in using Vaponefrin, with cardiac monitoring and emergency airway procedures available.

Follow-Up:

- Severe cases require ICU care
- **Watch for:** signs and symptoms of
    - Subglottic stenosis
    - Bacterial tracheitis (superinfection)
    - Pneumonia

ACUTE BRONCHITIS

Presenting Symptoms:

SUBJECTIVE	OBJECTIVE
Upper respiratory symptoms with coryza, malaise, chills, fever, cough	Rales Rhonchi Wheezes Injected pharynx NO pulmonary consolidation
Fatigue	
Muscle aches	
Hemoptysis (occasionally)	
Dyspnea	

Differential Diagnosis:

Influenza
Bronchopneumonia
Bronchiectasis
Sinusitis
Mycoplasma infection
Mycobacterium tuberculosis infection
Aspiration of foreign body
Cystic fibrosis
Reactive airways disease
Tracheitis

Suggested Workup:

- Diagnosis made based on History and Physical
- Chest radiograph (CXR):
  - Consolidation?
    ____Y: think bronchopneumonia
    ____N: normal CXR suggests bronchitis
- Sputum collection for Gram stain and culture: Expect:
  - *Bordetella pertussis*
  - *H. influenzae*
  - *S. pneumoniae*
  - *M. catarrhalis*
  - *Chlamydia*
- Viral titers/rapid antigen panel: Expect:
  - Adenovirus
  - Influenza and parainfluenza viruses
  - Herpes simplex virus
  - RSV
  - Coxsackievirus

Definitive Diagnosis:

Acute bronchitis   ICD-9-CM 466.0

Suggested Treatment:

- Antibiotic treatment is controversial
- Most reasonable approach is as follows:
  - Start antibiotics after sputum sample is obtained; if culture is positive for bacteria or if patient rapidly improves on antibiotics, continue
  - Start antibiotics if patient has history of chronic obstructive pulmonary disease (COPD) or other primary pulmonary disease
  - Withhold antibiotics until results of sputum culture is available if there is strong suspicion of viral etiology:

- —No purulent sputum produced
- —History of prodromal viral upper respiratory symptoms
- Empirical antibiotic therapy may be used:
  - Amoxicillin 250 mg orally every 8 hours for 7 to 10 days
  - Penicillin allergy: Erythromycin 250 mg orally every 6 hours for 10 days, or Tetracycline 250 mg orally every 6 hours for 10 days, or TMP-SMX DS orally twice a day for 10 days
- If influenza A is suspected: Amantadine 100 mg orally every 12 to 24 hours for 10 days
- In patients with COPD or other risk factors for chronic infection (e.g., smoking): Pneumococcal vaccine
- In elderly, immunocompromised patients, or those with cardiorespiratory disease: Influenza vaccine

Follow-Up:

- Monitor closely for 7 to 10 days
- **Watch for:** signs and symptoms of
  - Bronchopneumonia
  - Acute respiratory failure

BRONCHIOLITIS

Presenting Symptoms:

SUBJECTIVE	OBJECTIVE
Cough	Expiratory wheezes
Cyanosis	Inspiratory crackles
Fever	Intercostal retractions
Pharyngitis	Tachycardia
Anorexia	Tachypnea
Vomiting	

Differential Diagnosis:

Asthma
Emphysema
Foreign body aspiration
Pneumonia
Congestive heart failure (CHF)
Cystic fibrosis

Suggested Workup:

Pathognomonic CXR:
- Focal atelectasis
- Flattened diaphragms
- Increased Anteroposterior (AP) diameter
- Peribronchial cuffing

Definitive Diagnosis:

Acute bronchiolitis   ICD-9-CM 466.1

Suggested Treatment:

- Antibiotics given only in rare instances of secondary bacterial superinfection
- In pediatric cases where patient is hospitalized and there is:
  - Underlying pulmonary disease
  - Age younger than 6 weeks
  - Severe RSV infection with increased partial pressure of carbon dioxide (pCO_2) or requiring ventilatory support, may give: Ribavirin inhaler against RSV and influenza types A & B; aerosol for 20 hours/day for 3 to 5 days

Follow-Up:

- Follow closely for 2 to 4 days or until clinically improved
- **Watch for:** signs and symptoms of
  - Bacterial superinfection
  - Bronchiolitis obliterans
  - Respiratory failure
  - Reactive airways disease

INFLUENZA

Presenting Symptoms:

SUBJECTIVE	OBJECTIVE
High fever	Rales
Myalgia	Rhonchi
Pharyngitis	Wheezes
Nonproductive cough	Conjunctivitis
Headache	
Chills	
Nasal congestion	
Malaise	
Rhinorrhea	
Sinus congestion	
Sneezing	

Differential Diagnosis:

Common cold
Bronchitis
Atypical pneumonia
Tonsillitis
Infectious mononucleosis
Coxsackievirus infection

Suggested Workup:

- History and Physical give high index of suspicion
- Chest radiograph: Fifty percent are normal; 50% show basilar streaking with patchy infiltrates

Definitive Diagnosis:

Influenza   ICD-9-CM 487

Suggested Treatment:

- For suspected influenza type A, patients with severe disease, or patients with underlying COPD:
  - Amantadine 100 mg orally 2 times a day for 3 to 5 days, or
    Rimantadine 100 mg orally 2 times a day for 3 to 5 days

- **SPECIAL WARNING: Amantadine** and **rimantadine** are absolutely contraindicated in pregnant women and nursing mothers, and relatively contraindicated in patients with a history of seizure disorder, CHF, neurosis, or psychosis
- Antibiotics are to used only if there is a high index of suspicion for bacterial superinfection
- After acute episode has resolved, polyvalent influenza vaccine should be given to high-risk patients:
  - COPD
  - Cardiovascular disease
  - Immunosuppression
  - Renal disease
  - Diabetic or other metabolic disease
  - Alcoholic
  - Asplenia
  - Age over 65 years

Follow-Up:

- Until symptoms are resolved
- **Watch for:** signs and symptoms of
  - Otitis media
  - Guillain-Barré syndrome (Influenza A only)
  - Viral or bacterial pneumonia
  - Reye's syndrome (Influenza B primarily)
  - Bronchitis

RESPIRATORY SYNCYTIAL VIRUS (RSV) INFECTION

Presenting Symptoms:

SUBJECTIVE	OBJECTIVE
Fever	Otitis media
Cough	Pulmonary congestion

Coryza	with rales and
Congestion	rhonchi
Malaise	Wheezing
Vomiting	Dyspnea
	Hypoxia (severe cases only)

Differential Diagnosis:

Upper respiratory infection
Allergic rhinitis
Viral croup
Asthma
Bronchitis
Pneumonia

Suggested Workup:

Pathognomonic chest radiograph:
- Hyperinflated lungs
- Interstitial infiltrates
- Pleural fluid
- Segmental or lobar consolidation (in severe cases with concomitant pneumonia)

Definitive Diagnosis:

RSV infection   ICD-9-CM 480.1

Suggested Treatment:

- Ribavirin inhaler; aerosol for 18 to 20 hours a day for 3 to 7 days
- Bronchodilators as needed
- Antibiotics given only for secondary bacterial infection

Follow-Up:

- None for adults
- Educate parents about sudden infant death syndrome (SIDS) in pediatric patients

- **Watch for:** signs and symptoms of
    - Pneumonia
    - Residual lung damage
    - SIDS in pediatric patients

ORAL (HAIRY) LEUKOPLAKIA

Presenting Symptoms:

SUBJECTIVE

White or yellow patch on tongue, roof of mouth, inside cheeks, or lips

OBJECTIVE

Macular or plaque-like lesions on:
—Tongue, mandibular alveolar ridge, and buccal mucosa (50%)
—Palate and lower lip (25% to 30%)
—Floor of the mouth and retromolar areas (less than 10%)
Lesions vary in appearance:
—Nonpalpable, faintly translucent white areas
—Thick, fissured, papillomatous, indurated lesions
Lesions feel rough and leathery
Lesions CANNOT be wiped off

Differential Diagnosis:

Candida (thrush)
Aspirin burn
Keratosis
Leukoderma

Lichen planus
Verrucous carcinoma
Lupus
Squamous cell carcinoma
Leukokeratosis nicotina palati

Suggested Workup:

- History may be revealing:
  - Ninety percent are in males over 40 years old
  - Human immunodeficiency virus-positive?
    ____Y: oral leukoplakia common
    ____N: less common without other risk factors
  - Tobacco and/or alcohol use?
    ____Y: positive risk factor
    ____N: less common without other risk factors
  - Oral sepsis?
    ____Y: positive risk factor
    ____N: look for other risk factors
  - Chronic trauma to oral cavity (e.g., dental appliances)?
    ____Y: positive risk factor
    ____N: look for other risk factors
- Physical exam is pathognomonic
- White plaques as described above CANNOT be wiped away (rules out *Candida* and aspirin burn)
- Biopsy lesions for pathology and viral culture (rarely needed):
  - Distinguish keratoses and carcinomas from leukoplakia
  - Presence of Epstein-Barr virus and/or human papillomavirus, types 11 and 15?
    ____Y: oral leukoplakia likely
    ____N: oral leukoplakia unlikely

Definitive Diagnosis:

Oral leukoplakia   ICD-9-CM 528.6

Suggested Treatment:

- Eliminate risk factors
  - Smoking
  - Alcohol
  - Dental trauma
- Cryosurgery for small, circumscribed lesions
- For Epstein-Barr virus-positive lesions that are resistant to conservative therapy:
  - Ganciclovir 500 mg orally 6 times a day for 7 to 10 days

Follow-Up:

- Regular, close follow-up, with immediate biopsy of recurrent lesions (6% to 60% may be carcinoma with invasive properties, especially on floor of mouth)
- **Watch for:** signs and symptoms of
  - Recurrent lesions
  - Carcinoma
  - Underlying immune deficiency

Lower Respiratory Tract and Mycobacterial Infections 4

INFECTIONS COVERED

ACUTE BACTERIAL PNEUMONIA

Presenting Symptoms:

<u>SUBJECTIVE</u>
Cough
Fever
Pleuritic chest pain
Sudden onset of chills
Dark, thick, or rust-
  colored sputum
Anorexia
Shortness of breath
Prostration
Rigors
Shoulder pain
Weakness

<u>OBJECTIVE</u>
Bronchial breath
  sounds
Rales
Chest dullness to
  percussion
Cyanosis
Diminished breath
  sounds
Dehydration
  (tachycardia and
  orthostatic changes)
Tachypnea
Dyspnea
Egophony
Pleural friction rub
Vocal fremitus
Whispered
  pectoriloquy
Elicit history of
  significant risk
  factors:
—Advanced age
—Cigarette smoking
—Institutionalization
—Dementia
—Malnutrition
—Chronic obstructive
  pulmonary disease
  (COPD)
—Alcoholism
—Chronic liver/
  kidney disease
—Congestive heart
  failure (CHF)

> —Immunosuppression (myeloma, lymphoma, human immunodeficiency virus [HIV] infection)
> —Asplenia (traumatic, systemic lupus erythematosus [SLE], postmarrow transplant)
> —Diabetes mellitus
> —Malignancy
> —Cerebrovascular disease
> —Neuromuscular disease

Differential Diagnosis:

Viral or atypical pneumonia
Fungal infection of the lung
Pneumocystis carinii pneumonia
Tuberculosis (TB)
Pulmonary embolus with infarction
Bronchiolitis obliterans
Pulmonary contusion
Pulmonary vasculitis
Pulmonary sarcoid
Hypersensitivity pneumonitis
Pneumothorax
Upper respiratory infection (tracheobronchitis, bronchiolitis)
Asthma
Lung abscess
Pulmonary edema
Inhalation of noxious fumes
Peripheral airway obstruction (bronchiectasis)

Lung cancer
Cystic fibrosis (CF)
Amyloidosis
Goodpasture's syndrome
Wegener's granulomatosis
Pulmonary hemosiderosis
Primary pulmonary hypertension
Pericarditis
Mediastinitis
Pleural effusion
Empyema

Suggested Workup:

- History should be used to define:
  - Clinical setting in which pneumonia is taking place
  - Defects in host resistance that could predispose to development of pneumonia and could provide a clue as to the specific pathogen responsible, and
  - Possible exposure to specific pathogens
- Sputum examination:
  - Gram stain and culture of expectorated sputum are the mainstays of diagnosis, but controversial regarding their sensitivity and specificity because of the possibility of oropharyngeal contamination. Their use still allows a presumptive diagnosis in the majority of cases.
  - To decrease the possibility of contamination, where no sputum is produced, where there is no clear predominance of a potential pathogen on sputum Gram stain or culture, where there has been a poor response to antibiotics chosen on the basis of expectorated sputum, or where the possibility of a

superinfection exists, sputum may be obtained by:
— Induction by 15 minutes of 3% saline by nebulizer after patient has rinsed his or her mouth
— Nasotracheal suctioning
— Transtracheal aspiration (high risk of adverse reactions)
— Bronchoalveolar lavage or brushing via fiberoptic bronchoscopy; or
— Percutaneous transthoracic fine needle aspiration

- Examination of sputum should include observation of:
— Color: usually dark or rusty (rusty sputum suggests alveolar involvement and probable *Streptococcus pneumoniae* infection; dark-red, mucoid sputum ["currant-jelly"] suggests *Klebsiella pneumoniae* [Friedländer's bacillus pneumonia])
— Amount: usually copious
— Consistency: usually mucopurulent
— Odor: usually foul-smelling, especially in mixed anaerobic infections following aspiration (scant or watery sputum is more often associated with atypical or viral pneumonias)
— Number of neutrophils and epithelial cells (samples with more than 25 neutrophils and less than 10 epithelial cells/100X field are less likely to be contaminated with oropharyngeal flora)
— Gram-positive diplococci = *S. pneumoniae*
— Gram-negative coccobacilli = *Haemophilus influenzae*
— Gram-positive cocci in clusters = staphylococci

> —Mixed morphology = anaerobic infections
> —Scant bacteria = *Legionella, Mycoplasma,* or viral pneumonia
> —Giemsa, Gomori methenamine silver (GMS), or toluidine blue O stain (positive) = *P. carinii*

- Serologic tests:
  - Immunofluorescence or enzyme-linked immunosorbent assay (ELISA) assays can be used to detect the following in respiratory secretions:
    —Herpes simplex
    —Cytomegalovirus (CMV)
    —*Chlamydia* spp.
    —*Legionella* spp.
    —*Mycoplasma pneumoniae*
    —*Coxiella burnetii*
- Chest radiograph:
  - Patchy infiltrate representing bronchopneumonia is useful in making diagnosis of pneumonia, but not usually helpful in identifying the etiologic agent; however, several radiologic patterns may be suggestive:
  - Lobar consolidation, cavitation, and large pleural effusions: bacterial etiology
  - Bilateral diffuse involvement: *P. carinii, Legionella,* or viral pneumonia more suspect
  - Multiple nodular infiltrates: staphylococcal pneumonia
  - Pneumatoceles: *Staphylococcus, Klebsiella, H. influenzae, S. pneumoniae*
  - Cavitation: *Pseudomonas*
  - Primarily lower lobe pneumonia: *Pseudomonas,* Gram-negative bacteria, *Mycoplasma*

- Interstitial peribronchial pattern: *Mycoplasma*
  - Patchy interstitial or nodular lower lobe pattern that quickly involves more than two lobes: *Legionella* (distinguished from *Mycoplasma*, which rarely involves more than one or two lobes)
- Blood culture and serology:
  - Approximately 20% to 30% of patients with bacterial pneumonia are bacteremic, and blood cultures can offer definitive proof of the etiology of infection
  - Serologic assays using counterimmunoelectrophoresis, agglutination, or ELISA can be used to detect antibodies against pulmonary pathogens; their usefulness in making a rapid diagnosis is limited and of more help in confirming a clinical diagnosis
- Lung Biopsy:
  - May be percutaneous, transbronchial, or via thoracoscopy or open lung biopsy
  - Rarely indicated in a normal person with acute pneumonia
  - Reserved for cases in impaired hosts, in pediatric patients, or in patients where there is clinical worsening despite apparently adequate antimicrobial therapy
- Examination of pleural effusions:
  - Incidence of pleural effusions in pneumonia varies with the etiologic agent, from 10% (*S. pneumoniae*) to 70% (Gram-negative bacilli) up to 95% (Group A streptococci)
  - Pleural fluid collected for Gram stain and culture is specific for etiology of disease
  - Pleural fluid examination may also be used to exclude other causes of pulmonary

infiltrates that mimic pneumonia (e.g., TB, tumors, pulmonary emboli, and collagen vascular diseases)

Definitive Diagnosis:

Acute bacterial pneumonia	ICD-9-CM 482.9
Anaerobic pneumonia	ICD-9-CM 482.81
Aspiration pneumonia	ICD-9-CM 507.0
Friedländer's (*Klebsiella*) pneumonia	ICD-9-CM 482.0
H. influenza pneumonia	ICD-9-CM 482.2
Mycoplasma pneumonia	ICD-9-CM 483.0
Pneumococcal pneumonia	ICD-9-CM 481
Pseudomonas pneumonia	ICD-9-CM 482.1
Staphylococcal pneumonia	ICD-9-CM 482.4
Legionnaire's disease	ICD-9-CM 482.83
Chlamydial pneumonia	ICD-9-CM 078.88
P. carinii pneumonia	ICD-9-CM 136.3

Suggested Treatment:

- Empiric therapy for enigmatic community-acquired pneumonia in an immunocompetent adult (empiric therapy should be initiated upon the diagnosis of pneumonia and can be changed appropriately when a specific etiologic agent is identified by Gram stain, culture, or other testing):
  - **Outpatient** (mild case):
    —Clarithromycin 500 mg orally twice a day for 10 days, or

    Azithromycin 500 mg orally for 1 day, then 250 mg orally once daily for 4 days, and

    Cefuroxime 500 mg orally every 12 hours for 10 days, or

    Cefaclor 500 mg orally every 8 hours for 10 days, or

> Cefixime 400 mg orally once a day for
> 10 days, or
> Amoxicillin + clavulanate 500 mg
> orally every 8 hours, or
> Trimethoprim-sulfamethoxazole (TMP-
> SMX) DS 1 tablet orally twice a day
> for 10 to 14 days

—**NOTE:** Recent reports of *S. pneumoniae*
resistance to TMP-SMX makes this choice
less attractive

—**NOTE:** Because of the broad coverage of
clarithromycin and azithromycin against
*S. pneumoniae, H. influenzae, M.
pneumoniae,* and *Chlamydia,* they may be
used cautiously as monotherapy in mild
cases of outpatient pneumonia

- **Requiring hospitalization** (because of
having a moderate to severe case,
multilobar presentation, respiratory
distress, high fever, hypoxemia [partial
pressure of oxygen (PO_2) less than 55 mm
Hg on room air], hypotension [systolic
blood pressure (BP) less than 100 mm Hg],
altered mental status, severe laboratory
abnormalities [metabolic acidosis, increased
blood urea nitrogen (BUN)/creatinine ratio,
hypernatremia [serum Na greater than
155 mEq/L], a significant comorbid illness,
or age extreme [consider anyone over
50 a good candidate for in-hospital
treatment]):

> Erythromycin 500 mg intravenously (IV)
> every 6 hours, and
> Cefuroxime 0.75 to 1.5 g IV every 8
> hours, or

> Cefotaxime 1 to 2 g IV every 6 hours, or
> Ceftriaxone 0.5 to 1.0 g IV once a day, or
> Ampicillin + sulbactam 1 to 2 g of
>> ampicillin IV every 6 hours for 7 days
>> or until significant clinical
>> improvement, then change to oral
>> regimen for 7 days

- Empiric therapy for enigmatic pneumonia in elderly, debilitated, and/or institutionalized patients:
  - Cefotaxime 1 to 2 g IV every 6 hours, or
  - Ceftriaxone 0.5 to 1.0 g IV once a day, or
  - Ceftazidime 1 to 2 g IV every 8 hours, or
  - Ticarcillin + clavulanic acid 1 to 6 g ticarcillin IV every 6 hours, and
  - Gentamicin 3 to 5 mg/kg/day IV given every 8 hours
- Empiric treatment for enigmatic nosocomial pneumonia in immunocompetent adults (see Chapter 12 Nosocomial Infections and Fevers of Unknown Origin for further recommendations):
  - Cefotaxime 1 to 2 g IV every 6 hours, or
    > Ceftizoxime 1 to 2 g IV every 8
    >> hours, and
    > Vancomycin 1 g IV every 12 hours, or
  - Ceftazidime 1 to 2 g/day IV given every 8 hours, or
    > Piperacillin 6 to 24 g/day IV given every
    >> 6 hours, and
    > Gentamicin 3 to 5 mg/kg/day IV given
    >> every 8 hours
  - Clindamycin 1.8 to 2.7 g/day IV given every 6 hours, and
    > Aztreonam 1 to 2 g IV every 8 hours, or

Ciprofloxacin 400 mg IV every 12
hours, or
Gentamicin 3.5 mg/kg/day IV given
every 8 hours
(Use of any of the three regimens above
is necessary where *Pseudomonas
aeruginosa* is a concern)
- Where Gram-negative and anaerobic
infections are a concern, use:
Imipenem 0.5 to 0.75 g IV every 6
hours, or
Ticarcillin + clavulanate 1 to 4 g
ticarcillin IV every 6 hours, or
Clindamycin 1.8 to 2.7 g/day IV given
every 6 hours, and
Ceftazidime 1 to 2 g IV every 8 hours
- **NOTE:**
—Enigmatic pneumonia: no identified
pathogen according to common
sampling and culture techniques
described above;
—In the regimens outlined above,
ticarcillin, piperacillin, and mezlocillin
can be used interchangeably
- Specific treatment according to pathogens
identified (oral doses for mild disease;
intravenous doses for severe disease):
- *S. pneumoniae:*
—Penicillin (PCN) G or V 1 to 2 g orally
every 6 hours (PCN G 0.5 million units
[U] IV every 4 hours), or
Cefuroxime 500 mg orally every 12
hours (Cefuroxime 750 mg IV every
8 hours), or
Cefotaxime 2 g IV every 6
hours, or

    Ceftriaxone 2 g IV every 24
        hours
—For areas with high incidence of
penicillin resistance:
    Erythromycin 1 to 2 g/day orally
        given every 6 hours
    (Erythromycin 2 to 4 g/day IV given
        every 6 hours), or
    Clarithromycin 500 mg orally every 12
        hours, or
    Azithromycin 500 mg orally once,
        then 250 mg orally once a day for
        4 days, or
    Doxycycline 100 mg orally every 12
        hours (Doxycycline 100 mg IV every
        12 hours), or
    (Vancomycin 1 g IV every 12 hours)
- *H. influenzae:*
    Amoxicillin + clavulanate 500 mg orally
        every 8 hours, or
    Clarithromycin 500 mg orally every 12
        hours, or
    Azithromycin 500 mg orally once, then
        250 mg orally once a day for 4
        days, or
    Tetracycline 500 mg orally every 6 hours
        for 2 weeks, or
    Cefotaxime 2 g IV every 6 hours, or
    Ceftriaxone 2 g IV every 24 hours until
        clinical improvement, then change to
        oral therapy for 10 to 14 days
- *Staphylococcus aureus:*
—Dicloxacillin 500 mg orally every 6
    hours (Nafcillin 1 to 2 g IV every 6
    hours), or
—For **Methicillin-resistant S. *aureus*** (10%
    of community acquired strains and 30%

to 40% of nosocomial infections) or
for penicillin allergy, can give:
Vancomycin 1 g IV every 12 hours for 2
weeks
- *Klebsiella* spp. or *Escherichia coli:*
    Cefoxitin 1 to 2 g IV every 6 hours, or
    Cefuroxime 1.5 g IV every 8 hours, or
    Cefotaxime 2 g IV every 6 hours, or
    Ceftriaxone 2 g IV every 24 hours, and
    Gentamicin 3 to 5 mg/kg/day IV given
        every 8 hours
- Anaerobes:
    Clindamycin 1.8 to 2.7 g/day IV given
        every 6 hours, or
    PCN G 2 million U IV every 6
        hours, and
    Metronidazole 1 g IV every 12
        hours
- *Pseudomonas:*
    Gentamicin 3 to 5 mg/kg/day IV given
        every 8 hours, and
    Ticarcillin 1 to 3 g IV every 6
        hours, or
    Piperacillin 2 to 3 g IV every 6
        hours, or
    Mezlocillin 1 to 3 g IV every 6
        hours, or
    Ceftazidime 1 to 2 g IV every 8
        hours, or
    Cefoperazone 1 to 4 g IV every 12
        hours, or
    Aztreonam 0.5 to 2.0 g IV every 8
        hours, or
    Imipenem 0.5 to 1.0 g IV every 6 hours
- *Moraxella catarrhalis:*
    Cefaclor 500 mg orally every 8 hours, or
    Cefuroxime 500 mg orally every 12
        hours, or

Cefixime 200 mg orally every 12 hours or
400 mg orally once a day, or
Erythromycin 500 mg orally 4 times a
day or 1 g orally twice a day

- *Chlamydia pneumoniae:*
    Doxycycline 100 mg orally every 12
    hours, or
    Ciprofloxacin 500 to 750 mg orally every
    12 hours, or
    Ofloxacin 400 mg orally every 12 hours
    for 2 weeks

- *M. pneumoniae*
    Erythromycin 500 mg orally 4 times a
    day or 1 g orally twice a day
    (Clarithromycin or azithromycin may
    be substituted), or
    Tetracycline 500 mg orally every 6
    hours, or
    Ciprofloxacin 500 to 750 mg orally every
    12 hours, or
    Ofloxacin 400 mg orally every 12 hours
    for 2 weeks

- *Legionella pneumophila:*
    Erythromycin 1 g IV every 6 hours until
    improved, then
    Erythromycin 500 mg orally 4 times a
    day or 1 g orally twice a day for a
    total of 3 weeks

- *P. carinii:*
    —TMP-SMX 15 mg/kg/day of
    trimethoprim orally/IV given 3 times a
    day for 21 days, and
        Prednisone 30 to 40 mg orally once a
        day started within 72 hours of
        antibiotic
    —If patient is **intolerant of TMP-SMX,**
    may use:

Pentamidine 4 mg/kg/day IV for 21 days, or

Dapsone 100 mg orally once a day plus trimethoprim 15 mg/kg/day orally given 4 times a day, or

Clindamycin 600 mg orally 3 times a day plus primaquine 30 mg orally once a day for 21 days, or

Atovaquone 750 mg orally 3 times a day for 21 days (mild/moderate cases), or

Trimetrexate glucuronate 45 mg/m^2 IV once a day infused over 60 to 90 minutes for 21 days plus

Leucovorin 20 mg/m^2 IV/orally given every 6 hours for 24 days (severe cases)

Follow-Up:

- Daily assessment of patient's progress until there is significant clinical improvement
- Repeat chest radiograph 6 weeks after recovery to verify that pneumonia was not caused by obstructing endobronchial lesion
- Consider pneumovax and influenza vaccines after recovery
- For hospitalized patients: chest physical therapy and deep breathing and coughing exercises; incentive spirometry
- For *Pneumocystis* pneumonia patients: *Pneumocystis* prophylaxis after recovery; appropriate treatment of underlying immune deficiency (see Chapter 10 on Immunocompromised Hosts, section on acquired immunodeficiency syndrome [AIDS])
- **Watch for:** signs and symptoms of
  - Empyema
  - Pulmonary abscess

- Purulent pericarditis
- Pleurisy
- Respiratory failure
- Pneumothorax (especially severe infections and *Pneumocystis* pneumonia)

CHRONIC PNEUMONIA

Presenting Symptoms:

SUBJECTIVE	OBJECTIVE
Fever	Generalized wheezing
Chills	Signs of bronchospasm
Malaise	Localized wheezing
Progressive anorexia and weight loss	Cyanosis
Nonspecific constitutional complaints	Clubbing
Persistent cough with sputum	
Hemoptysis	
Pleuritic chest pain	
Dyspnea	

Differential Diagnosis:

Extrinsic allergic alveolitis
Allergic bronchopulmonary aspergillosis
Churg-Strauss syndrome
Endobronchial tumor
Cardiovascular disease (cardiac asthma)
TB
Pulmonary sarcoid
Hypersensitivity pneumonitis
Asthma
Lung abscess
Pulmonary edema

Inhalation of noxious fumes or irritants
Bronchiectasis
Lung cancer
CF
Amyloidosis
Goodpasture's syndrome
Wegener's granulomatosis
Pulmonary hemosiderosis
Primary pulmonary hypertension
Pericarditis
Mediastinitis
Pleural effusion
Hepatic disease with ascites
Chronic bronchitis
Pulmonary embolus
Loeffler's syndrome
Chronic eosinophilic pneumonia
Polyarteritis nodosa
Angioneurotic edema
Carcinoid syndrome
Hyperthyroidism
Emphysema
Interstitial lung disease
Drug reaction
Pulmonary fibrosis
Collagen vascular disease
HIV infection
Vasculitides
Myeloma
Lymphoproliferative neoplasms

Suggested Workup:

- Complete blood count (CBC):
  - Pancytopenia:
    —Miliary TB
    —Disseminated histoplasmosis
    —Metastatic lung cancer in bone marrow

- Normal CBC: mycotic chronic pneumonia
- Leukopenia:
  —HIV infection
  —Sarcoidosis
  —SLE
  —TB
  —Histoplasmosis
  —Tumor
- Leukocytosis: bacterial infection
- Liver function studies, urinalysis, BUN, serum creatinine to rule out multiple organ diseases:
  —Disseminated histoplasmosis
  —Disseminated mycobacteriosis
  —Vasculitides
  —Sarcoidosis
  —Lymphoproliferative neoplasms
- Serum globulin to rule out myeloma or another gammopathy
- Serology for antinuclear antibody (ANA), rheumatoid factors, and antineutrophil cytoplasmic autoantibody to rule out vasculitis and/or collagen vascular disease
- Chest radiograph and computed tomography (CT) exam of chest will often distinguish between infectious and noninfectious processes, and may discern the etiology of infectious processes: (Table 4.1)
- If patient has radiograph/CT scan evidence of localized infiltrates and/or cavitation:
  - **First: Sputum Examination:**
    —Sample must be a deep, coughed specimen, of adequate volume, and with more than 25 neutrophils and fewer than 10 epithelial cells/100X field
    —If adequate sputum specimen cannot be obtained, consider:

Table 4.1

Discerning the Etiology of Infectious and Non-infectious Pulmonary Processes

Radiologic Finding	Infectious	Noninfectious
Patchy infiltrates	Aspirin PN Necrotizing PN Actinomycosis Nocardiosis Tuberculous PN Blastomycosis Cryptococcosis Paracoccidioidomycosis	Eosinophilic PN Bronchiolitis obliterans
Pulmonary cavitation	Pyogenic abscess TB Atypical mycobacteria Melioidosis Rhodococcus Chronic histoplasmosis Coccidioidomycosis Sporotrichosis Aspergillosis Paragonimiasis Echinococcosis	Wegener's granulomatosis Lymphomatoid granulomatosis Silicosis Bronchogenic CA Lymphoma (especially Hodgkin's disease)

continued

Diffuse infiltration		Alveolar cell CA
Alveolar pattern		Goodpasture's syndrome
		Alveolar proteinosis
Ground-glass interstitial pattern		Sarcoidosis
		Asbestosis
		Berylliosis
		Bronchiolitis obliterans
Nodular interstitial pattern	Miliary TB	Sarcoidosis
	Disseminated histoplasmosis	Lymphangitic carcinomatosis
		Wegener's granulomatosis
		Churg-Strauss syndrome
		Rheumatoid lung disease
		Pneumoconioses
Linear interstitial pattern		Hypersensitivity pneumonitis
		Pulmonary hemosiderosis
		Chronic radiation
		Progressive systemic sclerosis
		Sarcoidosis
Coarse reticular pattern	Granuloma	Fibrosing alveolitis
		Bronchiectasis
		Sarcoidosis

PN = pneumonia; CA = cancer; TB = tuberculosis

183

> –Inducing sputum with hypertonic aerosols or ultrasonic nebulizers, chest physiotherapy, or postural drainage
> –Bronchoscopy for bronchial brushing
> –Transbronchial biopsy
> –Bronchoalveolar lavage
> —Examination should include:
> > –Gram stain for bacteria and actinomyces
> > –Acid-fast stain for *Mycobacteria* and *Nocardia*
> > –Wet mounts and potassium hydroxide (KOH) preparations for fungi
> > –GMS stain or periodic acid-Schiff (PAS) stain for fungi
> > –Cytologic preparations for neoplastic cells, eosinophils, and fungi
> > –Samples for culture of bacteria, fungi, and mycobacteria

- **Second: Culture** of blood, urine, pleural fluid (in those patients with pleural effusion), cerebrospinal fluid (CSF) (for patients with central nervous system [CNS] symptoms or signs), synovial fluid (in patients with a joint effusion)
- **Third: Skin testing** with purified protein derivative (PPD) and coccidioidin antigen
- **Fourth: Serology** (especially where there is a suspicion of coccidioidomycosis, cryptococcosis, histoplasmosis, and paracoccidioidomycosis)
- **Fifth: Immunologic studies** for precipitating antibodies to inhalant antigens, total serum immunoglobulin (Ig)E, and anti-*Aspergillus* antibody
- Bronchoscopy with a flexible fiberoptic bronchoscope, should be reserved for patients

- in whom a more aggressive diagnostic approach is needed
- Thoracentesis and pleural biopsy may be required in patients with extensive pleural involvement
- Open lung biopsy or percutaneous/ transthoracic needle aspiration may be considered where lung tissue is necessary for diagnosis
- Pulmonary function studies may be advisable in patients with a predominantly diffuse infiltrative pattern on chest radiograph to delineate the disease process and quantify the degree of pulmonary insufficiency

Definitive Diagnosis:

Chronic pneumonia   ICD-9-CM 515

Suggested Treatment:

- Stable patient with chronic indolent illness:
  - No immediate empiric therapy is required
  - Await results of diagnostic testing before initiating therapy
- In the nonseriously ill, otherwise healthy young patient with pneumonia for 2 to 3 weeks, empiric therapy is indicated until results of diagnostic tests are obtained:
  - Clarithromycin 500 mg orally twice a day for 10 days, or
  - Azithromycin 500 mg orally once, then 250 mg orally once a day for 4 days
- Patient with chronic pneumonia following thoracotomy, or has more serious illness, is elderly, or has other underlying medical problems should receive broad coverage:
  - Cefotaxime 1 to 2 g IV every 6 hours, or Ceftizoxime 1 to 2 g IV every 8 hours, and Vancomycin 1 g IV every 12 hours, or

- Ceftazidime 1 to 2 g/day IV given every 8 hours, or
    - Piperacillin 6 to 24 g/day IV given every 6 hours, and
    - Gentamicin 3 to 5 mg/kg/day IV given every 8 hours
- Patient with a positive PPD skin test and fever should receive presumptive therapy for TB for at least 8 weeks, pending final results of mycobacterial cultures (for specific anti-TB therapy recommendations, see section on *Mycobacterium tuberculosis*)
- Corticosteroids:
    - Usually NOT indicated where cause of illness is infectious agent
    - Beneficial where cause is noninfectious
        —Vasculitides
        —Sarcoidosis
        —Chronic eosinophilic pneumonia
        —Radiation injury
        —Bronchiolitis obliterans
        —Fibrotic lung diseases
        —Chronic hypersensitivity pneumonitis
- Supportive measures:
    - Bronchopulmonary hygiene
    - Hydration
    - Humidified air
    - Postural drainage or chest vibropercussion
- Bronchoscopy and surgery:
    - May be used as therapeutic adjunct
    - Therapeutic bronchoscopy may be used to clear mucus plugs or foreign bodies and to expand a collapsed lung
    - Lobectomy or pneumonectomy should be considered in a patient with chronic destructive pneumonia and multiple macro- or microabscesses involving an

entire lobe or lung, and a V/Q scan indicating nonfunction of the involved lung
- Thoracotamy may be indicated for purposes of decortication of pleura in a patient whose chronic pneumonia has involved the pleura with resulting restrictive lung disease

Follow-Up:

- Physical examinations and repeat chest radiographs until resolved
- Frequency and level of aggressiveness of approach must be individualized to the patient and will depend largely on severity of illness
- **Watch for:** signs and symptoms of
  - Empyema
  - Pulmonary abscess
  - Purulent pericarditis
  - Pleurisy
  - Respiratory failure
  - Pneumothorax
  - Obstructing lesions (underlying malignancy)
  - Immunodeficiency state

EOSINOPHILIC PNEUMONIA

Presenting Symptoms:

SUBJECTIVE	OBJECTIVE
Mild fever	Decreased localized breath sounds
Cough	
Dyspnea at rest	Localized crackles
Wheezing	Diffuse rhonchi
Anorexia	Mucoid sputum
	Tachycardia
	Symptoms may be mild or life-threatening

Differential Diagnosis:

Loffler's syndrome
TB
Sarcoidosis
Hodgkin's disease
Lymphoproliferative disorder with pulmonary
  involvement
Eosinophilic granuloma of the lung
Desquamative interstitial pneumonitis
Collagen vascular disease
Hypereosinophilic syndrome
Wegener's granulomatosis
Asthmatic pulmonary eosinophilia
Drug-induced pulmonary eosinophilia
Churg-Strauss syndrome
P. carinii pneumonia (secondary to HIV infection)

Suggested Workup:

- History to determine noninfectious causes of
  pulmonary eosinophilia:
  - Has patient been exposed to drug/toxin
    known to cause pulmonary eosinophilia?
    —Penicillin
    —Isoniazid
    —Sulfonamides
    —Gold
    —Hydralazine
    —Nitrofurantoin
    —Chlorpropamine
    —Anti-TB therapy (PAS)
    —Aspirin
  - Has patient been living or traveling in
    certain geographical areas associated with
    so-called chronic tropical pulmonary
    eosinophilia?
    —India
    —Burma

- —Indonesia
- —South America
- —Sri Lanka
- —Malaysia
- —Tropical Africa
- —South Pacific
- CBC: leukocytosis with marked eosinophilia (usually between 20% to 40%)
- Sputum examination: parasites and *Aspergillus fumigatus*
- Serology:
  - —Elevated IgE levels
  - —Positive filarial complement fixation
  - —Elevated erythrocyte sedimentation rate (ESR)
- Stool examination: look for presence of parasites, including:
  - —*Ascaris*
  - —*Paragonoma*
  - —*Schistosoma*
  - —*Ancylostoma* spp.
  - —*Entamoeba histolytica*
  - —*Strongyloides*
  - —*Echinococcus*
  - —Visceral larva migrans *(Toxocara)*
  - —*Dirofilaria immitis*
- Chest radiograph:
  - —Pulmonary infiltrates are transient and migratory, and peripherally located
  - —There may be small pleural effusion
- Open lung biopsy reserved for those rare cases where clinical course is severe, or when diagnosis is uncertain
- Pulmonary function tests are nonspecific and not helpful in making a specific diagnosis

Definitive Diagnosis:

Eosinophilic pneumonia   ICD-9-CM 518.3

Suggested Treatment:

- *Ascaris* infestation: Piperazine 250 mg orally twice a day for 3 days, or mebendazole 100 mg orally in the morning and every night at bedtime for 3 days
  - Patient should be rechecked 3 weeks after treatment; if not cured, a second course of treatment is advisable
- Helminthic infections:
  - *Ancylostoma:* Mebendazole 100 mg orally in the morning and every night at bedtime for 3 days
  - *Strongyloides:* Thiabendazole 25 mg/kg orally twice a day for 2 days
  - *Schistosoma:* Praziquantel 20 mg/kg orally 2 to 3 times a day for 1 day
  - *Paragonimus:* Praziquantel 25 mg/kg orally 3 times a day for 1 day
  - *Echinococcus:* Mebendazole 100 mg orally in the morning and every night at bedtime for 3 days
  - *Toxocara:*
    - —Mebendazole 100 mg orally in the morning and every night at bedtime for 3 days, or
        Diethylcarbamazine 3 mg/kg orally 3 times a day for 2 weeks, or
        Prednisone 20 to 40 mg orally once a day alone
    - —**NOTE:** Most patients recover without any therapy at all; treatment with anti-inflammatory or antihelminthic drugs should be considered only for patients with severe lung disease and/or those

with spread of disease to the brain or heart

- *Dirofilaria:* No antimicrobial treatment is necessary; patient pulmonary symptoms are most likely due to development of eosinophilic granuloma(s) with resulting pulmonary infarct
- *E. histolytica:* Metronidazole 750 mg orally 3 times a day for 5 to 10 days, and Paromomycin 30 mg/kg/day orally given 3 times a day for 5 to 10 days
- Tropical pulmonary eosinophilia (primarily caused by *Wuchereria bancrofti* or *Brugia malayi*): Diethylcarbamazine 3 mg/kg orally 3 times a day for 3 weeks
- Corticosteroids:
  - Prednisone 20 to 40 mg orally once a day is indicated for chronic pulmonary eosinophilia
  - Prednisone 40 to 60 mg orally once a day is indicated in Churg-Strauss syndrome
  - Slow withdrawal should be possible after recovery

Follow-Up:

- Physical examinations and chest radiographs until clinical symptoms are resolved
- **Watch for:** signs and symptoms of
  - Recurrent infections
  - Small airways dysfunction
  - Pulmonary fibrosis
  - Pulmonary infarction
  - Pulmonary embolus
  - Systemic spread of infection, especially to heart, brain, gastrointestinal (GI) tract

VIRAL PNEUMONIA

Presenting Symptoms:

SUBJECTIVE	OBJECTIVE
Often prodrome of upper respiratory tract symptoms	Rales and rhonchi
Cough with or without sputum	History reveals more gradual onset of symptoms
Low grade or no fever	Characteristic exanthem if measles virus or VZV are etiologic agents
Myalgias	
Prostration	
Rash (varicella-zoster virus [VZV] pneumonia)	

Differential Diagnosis:

Acute bacterial pneumonia
Viral upper respiratory tract infection
Atypical pneumonia
Pulmonary embolus
Churg-Strauss syndrome
Loffler's syndrome
Pulmonary vasculitis
Pulmonary contusion
Pulmonary sarcoid
Hypersensitivity pneumonitis
Pneumothorax
Asthma
Pulmonary edema
Inhalation of noxious fumes
Bronchiectasis
Lung cancer
CF
Amyloidosis
Goodpasture's syndrome
Wegener's granulomatosis

Pulmonary hemosiderosis
Primary pulmonary hypertension
Pericarditis
Pleural effusion
Collagen vascular disease

Suggested Workup:

- History and epidemiology are valuable: (Table 4.2)
- Pneumonia caused by CMV, herpes simplex virus (HSV), and human herpesvirus 6 (HHV6) is seen primarily in immunocompromised patients
- Bacteriologic studies (sputum culture, blood culture) should be negative
- Chest radiograph: variable findings:
  - Small patchy infiltrates in nodular pattern to diffuse bilateral disease
  - Air trapping and hyperinflation common in respiratory syncytial virus (RSV) pneumonia
- CBC and serology:
  - Leukocytosis usually absent
  - RSV detection in respiratory secretions by rapid ELISA technique is useful clinically
- Virus isolation in tissue culture:
  - Human parainfluenza virus (HPIV), RSV, and influenza virus can be isolated from respiratory secretions and grown in tissue culture, but isolation and identification can take up to 2 weeks; thus, this technique is of limited clinical utility
- VZV pneumonia is accompanied by a pathognomonic vesicular dermatomal skin eruption

Definitive Diagnosis:

Viral pneumonia   ICD-9-CM 480.9
Adenoviral pneumonia   ICD-9-CM 480.0

Table 4.2

History and Epidemiology for Workup of Viral Pneumonia

	RSV	Influenza A&B	HPIV I-III	Adenovirus	VZV
Age	<5	Adults	<5	Adults	All
Season	W/Sp	W	I, II-F; III-all	Sp/Su	W/Sp
Exanthem	No	No	No	No	Yes

RSV = respiratory syncytial virus; HPIV = human parainfluenza virus; VZV = varicella zoster virus; W = winter; F = fall; Sp = spring; Su = summer

HPIV pneumonia   ICD-9-CM 480.2
RSV pneumonia   ICD-9-CM 480.1

Suggested Treatment:

- RSV:
    - Ribavirin 1.1 g/day by aerosol through oxygen mask, hood, mist tent, or endotracheal tube for 3 to 7 days
    - **NOTE:** may also be effective in treatment of pneumonia caused by influenza A & B and HPIV, but is not approved by the Food and Drug Administration (FDA) for these indications
- Influenza A:
    - Amantadine 100 mg orally twice a day for 5 days, or
    - Rimantadine 100 mg orally twice a day for 5 days
- HSV, VZV: Acyclovir 5 mg/kg IV every 8 hours or 10 to 12 mg/kg every 12 hours for 7 to 14 days
- CMV and acyclovir-resistant HSV/VZV:
    - Ganciclovir 5 mg/kg IV every 12 hours (CMV), or
      Foscarnet 90 mg/kg every 24 hours (acyclovir resistant HSV/VZV)
      [**NOTE:** this is EXPERIMENTAL therapy and not yet approved by the FDA for this indication]
    - Given for 14 days with close clinical monitoring and
    - CMV immune globulin 50 to 150 mg/kg intravenous infusion (CMV pneumonia)

Follow-Up:

- Outpatient follow-up every 2 to 3 days for mild disease
- In-hospital close clinical monitoring for more serious disease, ensuring:

- • Adequate maintenance of volume status
- • Oxygen supplementation as needed
- • Bronchodilators for evident bronchospasm
- • Fever suppression for markedly febrile patients
- • Secretion management
- **Watch for:** signs and symptoms of
  - • Bacterial superinfection
  - • Respiratory collapse requiring intubation and mechanical ventilation
  - • Development of viremia

MYCOPLASMA PNEUMONIA

Presenting Symptoms:

SUBJECTIVE	OBJECTIVE
Gradual onset (over 2 to 3 weeks) of upper respiratory symptoms that persist	Minimal rales and wheezes
	Bullous myringitis
	Pleural friction rub
	Injected pharynx
Cough productive of no or whitish sputum	Cervical lymphadenopathy
	Pleural effusion (5% to 20%)
Fever and chills	Variable dermatologic involvement (10% of cases):
Headache	
Sore throat	
Dyspnea at rest	—Macular, morbilliform, or papulovesicular rash
Myalgias	
Nasal congestion	
Nonpleuritic chest pain	
Skin rash (occasionally)	—Erythema nodosum
Polyarthralgias	—Urticaria
Malaise	—Stevens-Johnson syndrome
No GI complaints	—Raynaud's phenomenon

Cardiac manifestations (5% to 10% of cases):
—Arrhythmias
—Congestive heart failure
—Electrocardiogram (ECG) conduction defects

Neurologic manifestations (less than 1% of cases):
—Aseptic meningitis
—Meningoencephalitis
—Transverse myelitis
—Brainstem dysfunction
—Guillain-Barré syndrome
—Peripeheral neuropathy

Differential Diagnosis:

Viral pneumonia
Bacterial pneumonia
Fungal pneumonias
P. carinii pneumonia
Chlamydia pneumonia
Legionella pneumonia
Asthma
Chronic obstructive pulmonary disease
Pulmonary vasculitis (especially in sickle cell patients)
Collagen vascular disease

Suggested Workup:

- History and physical are suggestive
- Sputum examination by Gram stain and culture shows no bacteria

- CBC shows generally normal or slightly elevated WBC count with no significant immature leukocytosis
- ESR increased
- Cold agglutinins:
  - Positive in approximately 50% of patients with *Mycoplasma* pneumonia
  - Manifested by:
    - —Cold agglutinin titer greater than 1:258 (a titer of greater than 1:32 is highly suggestive of infection with *M. pneumoniae*), or
    - —A greater than fourfold rise in cold agglutinin titer
  - A bedside cold agglutinin test is available:
    - —Patient's blood (1 mL) is drawn into a tube containing anticoagulant (e.g., blue-top tube for prothrombin determination)
    - —The blood is cooled on ice or in a refrigerator for 3 to 4 minutes
    - —The tube is then examined for the presence of macroscopic agglutination
    - —The tube is rewarmed by exposing it to body heat; rewarming should cause dissociation of the agglutination
    - —A positive bedside agglutination test corresponds approximately to a 1:64 laboratory titer of cold agglutinins
- Serology:
  - False-positive Venereal Disease Research Laboratories (VDRL) test consistent with *M. pneumoniae* infection
  - Complement fixation: C-fixing antibodies may rise fourfold 2 to 4 weeks after onset of symptoms (not a useful assay for diagnostic purposes or to guide therapeutic decisions; mainly for epidemiological use)
- Culture of *M. pneumoniae* is laborious, time consuming, and not practical for clinical diagnostic purposes

- Chest radiograph:
  - Diffuse interstitial infiltrates, usually with small bilateral pleural effusions
  - These findings are nonspecific and suggestive of infection with *M. pneumoniae,* but confirmation with other tests is usually necessary
- New rapid diagnostic tests are now available:
  - ELISA for specific anti-*M. pneumoniae* IgM and IgG antibodies (greater than 99% specificity; 98% sensitivity)
  - Antigen capture, indirect enzyme immunoassay (ACIEI) for *M. pneumoniae* antigens isolated from patient sputum (greater than 99% specificity; 91% sensitivity)
  - Detection of *M. pneumoniae*-specific nucleotide sequences in patient sputum or nasopharyngeal aspirates (Gen-Probe Rapid Diagnostic System; San Diego, CA) (90% to 95% specificity; 85% to 90% sensitivity)

Definitive Diagnosis:

Mycoplasma pneumonia   ICD-9-CM 483

Suggested Treatment:

- Adults and children older than 9 years:
  - Erythromycin 500 mg orally every 6 hours, or
  - Tetracycline 500 mg orally every 6 hours, or
  - Doxycycline 100 mg orally every 12 hours, or
  - Clarithromycin 250 mg orally every 12 hours, or
  - Ciprofloxacin 500 mg orally twice a day, or
  - Ofloxacin 400 mg orally twice a day
    —Each for 10 to 14 days, or

- Azithromycin 500 mg orally on day 1, then 250 mg orally for 4 days
- Children under 8 years: Erythromycin 30 to 50 mg/kg/day orally given every 6 hours for 10 to 14 days

Follow-Up:

- Clinical monitoring may be done in follow-up visit or by phone 2 weeks after treatment
- Repeat chest radiograph 4 to 6 weeks after treatment is indicated for smokers and patients over 50 years of age
- **Watch for:** signs and symptoms of
  - Reactive airway disease
  - Hemolytic anemia
  - Erythema multiforme
  - Pleural effusion
  - Rare occurrences of:
    —Meningoencephalitis
    —Polyneuritis
    —Polyarthritis
    —Stevens-Johnson syndrome
    —Pericarditis
    —Myocarditis
    —Adult respiratory distress syndrome (ARDS)
    —Cerebral ataxia
    —Thromboemboli

CHLAMYDIA PNEUMONIA (TWAR[1])

Presenting Symptoms:

SUBJECTIVE	OBJECTIVE
Gradual onset with prodrome of sore	Rales, rhonchi Wheezing

[1] TWAR = Taiwan Acute Respiratory Agent; now renamed *Chlamydia pneumoniae*

throat and
hoarseness (first
phase)
Nonproductive cough
2 weeks later
(second phase)
Rhinitis
Headache
Malaise
Sinus congestion
Low-grade or no fever
Generally mild illness
not requiring
hospitalization

Pharyngeal edema
Sinus tenderness
Clinical symptoms of
coronary artery
disease[2]
Usually benign
course

Differential Diagnosis:

Acute bacterial pneumonia
Atypical pneumonia (*Mycoplasma; Legionella*)
Viral pneumonia

Suggested Workup:

- CBC: normal or low
- ESR: elevated
- Sputum examination: no pathogens found on
  routine Gram stain and culture

[2] Recent seroepidemiologic studies have associated
coronary artery disease, atherosclerosis, and acute
myocardial infarction with antibody to *C. pneumoniae.*
In addition, *C. pneumoniae* organisms were
demonstrated in atheromatous plaques of coronary
arteries and aorta but not in normal arterial tissue.
Although these studies clearly associate *C. pneumoniae*
organisms with atheromatous plaques, it is unclear
whether the bacteria contribute to the formation of
atheroma or colonize arterial tissue damaged by the
atheromatous process. Thus, the role of *C. pneumoniae*
infection in the pathogenesis of atherosclerosis is
unclear.

- Chest radiograph: pneumonitis evident, usually as a single subsegmental lesion, with a small pleural effusion found occasionally (these findings are generally indistinguishable from those seen with other atypical pneumonias)
- Serology:
  - Chlamydial complement fixation test: if positive, cannot distinguish between *C. pneumoniae* and *Chlamydia psittaci* and positive in only 25% of patients with TWAR infection
  - Microimmunofluorescence test for TWAR antibody (American Medical labs, MRL Diagnostics): IgM titer greater than 1:16 or IgG titer greater than 1:512 suggests an acute or recent infection
- Polymerase chain reaction (PCR):
  - Can identify TWAR-specific DNA from patient throat swabs and sputum
  - Not presently available in most diagnostic labs
- Diagnosis often made on the basis of clinical finding of pneumonitis with no pathogen isolated from the sputum and/or the failure of the patient to respond to beta-lactam antibiotics

Definitive Diagnosis:

Chlamydia pneumonia   ICD-9-CM 078.89

Suggested Treatment:

- Erythromycin 500 mg orally every 6 hours, or
- Tetracycline 500 mg orally every 6 hours, or
- Doxycycline 100 mg orally every 12 hours, or
- Clarithromycin 500 mg orally every 12 hours, each for 10 to 14 days, or

- Azithromycin 500 mg orally once, then 250 mg orally every 24 hours for 4 days

Follow-Up:

- Weekly outpatient monitoring until clinical symptoms have resolved
- Repeat chest radiograph 6 to 8 weeks after treatment
- **Watch for:** signs and symptoms of
  - Erythema nodosum
  - Otitis media
  - Asthma
  - Endocarditis
  - Myocarditis
  - Pericarditis
  - Sarcoidosis
  - Meningitis
  - Reactive arthritis

EMPYEMA AND PLEURAL EFFUSION

Presenting Symptoms:

SUBJECTIVE	OBJECTIVE
Dyspnea	Signs of pleural
Chest pain	effusion:
Fever and chills	—Flatness or
Weight loss	hyperresonance to
Night sweats	percussion over area
	of fluid
	accumulation
	—Breath sounds may
	be absent,
	diminished, or
	bronchial
	—Whispered
	pectoriloquy

—Tracheal deviation to
the unaffected side
—No rales
Dyspnea and
tachypnea
Tachycardia
Fever

Differential Diagnosis:

Bacterial, viral, or atypical pneumonia
TB
Fungal infection of the lung
SLE
Rheumatoid disease
Wegener's granulomatosis
Polyarteritis nodosa
Progressive systemic sclerosis
Bronchogenic carcinoma
Lymphoma
Mesothelioma
Multiple myeloma
Metastatic carcinoma, especially from breast,
liver, pancreas
Waldenström's macroglobulinemia
Meigs' syndrome
Pulmonary embolus or infarction
Asbestosis
Chest trauma
Myxedema
Postmyocardial infarction (MI) syndrome
Spontaneous pneumothorax
Pancreatitis
Uremic pleuritis
Lymphedema
Sarcoidosis
CHF
Pericarditis

Renal disease
Fistula
—Bronchopleural
—Bronchoesophageal
Mediastinal osteomyelitis
Subdiaphragmatic abscess (liver, pancreas,
  spleen)

Suggested Workup:

- Chest radiograph: pleural effusion as
  evidenced by:
  - Blunting of costophrenic angles
  - Fluid meniscus on lateral decubitus views
- CT and ultrasound:
  - Pleural effusion, including loculated
    empyema with fistula formation, and
    extension of pleural fluid from mediastinal
    or subdiaphragmatic disease
  - Can also distinguish pleural effusions
    caused by bronchopleural fistulas from
    lung abscesses
- Examination of pleural fluid aspirated under
  ultrasound guidance: (Table 4.3)
- Gram stain and culture of aspirated pleural
  fluid: If negative for bacteria, test for:
  - *Legionella* by direct fluorescent antibody
    stains
  - Anaerobes
  - Fungi
  - *Mycobacteria*
  - Amoebae
  - Acridine orange staining of pleural fluid
- Cytology of aspirated pleural fluid for
  malignant cells
- Blood culture
- Serology for collagen vascular diseases:
  - ANA
  - Rheumatoid factor

Table 4.3

Examination of Pleural Fluid Aspirated Under Ultrasound Guidance

	Appearance	WBC/mm^3	Predominant WBC Type	RBC/mm^3	pH
Transudates: (PF protein $<$3.0 g/dL with normal serum protein; PF-LDH $<$200 IU with PF/S ratio $<$0.6)					
CHF	Clear, straw	$<$1,000	Monos	0–1000	$>$7.4
Cirrhosis	Clear, straw	$<$500	Monos	$<$1000	$>$7.4
Exudates: (PF protein $>$3.0 g/dL with normal serum protein; PF-LDH $>$200 IU with PF/S ratio $>$0.6)					
Pulmonary embolus	Hemorrhagic	5–15,000	Polys	Bloody	$>$7.3
Pneumonia	Turbid	5–40,000	Polys	$<$5,000	$>$7.3
TB	Straw	5–10,000	Monos	$<$10,000	$<$7.3
Carcinoma	Turbid	$<$10,000	Monos	$>$100,000	$<$7.3
SLE	Turbid	Variable	Mixed	$<$1000	$<$7.3
Pancreatitis	Turbid	5–20,000	Polys	1–10,000	$>$7.3
Rupture of esophagus	Purulent	TNTC	Polys	TNTC	6.0
Empyema	Purulent	25–50,000	Polys	$<$5,000	$<$7.2

continued

	Glucose mg/dL	Glucose PF/S	Protein PF/S	LDH IU/L	LDH PF/S	Amylase PF/S
Transudates:						
CHF	>60	1	<0.5	<200	<0.6	<1
Cirrhosis	>60	1	<0.5	<200	<0.6	<1
Exudates:						
Pulmonary embolus	>60	1	>0.5	—	>0.6	<1
Pneumonia	>60	1	>0.5	—	>0.6	<1
TB	30–60	1	>0.5	—	>0.6	<1
Carcinoma	<60	1	>0.5	—	>0.6	<1
SLE	<60	—	>0.5	—	>0.6	>2
Pancreatitis	>60	1	>0.5	—	—	>2
Rupture of esophagus	NL	—	>0.5	—	>0.6	Sal*
Empyema	<40	<0.5	>0.5	>1000	>0.6	<1

WBC = white blood cells, **RBC** = red blood cells, **PF** = pleural fluid, **LDH** = lactate dehydrogenase, **PF/S** = pleural fluid/serum ratio, **CHF** = congestive heart failure, **TB** = tuberculosis, **SLE** = systemic lupus erythematosus, **TNTC** = too numerous to count. *Sal = salivary type

Definitive Diagnosis:

Empyema   ICD-9-CM 510.9
Empyema with fistula   ICD-9-CM 510.0

Suggested Treatment:

- Surgical drainage necessary in patients with:
  - Pleural fluid containing gross pus
  - A heavy growth of microorganisms visible by microscopy
  - Pleural fluid with pH of less than 7.2, glucose less than 40 mg/dL, and lactate dehydrogenase (LDH) greater than 1000 mg/dL
- Where surgical drainage is not performed, antibiotic treatment should be instituted and thoracentesis repeated in 12 to 18 hours to reassess need for surgical drainage
- Loculation of pleural fluid is indication for CT-guided chest tube placement or thoracoscopy and thoracostomy
- Antibiotics should be selected on the basis of their activity against the microorganisms causing the infection and isolated from the pleural fluid; empiric therapy may be instituted as follows:
  - Ticarcillin + clavulanate 1 to 6 g ticarcillin IV every 6 hours
    Penicillin allergy: Vancomycin 1 g IV every 12 hours, and
    Gentamicin 3 to 5 mg/kg/day IV given every 8 hours for 2 to 4 weeks
  - Where anaerobic infection is suspected:
    Clindamycin 1.8 to 2.7 g/day IV given every 6 hours for 2 to 4 weeks, or
    Imipenem 0.5 to 0.75 g IV every 6 hours for 2 to 4 weeks

- *Nocardia* empyema:
  Sulfadiazine 1.5 to 2.0 g IV every 6
    hours, or
  TMP-SMX 15 mg/kg/day TMP and
    75 mg/kg/day SMX IV given every 8
    hours for 4 to 6 weeks, then
  TMP-SMX DS 2 tabs orally every 8 hours
    for 3 months
- *Actinomycosis* empyema:
  PCN G 18 to 24 million U/day IV given
    every 6 hours for 2 to 6 weeks, then
  Amoxicillin 250 to 500 mg orally every 6
    to 8 hours for 6 months, or
  Erythromycin 2 to 4 g/day IV given
    every 6 hours for 2 to 6 weeks, then
    250 to 500 mg orally every 6 hours for
    6 months, or
  Clindamycin 1.8 to 2.7 g/day IV given
    every 6 hours for 2 to 6 weeks, then
    0.6 to 1.8 g/day orally given every 6 to
    8 hours for 6 months
- Fungal empyema (especially *Aspergillus*):
  Amphotericin B 0.5 mg/kg/day IV
    infused over 2 to 6 hours, with
    frequent clinical monitoring to assess
    required duration of treatment
    (treatment for a period up to 11
    months with a total dose of 3.6 g has
    been reported), or
  Itraconazole 300 mg orally twice a day
    for 3 days, then 200 mg orally twice a
    day for 3 months, with frequent
    clinical and laboratory monitoring to
    verify that the infection has subsided
    (oral therapy may be given in the more
    indolent, non–life-threatening
    infections)

Follow-Up:

- Inpatient care required with close daily monitoring of clinical response to antimicrobial therapy
- If surgical drainage or thoracostomy with chest tube placement are performed, proper surgical follow-up is required
- If only thoracentesis is performed, a repeat evaluation should be made in 12 to 18 hours and thoracentesis repeated as needed, or surgical drainage/thoracostomy performed
- **Watch for:** signs and symptoms of
    - Lung abscess
    - Reaccumulation of pleural effusion
    - Pleural fibrosis and restrictive lung disease
    - Pericarditis
    - Myocarditis
    - Mediastinal extension and osteomyelitis
    - Pleurobronchial fistula
    - Pleuroesophageal fistula
    - Respiratory collapse

LUNG ABSCESS

Presenting Symptoms:

SUBJECTIVE	OBJECTIVE
Cough	Diminished breath sounds
Purulent, foul-smelling sputum	Rales
Fever	Wheezing
Chest pain	Tachypnea

Dyspnea
Chills, rigors
Malaise
Weakness
Weight loss
Anorexia
Night sweats
Hemoptysis

Tachycardia
Diaphoresis
Dullness to percussion
Consolidation by auscultation with amphoric or cavernous breath sounds over abscess area
Asymmetric chest movement
Clubbing
Fever: 101° to 102°F
Elicit history of:
—Presumed aspiration due to altered consciousness as a result of:
  –Alcoholism
  –Stroke
  –Drug overdose
  –Seizure
  –Diabetic coma
  –Shock
—Aspiration due to dysphagia as a result of:
  –Neurologic disorder
  –Esophageal disease
  –Intestinal obstruction
  –Dental or oropharyngeal surgery
—Periodontal disease

—Immunocompromise
–Drug-induced
–HIV infection

Differential Diagnosis:

Bronchogenic carcinoma
Bronchiectasis
Empyema with bronchopulmonary fistula
TB
Mycotic lung infections
Actinomycosis
Nocardiosis
Infected pulmonary bulla
Wegener's granulomatosis
Pulmonary sequestration
Silicotic nodule
Subphrenic or hepatic abscess with bronchial
  perforation
Bronchogenic or parenchymal cyst
Anaerobic necrotizing pneumonia
Pulmonary embolus
Immunosuppression

Suggested Workup:

- Chest radiograph:
  - Presence of a cavity with air-fluid level
  - Pleural effusion may be present
  - Multiple small excavations located in the
    dependent segment may be seen
- Laboratory:
  - CBC: leukocytosis with anemia
  - Hypoalbuminemia
- Expectorated sputum examination is generally
  of little diagnostic value because of
  contamination with oral flora
- Invasive sampling generally necessary:
  - Thoracentesis of empyema fluid, if
    available

- - Percutaneous transtracheal aspiration (best suited for obtaining specimens in children)
  - Fiberoptic bronchoscopy with protected brushing (most commonly used method today)
  - Fiberoptic bronchoscopy with bronchoalveolar lavage
- Specimens obtained by invasive sampling should be examined by:
  - Gram stain
  - PAS stain
  - Giemsa stain
  - GMS stain
  - Toluidine blue O stain
  - Cytology
  - Aerobic and anaerobic culture
- Blood cultures
- Serology: Hemagglutinating or complement-fixing antibodies for amoebae
- CT of the chest can be used to define the exact location and extent of the abscess

Definitive Diagnosis:

Abscess of lung   ICD-9-CM 513.0

Suggested Treatment:

- Presumptive anaerobic infection:
  - PCN G 10 to 20 million U/day IV given every 6 hours, and
       Metronidazole 1 g IV every 12 hours for 2 to 3 weeks (or until clinical symptoms are significantly improved), then
       PCN G 750 mg (1.2 million U) orally every 6 hours for 2 to 4 months
  - Penicillin allergy: Substitute for PCN G: Clindamycin 1.8 to 2.7 g/day IV given every 8 hours, then

- Clindamycin 900 mg orally every 8 hours for 2 to 4 months, or
  - Imipenem 1 to 4 g/day IV given every 6 hours, then oral therapy as above, or
  - Ticarcillin + clavulanate 4 to 24 g/day IV given every 6 hours, or
    - Ampicillin + sulbactam 4 to 8 g/day IV given every 6 hours for 2 to 3 weeks, then oral therapy as above
- Staphylococcal infections:
  - Penicillinase-resistant PCN IV for 2 to 3 weeks or until clinical improvement, then orally for 2 to 4 months:
  - Nafcillin 2 to 12 g/day IV given every 6 hours, then Dicloxacillin 1 to 2 g/day orally given every 6 hours, or
    - Oxacillin 2 to 12 g/day IV given every 6 hours, then 2 to 4 g/day orally every 6 hours
  - Penicillin allergy: Vancomycin 1 to 2 g/day IV given every 12 hours, then 0.5 g/day orally every 6 hours
  - **NOTE:** Vancomycin is also the drug of choice for methicillin-resistant *S. aureus*
- Group A Streptococcal infection:
  - PCN G 6 to 12 million U/day IV given every 6 hours for 2 to 3 weeks, then 1.2 million U (750 mg) orally every 6 hours for 2 to 4 months, or
  - Penicillin allergy: Erythromycin 2 to 4 g/day IV given every 6 hours for 2 to 3 weeks, then 500 mg orally every 6 hours for 3 to 4 months
- Aerobic gram negative bacterial infection:
  - Gentamicin 3 to 5 mg/kg/day IV given every 8 hours, or
  - Amikacin 15 mg/kg/day IV given every 12 hours, or

- Imipenem 1 to 4 g/day IV given every 6 hours, each for 2 to 3 weeks with close monitoring of clinical symptoms
- Postural drainage is an important aspect of the therapy for a lung abscess
- Bronchoscopy may be helpful in effecting drainage and for removal of foreign bodies and biopsy diagnosis of tumors
- Surgical resection of lung abscesses is rarely required unless there is a coexisting malignancy; indeed, this is generally contraindicated because of the hazard of the spread of infection or asphyxiation from spillage of the abscess contents
- Surgical drainage of a lung abscess through the chest wall is also rarely indicated unless there is a complicating empyema

Follow-Up:

- Inpatient monitoring while patient is ill, then outpatient
- Postural drainage and pulmonary physiotherapy should be aggressive while in-hospital, but should be continued on outpatient basis
- Treatment and careful clinical monitoring should be continued until cavity has disappeared or stabilized on serial radiographs (repeated initially at 1-week intervals, then 2- to 3-week intervals for several weeks or months)
- Treat underlying condition
  - Subphrenic abscess
  - Malignancy
  - Periodontal disease
  - Alcoholism
  - Epilepsy

- TB
- Fungal disease
- Neurologic disorder
- **Watch for:** signs and symptoms of
    - Extension of abscess
    - Brain abscess
    - Meningitis
    - Empyema
    - Pneumothorax
    - Massive hemoptysis

CYSTIC FIBROSIS

Presenting Symptoms:

SUBJECTIVE	OBJECTIVE
Chronic cough	Chronic cough with:
Episodic exacerbations:	—Wheezing
—Increased volume of sputum	—Dyspnea
—Foul-smelling sputum	—Tachypnea
—Dyspnea	—Recurrent bronchitis and pneumonia leading to bronchiectasis (98% of the recurrent pneumonias are from infection with *S. aureus* or *P. aeruginosa*)
—Anorexia	
—Weight loss	
—Low-grade fever (usually in adults only)	
—Hemoptysis	
—Vomiting	Barrel chest
—Disturbed sleep	Digital clubbing and cyanosis
	Nasal polyposis
	Positive history of autosomal recessive genetic defect for CF gene with classic extrapulmonary manifestations:

—Chronic abdominal pain caused by esophageal and colonic disease, intestinal obstruction, and pancreatic insufficiency

—Endocrine disturbances (male infertility, delayed sexual development, retarded bone growth)

—Exocrine sweat gland abnormalities (increased sodium and chloride excretion)

—Vitamin A, D, E, K deficiencies

Recurrent spontaneous pneumothorax

Pulmonary hypertension leading to right heart failure (adults only)

Differential Diagnosis:

Recurrent pneumonias
Immunodeficiency
Bronchiectasis
Asthma

Suggested Workup:

- Sputum examination: Gram stain and culture → normally positive for *S. aureus* and *P. aeruginosa*

- Chest radiograph:
  - Hyperaeration
  - Airway wall thickening
  - Hilar lymphadenopathy
  - Cystic bronchiectasis
  - Retained secretions
  - Typical predominance of right upper lobe involvement
  - Occasional pneumothorax
- Pulmonary function tests:
  - Falling forced expiratory volume in 1 second (FEV_1) values, eventually to less than 40% of the predicted value
  - Results consistent with obstructive airway disease
  - Hypoxemia and carbon dioxide retention are rare until the terminal stages of the disease
- Laboratory evaluation:
  - White blood cell (WBC) count may be mildly elevated during exacerbation
  - Blood cultures are usually negative
  - Glucose tolerance test and/or fasting blood sugar are abnormal in 15% to 20% of patients
- Special tests for CF diagnosis:
  - Quantititative pilocarpine iontophoresis sweat test : [Na] or [Cl] concentration greater than 60 mEq/L confirms the diagnosis of CF
  - Genetic testing for CF gene (required only where sweat test is inconclusive)
  - Stool trypsin or chymotrypsin absent or diminished
  - Seventy–two-hour fecal fat markedly increased

Definitive Diagnosis:

Cystic fibrosis   ICD-9-CM 277.0
Fibrotic lung disease   ICD-9-CM 515

Suggested Treatment:

- Oral antibiotics for mild to moderate exacerbations of pulmonary disease:
  - Adult:
    - Ciprofloxacin 500 to 750 mg orally every 12 hours, or
    - Ofloxacin 400 mg orally every 12 hours for 14 to 21 days
  - Pediatric: (Pediatric = child younger than 10 years old)
    - Cephalexin 12.5 mg/kg orally every 6 hours for 14 to 21 days, or
    - Amoxicillin + clavulanate 10 to 15 mg amoxicillin/kg orally every 6 hours for 14 to 21 days
- Parenteral antibiotics (for serious respiratory illness or where infection has not responded to oral antimicrobials) are given for 10 to 14 days (longer if necessary to achieve a full clinical response):
  - Adult:
    - —Tobramycin 3 mg/kg IV given every 8 hours, or
      - Gentamicin 6 to 15 mg/kg/day given every 8 hours, and
      - Ceftazidime 2 g IV every 8 hours, or
      - Ticarcillin + clavulanate 3 g ticarcillin + 0.1 g clavulanate IV every 6 hours, or
      - Imipenem 0.5 to 1.0 g IV every 6 hours,
    - —and (if *S. aureus* is present or suspected)
      - Cephalothin 1 g IV given every 6 hours, or
      - Nafcillin 1 g IV every 6 hours, or
      - Vancomycin 500 mg IV every 6 hours

- Pediatric:
  —Tobramycin 3 mg/kg IV every 8 hours, and
    Ceftazidime 50 to 75 mg/kg IV every 8 hours, or
    Ticarcillin + clavulanate 100 mg ticarcillin/kg + 3.3 mg clavulanate/kg IV every 6 hours, or
    Imipenem 15 to 25 mg/kg IV every 6 hours,
  —and (if *S. aureus* is present or suspected)
    Cephalothin 25 to 50 mg/kg IV every 6 hours, or
    Nafcillin 25 to 50 mg/kg IV every 6 hours, or
    Vancomycin 15 mg/kg IV every 6 hours
- Aerosolized antibiotics can be used for subacute pulmonary exacerbations to help maintain a stable clinical status:
  - Tobramycin 60 to 80 mg per aerosol 3 times a day
  - Colistin sulfate inhalation therapy
- Maintenance antibiotic therapy:
  - The long-term administration of oral antibiotics to patients with CF aimed at reducing the frequency of exacerbations of pulmonary infections has recently come into question; two well-controlled studies showed no benefit from such therapy compared with treatment of exacerbations, and suggested that such treatment may select for antibiotic-resistant bacteria.
  - If the practitioner wishes to institute chronic suppressive therapy, reference is made to the antibiotic selection guidelines in: Ramsey W. N Engl J Med 1996; 335:179-188.

- General measures:
  - Annual influenza vaccinations
  - Pneumococcal vaccine not recommended
  - Postural drainage and chest physiotherapy
  - Aerosolized mucolytics
  - Aerosolized B2 agonists
  - High protein, high fat diet
  - Oxygen therapy as needed

Follow-Up:

- Long-term care requires team approach:
  - Physician
  - Respiratory therapist
  - Nurse
  - Nutritionist
  - Physical therapist
  - Genetic counselor
  - Psychologist (median survival of patients with CF is to age 29)
  - Social worker
- In-hospital care may be required for severe exacerbations of pulmonary disease
  - May need assisted ventilation (intermittent positive pressure breathing [IPPB] strictly contraindicated)
  - May need supplemental oxygen
  - May consider lung transplant for severe, progressive, and debilitating disease
- Otherwise, outpatient care with office visits at least every 3 to 4 months
- Advisability of pregnancy in patient with CF depends on:
  - Adequate genetic counseling
  - Adequate nutrition and pulmonary function at start of pregnancy
- **Watch for:** signs and symptoms of
  - Atelectasis

- Pneumothorax
- Hemoptysis
- Right heart failure
- Pulmonary hypertension
- Emphysema
- Hypertrophic pulmonary osteodystrophy
- Diabetes mellitus
- Metabolic alkalosis
- Volume depletion
- Bleeding esophageal varices
- Biliary cirrhosis
- Intestinal obstruction
- Anovulation
- Malnutrition
- Retarded growth
- Psychosocial problems

ASPERGILLOSIS (ASPERGILLOMA OF THE LUNG)

Presenting Symptoms:

SUBJECTIVE	OBJECTIVE
Cough	Rales, rhonchi
Wheezing	Wheezing
Fever	Fever
Dyspnea	Tachypnea
Manifestations of underlying lung disease	Localized area of dullness to percussion and diminished breath sounds
Hemoptysis	Elicit history of:
	—COPD
	—TB
	—Bronchiectasis
	—Malignancy

—Sarcoidosis
—Histoplasmosis
—Anthracosilicosis
—Lung abscess
—Immunodeficiency state especially with granulocytopenia

Differential Diagnosis:

Asthma
Hypersensitivity pneumonitis
Allergic bronchopulmonary aspergillosis
TB
Lung cancer
Bacterial pneumonia
Pulmonary hemorrhage
Pulmonary embolus
Drug toxicity
Eosinophilic pneumonia

Suggested Workup:

- Chest radiograph: visualization of air or fleeting infiltrates around a cavitary mass; the patchy infiltrates may later consolidate and extend cavitation (practitioner may wish to confirm with CT or MRI of chest, where pathognomonic "fungus ball" in the lung is sometimes better visualized)
- Sputum examination: PAS stain and fungal culture on Sabouraud's agar: positive for *Aspergillus*
- Serology:
  - High titers of IgG and IgE antibody to *A. fumigatus*
  - CBC shows marked eosinophilia
  - Precipitins against *Aspergillus* antigens
- Skin testing: Positive immediate-type sensitivity to *Aspergillus* antigen

- Bronchoscopy with bronchial washings:
  - Helpful in isolating organism in invasive disease, but risk/benefit ratio makes this test generally not recommended
- Transthoracic needle aspiration: Same comment as above

Definitive Diagnosis:

Aspergillosis   ICD-9-CM 117.3

Suggested Treatment:

- Antimicrobial therapy:
  - Amphotericin B 0.5 mg/kg/day IV (1.0 to 1.5 mg/kg/day IV in markedly neutropenic patients); follow clinically, but total cumulative dose should not exceed 1.5 to 2.5 g
  - Patients with more indolent infection and no remote spread (i.e., no invasive aspergillosis) may be treated with: Itraconazole 300 mg orally twice a day for 1 day, then 200 mg orally twice a day; follow clinically for 6 months
- Surgical resection: Surgical resection of a single, isolated pulmonary lesion may be beneficial. This is EXPERIMENTAL and has been used primarily in neutropenic patients at high risk for hemoptysis or pneumothorax (Moreau P, et al. Cancer 1993;72:3223-3226)
- Intracavitary antimicrobial therapy: Transthoracic intracavitary instillation of amphotericin B has been used in patients with inoperable cases and intolerance to systemic amphotericin B; this is EXPERIMENTAL and is associated with a high rate of complications with questionable benefit (Jackson M, et al. Thorax 1993; 48:928-930; Lee KS et al. Am J Radiol 1993; 161:727-731; Giron JM et al. Radiol 1993; 188:825-827)

Follow-Up:

- In-hospital care for aspergilloma patients with good clinical monitoring, repeat CBC, and chest radiographs
- Aggressive treatment of underlying disease and/or immunodeficiency
- **Watch for:** signs and symptoms of
    - Hemoptysis
    - Pneumothorax
    - Metastatic invasion of
      —CNS
      —GI tract
      —Heart valves
      —Ear and sinuses
      —Eye
      —Bone (especially ribs and thoracic vertebra, which may lead to spinal cord compression)
      —Skin
      —Kidneys
  - Empyema
  - Bronchopleural fistula
  - Amphotericin-induced nephrotoxicity, electrolyte disturbances, or anemia

BLASTOMYCOSIS

Presenting Symptoms:

SUBJECTIVE	OBJECTIVE
Onset of symptoms may be abrupt or insidious	Diffuse rales and rhonchi
Symptoms may range from mild to	Mild wheezing
	Low grade fever
	May elicit history of

bordering on respiratory failure

Cough, may be productive

Hemoptysis

Weight loss

Pleuritic chest pain

Myalgias

Arthralgias

Low-grade fever and chills

—Occupational/ recreational exposure to soil containing spores of *Blastomyces dermatitidis*

—Residence in endemic area

—Rare association with AIDS

Differential Diagnosis:

Chronic pneumonia

Acute bacterial pneumonia

TB

Fungal lung disease

Lung abscess

Empyema

Bronchogenic carcinoma

Coccidioidomycosis

Sporotrichosis

Suggested Workup:

- Chest radiograph:
  - Variable findings
  - Lobar or segmental alveolar infiltrates, with or without cavitation
  - Upper lobe fibronodular infiltrates with consolidation are most common
  - Mass lesions seen occasionally
  - Pleural thickening
  - Hilar adenopathy variably seen
  - Small pleural effusions may be noted
- Sputum examination:
  - Yeast forms demonstrable on KOH wet mount or special stains (GMS stain, PAS stain, and mucicarmine stain will identify

> *B. dermatitidis* and help differentiate it from encapsulated *Cryptococcus*)
> - Culture of *B. dermatitidis* on Sabouraud's agar
- Serology:
  - Complement fixation and precipitins are not helpful in diagnosis because of low sensitivity and specificity
  - ELISA test for specific antibodies to *B. dermatitidis* has variable sensitivity and specificity; not cost effective
- Special tests to evaluate extra-pulmonary disease:
  - CT scan of head for CNS lesions
  - CT scan of spine for vertebral lesions
  - Bone scan for skeletal lesions

Definitive Diagnosis:

Blastomycosis, pulmonary   ICD-9-CM 116.0

Suggested Treatment:

- Severe disease: Amphotericin B 0.5 to 0.8 mg/kg/d IV given over 6 hours; follow clinically, but total cumulative dose should not exceed 1.5 to 2.5 g
- Milder forms:
  - Itraconazole 200 mg orally twice a day for 6 months, or
  - Ketoconazole 400 to 800 mg orally once a day for 6 months

Follow-Up:

- Monitor closely during early therapy, depending on severity of disease
- Post-therapy follow-up every 3 months for 2 years, then every 6 months for life
- **Watch for:** signs and symptoms of
  - Spread of infection to
    —CNS

      —Bone and joints
      —Skin
      —Pericardium
      —GI tract and liver
      —Spleen
      —Adrenal glands
- Respiratory collapse
- Amphotericin-induced nephrotoxicity, electrolyte disturbances, or anemia

MYCOBACTERIUM TUBERCULOSIS

Presenting Symptoms:

SUBJECTIVE	OBJECTIVE
Early on, infection may be asymptomatic	Physical findings are not specific:
Course of disease is variable and symptoms generally progress slowly so that they are sometimes not even noticed by the patient (see note below)	Dullness to percussion Increased fremitus Post-tussive rales Signs of consolidation may be present late in disease
Eventually the following symptoms are reported:	—Whispered pectoriloquy —Tubular breath sounds —Amphoric breath sounds
Cough	Lymphadenopathy
Mucopurulent sputum	Hepatosplenomegaly
Hemoptysis	History of prominent risk factors helps increase the index of suspicion for the disease:
Fever and night sweats	
Anorexia	
Weight loss	
Decreased activity and fatigue	—Urban, homeless,

Pleuritic chest pain

Note: Progression and course of the disease will be largely determined by several factors, including size of the inoculum, virulence of the organism, competence of host defense, presence of other diseases (especially HIV infection and diabetes mellitus), and use of chronic corticosteroid therapy

- minority group patient
—Institutionalized (especially correctional facilities and homeless shelters)
—Immunosuppressed (especially HIV-positive)
—Hodgkin's disease
—Lymphoma
—Diabetes mellitus
—Chronic renal failure
—Malnutrition
—Chronic high-dose steroids
—Close contact with infected individual
—Intravenous drug users

Differential Diagnosis:

Acute bacterial pneumonia
Atypical pneumonia
Viral pneumonia
Fungal pneumonia (especially *Nocardia*)
Lymphoma

Suggested Workup:

- Chest radiograph findings may be highly suggestive of TB:
  - A pneumonic lesion with enlarged hilar nodes should suggest primary TB, regardless of other factors
  - Patchy or nodular infiltrates in the apical or subapical posterior areas of the upper

lobes, or in the superior segment of a lower lobe, especially if it is bilateral or associated with cavity formation are virtually pathognomonic for pulmonary TB
- Hilar adenopathy is common
- Pleural effusion may be present or absent
- Air-fluid levels may be seen, especially with lower lobe disease
- Chronicity and nature of the disease may be ascertained from radiograph findings:
  —Productive, granulomatous lesions tend to be small and nodular with sharply defined margins
  —Exudative, pneumonic lesions tend to have soft, indistinct borders
  —Fibrotic scars have sharp margins and tend to contract over time
  —Caseation causes increased density
- Sputum examination:
  - Three daily collections should be made; especially important is a good early-morning sample
  - If sputum is unobtainable, an early-morning gastric aspiration should be collected from hospitalized patients, or heated saline aerosol induction for sputum attempted in ambulatory patients
  - Specimens should be stained with Ziehl-Neelsen or auramine-rhodamine stain for presence of acid-fast bacillus (AFB)
  - Specimens should be cultured by the BACTEC radiometric broth system for *Mycobacteria* (still requires 9 to 16 days for detection of mycobacterial metabolism)
  - **NOTE:** Because of the increased incidence of mycobacterial strains that are resistant to

antimicrobials, drug sensitivity testing should be routinely incorporated into all culture techniques
- Tuberculin skin testing:
  - PPD can be used as antigen
  - Five tuberculin units (TU) of intermediate strength PPD in 0.1 mL of buffer is injected intradermally in volar aspect of forearm with a No. 26 or 27 needle; a raised, blanched wheal should be produced by the injection
  - Reaction is read as area of induration, NOT erythema at 48 to 72 hours
    —Greater than 5 mm: positive for HIV patient, immunosuppressed patient, exposed household contact, or patient with clinical evidence of disease
    —Greater than 10 mm:
      –90% of persons demonstrating 10 mm and virtually all persons with 15 to 20 mm of induration to 5 TU are infected with *M. tuberculosis*
      –Lesser induration, or reactions requiring up to 250 TU to be elicited, are frequently nonspecific cross-reactions from infection with other mycobacterial species
      –Reactions of 5 to 10 mm should be regarded as suspicious for tuberculous infection
      –False-negative reactions may be observed on first testing in over 20% of patients with active TB and may be due to general immunosuppression caused by illness; retesting 2 to 3 weeks after treatment is initiated is indicated
- Laboratory and serology evaluation show nonspecific results:

- CBC: anemia, monocytosis, thrombocytosis
- Serum protein electrophoresis: hypergammaglobulinemia
- Renal function may show electrolyte pattern consistent with syndrome of inappropriate secretion of antidiuretic hormone (SIADH)
- Rapid diagnostic methods:
  - Nucleic acid hybridization with DNA probes (GenProbe, San Diego, CA)
    —Advantage: complete in several hours
    —Drawback: suitable only for organisms in pure culture
  - PCR for *M. tuberculosis*
    —Advantage: specific identification possible from clinical specimens within 24 hours
    —Disadvantage: not yet widely available commercially
- Fiberoptic bronchoscopy with transbronchial biopsy and bronchial washings is an efficient way to obtain diagnostic materials when sputum does not suffice
- Extrapulmonary infections:
  - Lumbar puncture if mycobacterial meningitis is suspected
  - Blood culture, bone marrow biopsy, renal biopsy, and liver biopsy if miliary TB is suspected

Definitive Diagnosis:

Tuberculosis   ICD-9-CM 011.9
(There are multiple modifiers for this disease category; specific type or subtype may have a different ICD-9-CM code)

Suggested Treatment:

- Whom to treat (Centers for Disease Control and Prevention [CDC] guidelines) (Table 4.4)

Table 4.4

**Whom to Treat for Tuberculosis—
CDC Guidelines**

Risk Factor*	Incidence Group[†]	Age	
		<35	35 or Older
Present	High or Low	Treat all ages if >10 mm PPD reaction to 5 TU or >5 mm and patient is: • Recent contact • HIV-infected • Has CXR showing old TB	
Absent	High	Treat if PPD >10 mm	Do not treat
Absent	Low	Treat if PPD >15 mm	Do not treat

* Risk factors: HIV infection; recent exposure to TB; recent skin test conversion; abnormal chest radiograph; IV drug use.

[†] High-incidence groups: immigrants from high incidence areas; medically underserved populations; residents of long-term care facilities

PPD = purified protein derivative; TU = tuberculin units; CXR = chest radiograph (x-ray)

- How to treat
  - Standard therapy for *M. tuberculosis* (9-month regimen):
    Isoniazid (INH) 300 mg orally once a day, and
    Rifampin 600 mg orally once a day
  - Fortified regimen recommended by most experts as the regimen of choice pending drug sensitivity results (9-month regimen):
    —INH PLUS rifampin as in standard therapy, and
        Pyrazinamide 20 to 35 mg/kg/day orally given once a day or twice a day,

  —and (if INH resistance is suspected)
    Ethambutol 15 mg/kg/day orally (up
     to 25 mg/kg/day may be given for
     the first 60 days), or
    Streptomycin 0.5 to 1.0 g
     intramuscularly once a day, up to
     1 g intramuscularly twice weekly

- Intermittent 9-month regimen to be used only where there is no substantial likelihood of antimicrobial resistance:
  - —INH PLUS rifampin as in standard therapy for 1 to 2 months, then
  - —INH 900 mg PLUS rifampin 600 mg orally twice weekly for the remaining 7 to 8 months
- CDC 6-month regimen:
  - —INH PLUS rifampin PLUS pyrazinamide PLUS ethambutol or
    - Streptomycin as in the fortified regimen for 2 months, then
  - —INH PLUS rifampin as in the standard therapy daily or 2 to 3 times weekly for 4 months
- Directly observed therapy (DOT) in noncompliant patients. All doses are observed and provided in the practitioner's office:
  - —Once daily dose for 2 weeks of INH 300 mg PLUS rifampin 600 mg PLUS pyrazinamide 1.5 to 2.5 g PLUS streptomycin 750 mg to 1.0 g
  - —Then, twice weekly doses for 6 weeks of INH 15 mg/kg PLUS rifampin 600 mg PLUS pyrazinamide 3 to 4 g PLUS streptomycin 1 to 1.5 g
  - —Then, twice weekly doses for 4 months of INH 15 mg/kg PLUS rifampin 600 mg

- Pediatric patients:
  - —INH 10 mg/kg orally once a day (up to maximum of 300 mg daily), and
    - Rifampin 15 mg/kg orally once a day (up to a maximum of 600 mg daily) for 1 year
  - —Streptomycin 20 mg/kg/day intramuscularly (up to a maximum of 1.0 g daily) or 25 to 30 mg/kg intramuscularly twice weekly, or
    - Ethambutol 15 mg/kg/day orally, may be added if extensive disease is present (Ethambutol should be avoided in very young children because of the inability to adequately monitor visual acuity limits in this patient population)
- Pregnant patients:
  - —INH 300 mg orally once a day, and
  - —Ethambutol 15 mg/kg/day, or
  - —Rifampin 600 mg orally once a day for 6 to 9 months
- Patients with AIDS:
  - —Begin with fortified regimen above
  - —Continue for 9 months or at least 6 months beyond sputum culture conversion, whichever is longer
  - —Patients with fever beyond 7 to 14 days of antituberculous therapy suggests drug resistance and the need to add more agents (see section on MDR-TB)
- MDR-TB (Multiple drug-resistant *M. tuberculosis*):
  - —MDR-TB strains have various combinations of resistance to INH, rifampin, streptomycin, or ethambutol

—Resistance to rifampin is often a good marker for the presence of MDR-TB
—CDC guidelines provide general recommendations to help prevent the emergence of MDR-TB (see JAMA 1993; 11:270)
  –*M. tuberculosis* isolates from ALL patients should be tested for antibiotic susceptibility immediately upon collection
  –Initial treatment regimens with first-line drugs should include four drugs (as in the fortified or the CDC 6-month regimens above)
  –DOT (above) should be considered for ALL patients initially and certainly for patients suspected of being recalcitrant or noncompliant
  –Treatment of MDR-TB should be based on in vitro drug susceptibilities of the patient's isolate and should include AT LEAST TWO additional drugs to which the isolate is sensitive; adding only one second-line drug to an already failing regimen is NOT advisable
—The following second-line drugs should be considered as additions to an initial regimen that is failing to eradicate the disease, or where MDR-TB is otherwise evident; selection of specific drugs should be guided by in vitro susceptibility testing of the patient's bacterial isolate and local patterns of resistance and susceptibility:
  –Cycloserine 250 to 500 mg orally twice a day

 –Ethionamide 250 mg orally twice a day initially, titrated to as high as 1 g/day in divided doses as tolerated
 –Rifabutin 300 mg orally once a day or 150 mg orally twice a day
 –Capreomycin 500 mg to 1 g intramuscularly 5 times weekly for 2 to 4 months, then 1 g intramuscularly 2 to 3 times a week
 –Amikacin 10 mg/kg intramuscularly 5 times a week
 –Kanamycin 10 mg/kg/day intramuscularly
 –Viomycin 2 g (1 g 12 hours apart) intramuscularly twice a week
 –Amithiozone 150 mg orally once a day or 450 mg orally 2 times a week
 –Ciprofloxacin 500 to 750 mg orally twice a day
 –Ofloxacin 400 mg orally every 12 hours
 –Lomefloxacin 400 mg orally every night at bedtime
 –Amoxicillin + clavulanate 1 to 1.5 g amoxicillin/day orally given every 8 hours
- Miliary TB (6 to 9 months of therapy):
  —INH 300 mg orally once a day, and
    Rifampin 600 mg orally once a day, and
    Pyrazinamide 20 to 35 mg/kg/day orally given once or twice a day,
  —and (in debilitated patients with poor initial response to therapy or with fulminant disease): Prednisone 60 to 80 mg orally once a day

Follow-Up:

- See patients every 2 to 3 months for duration of treatment

- Repeat chest radiograph every 2 to 3 months and if symptoms change
- Repeat PPD skin test 12 months after treatment and annually thereafter
- Check liver enzymes every 2 to 3 months; if changes occur, modify drugs as outlined above and in Drug Index
- Treat any underlying diseases or immunodeficiencies
- Notify public health department if patient has had significant close contacts with others
- **Watch for:** signs and symptoms of
    - Secondary infections, especially if there is cavitary lesion in lung
    - Hematogenous spread: miliary TB
    - Spread to susceptible persons
    - Development of drug resistance

Cardiac Infections   5

INFECTIVE ENDOCARDITIS

Presenting Symptoms:

<u>SUBJECTIVE</u>

Fever

Night sweats

Chills

Malaise and weakness

Myalgia and arthralgia

Joint pain

Back pain (may be
  severe)

Anorexia, weight loss

Stiff neck

Headache

Delirium

Paralysis or
  hemiparesis

Aphasia

Muscle weakness

Cold, painful extremity

Blood in urine or
  sputum

Petechiae

Conjunctival
  hemorrhage

Chest pain

Shortness of breath

Pain in tip of finger/
  toe

Various skin lesions

Symptoms are variable
  in course and
  development:

—Aggressive, rapidly
  progressive, and
  fulminant (acute)

<u>OBJECTIVE</u>

Fever (95% of cases)

Heart murmur, new or
  changing (85% of
  cases), usually aortic
  insufficiency

Physical findings of
  congestive heart
  failure

Clubbing

Splinter hemorrhages

Conjunctival petechiae

Petechiae on buccal
  mucosa, palate, or
  extremities

Osler nodes (small,
  painful, nodular
  lesions on pads of
  fingers or toes)

Janeway lesions
  (hemorrhagic,
  macular, painless
  plaques, usually on
  palms and soles)

Roth's spots (oval,
  pale, retinal lesions
  surrounded by
  hemorrhage and
  located near the
  optic disk)

Splenomegaly

Major embolic
  phenomena

—Splenic artery

—Slow, indolent course over weeks to months (subacute/chronic)

—Distinction between these forms is less useful today except to focus attention on possible etiologic agents:

Acute: *Staphylococcus aureus, Streptococcus pyogenes, Streptococcus pneumoniae, Neisseria gonorrhoeae, Enterococci*

Subacute: *Streptococcus viridans, Enterococci*

emboli

—Renal infarction → hematuria

—Pulmonary emboli

—Septic pulmonary emboli → pneumonia

—Coronary artery emboli →
  –Myocarditis
  –Cardiac arrhythmia
  –Myocardial infarction

—Major vessel emboli (femoral, brachial, popliteal, radial arteries)

—Stroke (20% to 40% of cases) →
  –Hemiplegia
  –Sensory loss
  –Ataxia
  –Aphasia
  –Altered mental status

—Septic cerebral emboli → meningitis

—Retinal artery → loss of vision

Signs of renal failure (10% of patients)

Differential Diagnosis:

Brain abscess
Cerebral embolus
Cerebral hemorrhage
Collagen vascular disease

Glomerulonephritis
Intra-abdominal infection
Meningitis
Myocardial infarction
Osteomyelitis
Pericarditis
Rheumatic fever
Salmonellosis
Tuberculosis
Septic pulmonary infarcts
Pulmonary embolus
Thrombotic thrombocytopenic purpura

Suggested Workup:

- History is critical in eliciting predisposing factor(s) for bacterial endocarditis:
  - Prosthetic heart valve
  - Previous bacterial endocarditis, even in the absence of other predisposing factors
  - Congenital cardiac malformation
  - Rheumatic valvular dysfunction
  - Valvular surgery
  - Hypertrophic cardiomyopathy
  - Mitral valve prolapse with mitral regurgitation and/or redundant mitral valves
  - Indwelling intravascular device
  - Intravenous drug use
  - Recent dental or surgical procedure that may have caused transient bacteremia (in susceptible hosts), including:
    —Dental extraction
    —Periodontal surgery
    —Tonsillectomy
    —Bronchoscopy
    —Upper gastrointestinal endoscopy
    —Barium enema

—Sigmoidoscopy/colonoscopy
—Urethral dilatation
—Cystoscopy
—Transurethral prostatic resection (TURP)
—Normal vaginal delivery
—Vaginal hysterectomy

- Laboratory:
  - Normochromic, normocytic anemia (70% to 90% of cases)
  - Low serum iron concentration
  - Low iron-binding capacity
  - Thrombocytopenia (5% to 15%)
  - Leukocytosis (especially in acute infectious endocarditis)
  - Peripheral smear histiocytes
  - Elevated erythrocyte sedimentation rate (ESR) (90% to 100%)
  - Hypergammaglobulinemia (20% to 30%)
  - Positive rheumatoid factor (RF) (40% to 50%)
  - Hypocomplementemia (5% to 15%)
  - False-positive Venereal Disease Research Laboratories (VDRL) test uncommon (less than 1%)
  - Proteinuria (50% to 65%)
  - Microscopic hematuria (30% to 60%)
  - Red cell casts (10% to 15%)
  - Circulating immune complexes (levels greater than 100 μg of aggregated human gamma-globulin equivalent per mL is virtually pathognomonic for infectious endocarditis)
  - Cryoglobulins, mixed type (85% to 95%)
- Blood cultures typically show a continuous and low-grade bacteremia (95% to 98% of patients)
  - Sets of two cultures should be taken at different times

- At least three sets should be obtained in the first 24 hours and before antibiotics are started
- The first two blood cultures will yield the etiologic agent 90% of the time
- In patients with culture-negative endocarditis, intraleukocytic bacteria may be detected in peripheral blood (50% of cases)
- Imaging studies:
  - Echocardiography can be used to identify vegetations on all valves
    —Two-dimensional (2D) cross-sectional real-time techniques are preferred over M-mode
    —2D echocardiogram with digital image processing may be able to differentiate active from healed lesions (still EXPERIMENTAL)
    —Transesophageal echocardiography (TEE) appears to have higher sensitivity (95%) compared with transthoracic techniques (60% to 65%); both techniques have high specificity (98%)
  - Magnetic resonance imaging (MRI) appears useful in locating vegetations
  - Axial computed tomography (CT) scan may be useful in locating abscesses
  - Pulmonary V/Q scan may be useful in right-sided endocarditis
  - Colonoscopy in patients with *Streptococcus bovis* bacteremia/endocarditis to rule out colon cancer
- Cardiac catheterization:
  - Aids in determining the extent of valvular damage
  - Allows collection of quantitative blood cultures proximal and distal to suspected

sites of infection to localize vegetations in both right- and left-sided endocarditis
- Indicated when considering surgical intervention
- Cineangiography performed at catheterization is the definitive procedure in determining the anatomic alterations resulting from the infection:
  —Determine the degree of aortic regurgitation
  —Determine the degree of left ventricular dysfunction as a contributing factor to congestive heart failure
  —Visualize ventricular and aortic aneurysms
  —Gauge the patency of the coronary arteries

CLINICAL CRITERIA FOR DIAGNOSIS OF INFECTIVE ENDOCARDITIS (according to von Reym as adapted by Durack)

- Definite[1]:
  - Two major criteria, or
  - One major plus three minor criteria, or
  - Five minor criteria
- Possible: clinical findings consistent with infective endocarditis that fall short of Definite, but not Rejected
- Rejected:
  - Firm alternate diagnosis, or

[1] Pathologic criteria may be substituted for clinical criteria in making diagnosis of definite infective endocarditis: (1) Microorganisms demonstrated by culture or histology in a vegetation, embolized vegetation, or abscess; or (2) presence of a vegetation or intracardiac abscess, confirmed by histology, showing active endocarditis

- Resolution of endocarditis syndrome with antibiotic therapy for 4 days or less
- Major Criteria:
  - Positive culture for microorganism typical for infective endocarditis:
    - —From two separate blood cultures drawn more than 12 hours apart, or
    - —All of three or three of four separate blood cultures, with first and last cultures drawn at least 1 hour apart
  - Evidence of endocardial involvement by:
    - —Positive echocardiogram for infective endocarditis (intracardiac mass, abscess, or new partial dehiscence of prosthetic valve), or
    - —New valvular regurgitation (increase or change in preexisting murmur is not sufficient)
- Minor Criteria:
  - Predisposing heart condition or intravenous drug use, or
  - Fever over 38°C, or
  - Embolic vascular phenomena (arterial embolism, septic pulmonary infarcts, mycotic aneurysm, intracranial hemorrhage, Janeway lesions), or
  - Immunologic phenomena (glomerulonephritis, Osler nodes, Roth's spots, RF), or
  - Echocardiogram consistent with infective endocarditis but not meeting major criteria, or
  - Microbiologic evidence (positive blood culture, but not meeting major criteria, serologic evidence of active infection with organism consistent with infective endocarditis)

Definitive Diagnosis:

Infective endocarditis   ICD-9-CM 421.0
Prosthetic valve endocarditis   ICD-9-CM 996.61
Aortic valve endocarditis   ICD-9-CM 424.1
Mitral valve endocarditis   ICD-9-CM 394.9
Pulmonary valve   ICD-9-CM 424.3
   endocarditis
Tricuspid valve endocarditis   ICD-9-CM 397.0

Suggested Treatment:

- **Antimicrobial treatment monitoring:** In every case of infective endocarditis, the following protocols should be followed to help monitor treatment and aid in therapeutic decisions:
  - Etiologic agent must be isolated in pure culture
  - Minimal inhibitory concentration (MIC) and minimal bactericidal concentration (MBC) must be determined for antibiotics to be used (standard disc sensitivity testing is unreliable and should not be used)
  - During therapy, patient's serum should be monitored for bactericidal activity against the etiologic organisms and the serum bactericidal titer (SBT) should be determined, especially when the organism appears to be resistant or tolerant to one of the drugs used or the patient's response to therapy is suboptimal (**NOTE:** the utility and clinical correlation of the SBT is **CONTROVERSIAL,** but it seems reasonable to attempt to achieve SBT levels of 1:8 to 1:16 if not precluded by drug toxicity)
  - Serum aminoglycoside and vancomycin levels should be monitored for peak and trough levels, and doses adjusted accordingly

- **Penicillin-sensitive streptococcal endocarditis:** (*S. viridans*, *S. pyogenes*, group D *Streptococcus* [*S. bovis*] with MBC = [Penicillin (PCN)] 0.1 to 1.0 μg/mL; [cephalothin] 0.15 to 1.25 μg/mL; [vancomycin] 0.15 to 0.4 μg/mL; [streptomycin] 6.25 to 50 μg/mL; [gentamicin] 1.56 to 3.12 μg/mL;)
  - PCN G 18 to 24 million units (U)/day intravenously (IV) given every 4 to 6 hours, and
    - Gentamicin 3 mg/kg/day IV given every 8 hours, or
    - Streptomycin 0.5 g intramuscularly given every 12 hours
  - This regimen is given for 2 weeks in patients with uncomplicated native valve endocarditis and for 6 weeks for patients with prosthetic valve endocarditis
  - Penicillin allergy: Cephalothin 2 g IV every 4 hours, or
    - Cefazolin 1 to 2 g IV every 8 hours for 4 weeks, and
    - Gentamicin 3 mg/kg/day IV given every 8 hours, or
    - Streptomycin 0.5 g intramuscularly every 12 hours for the first 2 weeks, or
    - Ceftriaxone 2 g IV daily alone for 4 weeks, or
    - Vancomycin 1 g IV every 12 hours alone for 4 weeks
  - In patients with native valve endocarditis and who:
    - —Are older than 65 years
    - —Have renal impairment
    - —Have cranial nerve (CN) VIII impairment
    - —Have central nervous system (CNS) involvement, use PCN G or ceftriaxone, or vancomycin alone for 4 weeks

- **Penicillin-resistant and enterococcal endocarditis:** (MBC = [PCN] greater than 100 μg/mL; [cephalothin] greater than 100 μg/mL; [vancomycin] greater than 100 μg/mL; [streptomycin] greater than 25 μg/mL; [gentamicin] greater than 25 μg/mL)
  - PCN G 20 to 40 million U/day IV given every 4 hours, and
    Streptomycin 0.5 g intramuscularly every 12 hours, or, if MIC for streptomycin is 2000 μg/mL or higher,
    Gentamicin 3 mg/kg/day IV given every 8 hours for 4 to 6 weeks
  - Penicillin allergy: Vancomycin 1 g IV every 12 hours, and
    Streptomycin or gentamicin as above for 4 to 6 weeks, or
    PCN desensitization followed by use of PCN plus an aminoglycoside
  - Vancomycin-resistant enterococcal endocarditis (EXPERIMENTAL treatment):
    PCN G 20 to 40 million U/day IV given every 4 hours, and
    Vancomycin 1 g IV every 12 hours, and
    Gentamicin 3 mg/kg/day IV given every 8 hours for 4 to 6 weeks
- **Staphylococcal endocarditis:**
  - Nafcillin 1.5 to 2.0 g IV every 4 hours, or
    Oxacillin 1.5 to 2.0 g IV every 4 hours, or
    Cephalothin 2 g IV every 4 hours, or
    Cefazolin 1 to 2 g IV/intramuscularly every 8 hours for 4 to 6 weeks
  - Gentamicin 3 mg/kg/day IV given every 8 hours may be added for the first 3 to 5 days of therapy for a synergistic effect, but the literature suggests a poor risk/benefit ratio except in intravenous drug users (mortality is essentially unchanged)

- Penicillin allergy: Vancomycin 1 g IV every 12 hours for 6 weeks, and Rifampin 600 mg IV once daily may be added in patients with poor clinical response or poor SBT levels for the infecting organism
- Methicillin-resistant *S. aureus* (MRSA):
    Vancomycin alone or with rifampin, or
    Minocycline 200 mg IV given once, then 100 mg IV given every 12 hours, or
    Trimethoprim-sulfamethoxazole (TMP-SMX) 10 mg/kg/day (based on TMP) IV given every 6 hours, or
    Ciprofloxacin 500 mg IV every 12 hours and
    Rifampin 600 mg IV once daily for 6 weeks
- Prosthetic valve or *Staphylococcus epidermidis* endocarditis:
    Vancomycin 1 g IV every 12 hours for 6 weeks, and
    Rifampin 300 mg orally every 8 hours for 6 weeks, and
    Gentamicin 3 mg/kg/day IV given every 8 hours for 2 weeks
- **Gram-negative aerobic endocarditis:**
  - *Escherichia coli/Proteus:*
      Ampicillin 2 g IV every 4 hours, and
      Gentamicin 1.7 mg/kg IV every 8 hours, or
      Ceftriaxone 1 to 2 g IV every 24 hours for 4 to 6 weeks
  - *Klebsiella:*
      Ceftriaxone 2 g IV every 24 hours, and
      Gentamicin 1.7 mg/kg IV every 8 hours, or
      Amikacin 15 mg/kg/day IV given every 8 to 12 hours for 4 to 6 weeks

- *Pseudomonas:*
    - Tobramycin 8 mg/kg/day IV/ intramuscularly given every 8 hours (maintain peak concentration of 15 to 20 μg/mL and trough concentration of less than 2 μg/mL), and
    - Ticarcillin 4 to 24 g/day IV given every 4 to 6 hours, or
    - Piperacillin 6 to 24 g/day IV given every 4 to 6 hours, or
    - Penicillin allergy: Ceftazidime 3 to 6 g/ day IV given every 8 to 12 hours for 6 to 8 weeks
- *Haemophilus:*
    - Ampicillin 2 g IV every 4 hours for 4 weeks, or
    - Ceftriaxone 1 to 2 g IV every 24 hours for 4 weeks
- **Anaerobic endocarditis:** *Bacillus fragilis*
    - PCN G 20 million U/day IV given every 4 to 6 hours, or
    - Metronidazole 0.75 to 2 g/day IV given every 6 to 12 hours, or
    - Ticarcillin + clavulanic acid 4 to 24 g/day (ticarcillin) IV given every 4 to 6 hours, or
    - Imipenem 1 to 4 g/day IV given every 6 hours for 4 to 6 weeks
- **Pneumococcal, gonococcal, and meningococcal endocarditis:**
    - PCN G 20 million U /day IV given every 4 to 6 hours, or
    - Ceftriaxone 1 to 2 g IV every 24 hours for 4 weeks
- **Fungal endocarditis:**
    - Amphotericin B 0.3 to 0.5 mg/kg/day IV given over 2 to 4 hours for 6 to 8 weeks

- Surgery (tricuspid valvulectomy, or valve replacement in left-sided fungal endocarditis) should be performed after 1 to 2 weeks of treatment with amphotericin B
- If clinical response to amphotericin B is poor, or dose must be lowered because of toxicity, may add:
    - 5-Fluorocytosine 150 mg/kg/day orally given every 4 hours, or
    - Rifampin 300 mg orally every 8 hours, or may substitute:
    - Fluconazole 400 mg IV once, then 200 mg IV every 24 hours for 6 to 8 weeks
- *Chlamydia* **endocarditis:**
  - Tetracycline 300 mg orally every 12 hours for 3 months, and
  - Valve replacement
- **Culture-negative endocarditis:**
  - PCN G 20 million U/day IV given every 4 to 6 hours, or
      - Ampicillin 2 g IV every 4 hours for 6 weeks, and
      - Streptomycin 0.5 g intramuscularly every 12 hours, or
      - Gentamicin 1.7 mg/kg IV every 8 hours for 2 weeks
  - Penicillin allergy: Vancomycin 1 g IV every 12 hours, or
      - Ceftriaxone 1 to 2 g IV every 24 hours for 6 weeks, and
      - Streptomycin or gentamicin as above
- **Surgical therapy:**
  - Generally, valve replacement is performed
  - Used in 25% of cases

- Indications for surgical intervention:
  - —Refractory congestive heart failure
  - —More than one serious systemic embolic episode
  - —Uncontrolled infection
  - —Valve dysfunction as demonstrated by fluoroscopy
  - —Ineffective antimicrobial therapy (e.g., fungal endocarditis)
  - —Mycotic aneurysms present
  - —Prosthetic valve endocarditis
  - —Local suppurative complications
  - —Perivalvular/myocardial abscesses
  - —Conduction system abnormalities/heart block
  - —Aortic involvement

Follow-Up:

- Careful inpatient monitoring until clinically improved, then consider home parenteral therapy with close follow-up
- Gentamicin blood levels should be performed if the drug is used for more than 5 days and in all patients with renal dysfunction
  - —Peak should be approximately 3 μg/mL
  - —Trough should be less than 1 μg/mL
- Vancomycin blood levels should be performed in patients with renal dysfunction
  - —Peak should be approximately 30 to 45 μg/mL
  - —Trough should be less than 10 μg/mL
- Twice weekly serum blood urea nitrogen (BUN) and creatinine measurements while the patient is on gentamicin or vancomycin
- If long-term aminoglycoside therapy is considered, perform baseline and follow-up audiometry

- **Watch for:** signs and symptoms of
    - Congestive heart failure
    - Ruptured valve cusp
    - Aneurysm of sinus of Valsalva
    - Aortic root abscesses
    - Myocardial abscesses
    - Pericarditis
    - Cardiac arrhythmias
    - Meningitis
    - Cerebral emboli
    - Brain abscesses
    - Ruptured mycotic aneurysm
    - Septic pulmonary infarcts
    - Splenic infarcts
    - Arterial emboli and infarcts
    - Arthritis
    - Myositis
    - Glomerulonephritis
    - Acute renal failure
    - Mesenteric infarct

SUPPURATIVE THROMBOPHLEBITIS

Presenting Symptoms:

SUBJECTIVE	OBJECTIVE
Swelling, tenderness, redness, and warmth along the course of a vein (variable according to site)	**Burn Patients:** Predominantly lower extremity involved with plastic catheter
Swollen glands	Fever without rigors
Fever	Warmth, erythema, tenderness, swelling locally (32%)
Systemic symptoms (over 80% of	Regional lymphangitis
	Signs of systemic

patients)
—Chills
—Anorexia
—Vomiting
—Light-headedness
—Malaise
—Prostration
—Debilitation

sepsis (80%)
Secondary pneumonia
Pulmonary emboli

Medical/Postoperative Patients:

Predominantly upper extremity involved

Warmth, erythema, pain, swelling locally (over 90%)

Elderly, debilitated patients with intravenous catheter

Already receiving antibiotics

Critically Ill Patients:

Presence of central venous catheters

Patients receiving total parenteral nutrition (TPN)

Patients with long-standing Broviac or Hickman catheters

Signs of sepsis/ fungemia predominate

Postpartum/Postpelvic Surgery:

Symptoms occur 1 to 2 weeks postoperative/ postpartum

Fever, chills, anorexia, vomiting

Flank pain and percussive costovertebral tenderness

> Right sided abdominal
> tenderness (80%)
> Tender vein palpable
> on pelvic or
> abdominal
> examination (30%)
> Septic pulmonary
> emboli

Differential Diagnosis:

Cellulitis
Erythema nodosum
Cutaneous polyarteritis nodosa
Sarcoid
Kaposi's sarcoma
Hyperalgesic pseudothrombophlebitis
Aseptic superficial thrombophlebitis
Deep vein thrombosis
Buerger's disease
Mondor's disease
Aseptic catheter-related thrombophlebitis
Trousseau's syndrome
Behçet's disease
Systemic lupus erythematosus
Subperiosteal abscess
Acute appendicitis[2]
Ureteral obstruction[2]
Torsion of an ovarian cyst[2]
Pyelonephritis[2]
Broad ligament hematoma[2]
Parametritis/endometritis[2]
Perinephric abscess[2]
Pelvic abscess[2]
Small bowel volvulus[2]
Pelvic inflammatory disease[2]

[2] For pelvic suppurative thrombophlebitis only

Sickle cell crisis[2]
Ectopic pregnancy[2]

Suggested Workup:

- History and physical examination are highly suggestive
- Bacterial cultures:
  - Blood cultures positive in up to 90% of cases
  - Semiquantitative catheter culture:
    —Catheter removed under aseptic conditions
    —Catheter fragments plated on 5% sheep blood agar
    —Growth of greater than 15 colonies/plate is highly correlative with the presence of venous infection
- Imaging studies:
  - Indium (^{111}In)-labeled leukocyte imaging studies can detect superficial suppurative thrombophlebitis
  - Ultrasound: increased diameter of veins
    —Nonspecific; can occur in aseptic thrombophlebitis as well
    —Very helpful in diagnosis of pelvic suppurative thrombophlebitis and in delineating location and extent of thrombus
  - Bone and gallium (Ga) scan: will detect associated subperiosteal abscess
  - Chest radiograph: multiple peripheral densities and pleural effusion consistent with multiple pulmonary emboli, infarction, abscess, or empyema
  - CT scans:
    —Soft tissue swelling with obliteration of tissue planes (nonspecific and not helpful in determining infectious etiology)

> —Very sensitive in diagnosing pelvic and thoracic suppurative thrombophlebitis
> - Venography: helpful in diagnosis of deep central vein suppurative thrombophlebitis in the thorax

- Laboratory: nonspecific leukocytosis
- Invasive tests:
  - Exploratory venotomy: gross pus within vein lumen is pathognomonic
  - Needle aspiration of suspected vein for culture may also be diagnostic

Definitive Diagnosis:

Thrombophlebitis (nonspecific)   ICD-9-CM 451

Infection/inflammatory reaction caused by implantation of vascular device   ICD-9-CM 996.62

Suggested Treatment:

- Presumptive antimicrobial therapy:
  - Nafcillin 2 g IV every 4 to 6 hours (Penicillin allergy: Vancomycin 1 g IV every 12 hours), and Gentamicin 1.0 to 1.7 mg/kg IV every 8 hours
  - Duration of therapy is largely empirical and should be tailored to individual patient's clinical response
- Exploratory venotomy with surgical excision of affected vein segment and all its involved tributaries is strongly endorsed in patients with superficial suppurative thrombophlebitis
- Radical surgery with extensive excision is reserved for patients failing exploratory venotomy (i.e., persistence of systemic and/or local symptoms, bacteremia, and fever)

- Patient with suppurative thrombophlebitis of great central veins:
    - Vascular resection is technically impossible
    - Immediate catheter removal is indicated
    - Antimicrobial therapy as with presumptive antimicrobial therapy (see above) and/or suppurative thrombophlebitis from *Candida* spp. (see below)
    - Full-dose heparin anticoagulation
    - Tissue plasminogen activator therapy has been successful on a limited use basis and must be considered **EXPERIMENTAL**
- Pelvic suppurative thrombophlebitis requires different empiric antimicrobial therapy:
    - PCN G 20 million U IV daily
        (Penicillin allergy: Erythromycin 2 to
            4 g/day IV given every 6 hours), and
        Clindamycin 450 to 600 mg IV every 6
            hours, or
        Metronidazole 500 to 750 mg IV every 8
            hours
    - Concomitant anticoagulation with heparin is **CONTROVERSIAL**
    - Exploratory laparotomy may be necessary if medical therapy alone is not successful
- Suppurative thrombophlebitis from *Candida* spp.:
    - Superficial disease: most infections are cured by vein excision, but literature supports use of a short postoperative course of: Amphotericin B 0.3 to 1.0 mg/kg/day IV to a total dose of 200 mg
    - Disease of the great central veins or in any immunosuppressed patient or where there are signs of metastatic complications (e.g., endophthalmitis):
        Amphotericin B 0.7 mg/kg/day IV to a
            total dose of 22 mg/kg, and

> 5-Flucytosine 100 to 150 mg/kg/day
> orally given every 6 hours

Follow-Up:

- Suppurative thrombophlebitis requires inpatient treatment
- Routine white blood cell (WBC) count with differential
- Repeat blood cultures and cultures from phlebitic vein
- Avoid lower extremity cannulations for antibiotics
- Insertion of cannulae under aseptic conditions
- Replace cannulae, tubing, and intravenous fluid bottles every 48 to 72 hours
- **Watch for:** signs and symptoms of
  - Bacteremia and systemic sepsis
  - Septic pulmonary emboli
  - Metastatic abscess formation
  - Pneumonia
  - Subperiosteal abscess of adjacent bones

PROSTHETIC VALVE ENDOCARDITIS (PVE)

Presenting Symptoms:

SUBJECTIVE	OBJECTIVE
Fever and chills	History of prosthetic
Night sweats	valve insertion
Fatigability	—Within 60 days:
Malaise	"early" PVE
Weight loss	—After 60 days: "late"
Arthralgias	PVE
Gross hematuria	Fever
Signs of neurologic	New or changing
deficits	murmur

Clinical evidence of systemic embolization (lung, CNS)
—Focal neurologic deficits
—Petechiae
—Osler nodes
—Janeway lesions
—Roth's spots
Splenomegaly

Differential Diagnosis:

Brain abscess
Cerebral embolus
Cerebral hemorrhage with fever
Connective tissue diseases
Fever of unknown origin
Glomerulonephritis
Intra-abdominal infection
Meningitis
Myocardial infarction
Osteomyelitis
Pericarditis
Purulent meningitis
Rheumatic fever
Salmonellosis
Tuberculosis
Septic pulmonary infarcts

Suggested Workup:

- History and physical are usually pathognomonic
- Laboratory:
  - Anemia, frequently with hematocrit (HCT) less than 35
  - Leukocytosis, frequently with WBC greater than $12,000/mm^3$
  - Hematuria

- Blood cultures:
  - Ninety percent are positive for etiologic agent
  - Should be taken at different times
- Echocardiography:
  - Standard 2D transthoracic testing is not very helpful because of the intense echoes generated by the prosthesis that may obscure small vegetations
  - TEE is significantly more sensitive and effective in detecting the vegetations of PVE
  - Doppler echocardiography is also effective in detecting the regurgitation or obstruction associated with malfunctioning prosthetic valves
- Imaging studies: ^{111}In or ^{67}Ga scans with single photon emission computed tomography (SPECT) imaging have been used to detect PVE infections in small controlled studies
- Cardiac catheterization is usually unnecessary, unless it would be useful to know:
  - An estimate of valvular dysfunction
  - Location of the fistula
  - An evaluation of left ventricular function
  - Delineation of coronary artery anatomy
  - Assessment of multiple valve involvement
- CT scan of the head is indicated in all patients with PVE and focal neurologic deficits to evaluate for:
  - Infarction
  - Hemorrhage
  - Abscess
- Cerebral angiography is indicated in all patients with PVE, focal neurologic deficits, and a normal CT scan of the head to exclude the possibility of an intracranial mycotic aneurysm

Definitive Diagnosis:

Prosthetic valve endocarditis   ICD-9-CM 996.61

Suggested Treatment:

- *Streptococcus* or *Enterococcus:*
    - PCN G 24 million U /day IV given every 4 hours
    - Penicillin allergy: Vancomycin 1 g IV every 12 hours for 4 to 6 weeks, and
    - Gentamicin 1 mg/kg IV every 8 hours for 2 weeks, or
    - Streptomycin 1 to 2 g intramuscularly each day for 2 weeks (can be used for gentamicin-resistant isolates that show streptomycin MIC less than 1000 μg/mL)
- *S. aureus:*
    - Methicillin-susceptible:
        Nafcillin 2 g IV every 4 hours
        (Penicillin allergy: Vancomycin 1 g IV
            every 12 hours) for 6 to 8
            weeks, and
        Gentamicin 1 mg/kg IV every 8 hours
            for 2 weeks
    - Methicillin resistant: Vancomycin 1 g IV every 12 hours for 6 to 8 weeks
- *S. epidermidis:*
    - Vancomycin 1 g IV every 12 hours for 6 to 8 weeks, and
    - Rifampin 300 mg orally every 8 hours for 6 to 8 weeks, and
    - Gentamicin 1 mg/kg IV every 8 hours for 2 weeks
- Diphtheroids
    - PCN G 24 million U/day IV given every 4 hours

- (Penicillin allergy: Vancomycin 0.5 g IV every 6 hours) for 6 weeks, and
- Gentamicin 1 mg/kg IV every 8 hours for 2 weeks
- (Vancomycin alone can be given for infection with gentamicin-resistant strains)
- Aerobic Gram-negative bacilli (may need to be altered based on sensitivity results):
  - PCN G 24 million U /day IV given every 4 hours
  - (Penicillin allergy: Aztreonam 1 g IV every 6 hours, or
  - Ceftriaxone 2 g IV every 24 hours, or
  - Ceftazidime 1 g IV every 8 hours) for 6 to 8 weeks, and
  - Gentamicin 1 mg/kg IV every 8 hours for 2 weeks, or
  - Ciprofloxacin 400 mg IV every 12 hours for 6 to 8 weeks
- Empirical regimen before bacteria are identified or where cultures are equivocal:
  - Vancomycin 0.5 g IV every 6 hours for 6 to 8 weeks, and
  - Gentamicin 1 mg/kg IV every 8 hours for 2 weeks
- Fungal PVE:
  - Amphotericin B 1 mg/kg/day IV to a total dose of 3 to 5 g, and
  - 5-Flucytosine 100 to 150 mg/kg/day orally given every 6 hours
- Surgical removal of infected prosthesis is suggested in the following situations:
  - Moderate to severe heart failure due to valve dysfunction
  - Acute valve obstruction
  - Fungal etiology
  - Persistent bacteremia

- Presence of two or more emboli
- Ruptured ventricular septal defect or sinus of Valsalva
- Unstable prosthesis by fluoroscopy
- Surgical removal of infected prosthesis is suggested in the following situations where at least two of the conditions coexist:
  - Mild heart failure caused by valve dysfunction
  - Infecting organism other that penicillin-susceptible *Streptococcus*
  - Relapse after appropriate antimicrobial therapy
  - Vegetations observed by echocardiogram
  - Early PVE (within 60 days)
  - Paravalvular leak
- Surgical removal of infected prosthesis is not suggested unless absolutely necessary in a patient with a prior prosthetic valve replacement
- Anticoagulation: most studies suggest that long-term anticoagulation should be continued in a patient with active PVE; however, it is prudent to monitor patients closely and maintain clotting parameters at the lower end of the therapeutic range

Follow-Up:

- All patients should be hospitalized
- Careful monitoring of arrhythmias and hemodynamic deterioration
- Daily physical exams to detect heart failure, changes in murmurs, or evidence of embolization or aneurysm formation
- **Watch for:** signs and symptoms of
  - Congestive heart failure
  - Dysfunctional valve

- Sinus of Valsalva aneurysm
- Myocardial infarction
- Pericarditis
- Cardiac arrhythmia
- Meningitis
- Cerebral emboli
- Brain abscess
- Mycotic aneurysm
- Septic pulmonary infarcts
- Splenic infarcts
- Arterial emboli and infarcts
- Arthritis
- Myositis
- Glomerulonephritis
- Acute renal failure
- Mesenteric infarct
- Amphotericin B and 5-flucytosine toxicity

VASCULAR GRAFT INFECTIONS

Presenting Symptoms:

SUBJECTIVE	OBJECTIVE
Localized pain, swelling, warmth, and redness	**Graft Infection in Groin/Leg:**
	Localized abscess or draining sinus
Draining sinus at infected site	New or different bruit over graft site
Low-grade fever	Erythema, warmth, and tenderness at graft site
	Ischemic changes and loss of pulse in the distal part of the extremity

Exteriorization of the graft caused by overlying tissue breakdown

Intra-Abdominal Graft Infection:
Low-grade fever
Abdominal tenderness or mass
Retroperitoneal hemorrhage
Petechiae
Splinter hemorrhages
Aortoenteric fistula
Gastrointestinal bleeding (melena/hematemesis)

Differential Diagnosis:

Cellulitis
Abscess
Aneurysm
Thrombophlebitis
Inflammatory bowel disease
Intestinal obstruction
Mesenteric artery insufficiency or thrombosis
Peritonitis
Pancreatitis
Peptic ulcer
Bacterial endocarditis with septic emboli

Suggested Workup:

- History and physical are virtually pathognomonic
- Sinogram may reveal extent of underlying infectious process
- Ultrasound may demonstrate abscesses and aneurysms

- CT/MRI of graft area can delineate extent of perigraft infection
- ^{111}In-labeled leukocyte scanning has high sensitivity but low specificity in detecting vascular graft infection, especially in the perioperative period
- Arteriography can be used to document suture line leakage or graft thrombosis
- Microbiology:
    - Gram stain and culture all draining wound material
    - Blood cultures should be obtained —Persistently positive blood cultures suggest endovascular infection
    - If embolectomy is performed, removed material should be cultured

Definitive Diagnosis:

Infection of vascular device, implant, or graft   ICD-9-CM 996.62

Suggested Treatment:

- Surgical removal of entire graft and debridement of infected tissue is almost always necessary
- Empiric antibiotics pending culture and sensitivity testing of isolated bacteria should be given after the prosthetic device is removed:
    - Vancomycin 0.5 g IV every 6 hours for 4 to 6 weeks, and
    - Gentamicin 1 mg/kg IV every 8 hours for 2 weeks

Follow-Up:

- Inpatient care, requiring surgical consultation and strict medical management

- Graft replacement should await complete clearance of bacteremia
- **Watch for:** signs and symptoms of
    - Abscess formation
    - Aneurysm
    - Septic embolization (especially to lung, CNS, and spleen)
    - Graft thrombosis with ischemic complications distal to graft site
    - Acute renal failure

MYOCARDITIS

Presenting Symptoms:

SUBJECTIVE	OBJECTIVE
Fever	Unexplained heart failure and/or cardiac arrhythmias in a young patient
Malaise	
Arthralgias	
Upper respiratory symptoms	Cardiac abnormalities during the course of a systemic infection
Dyspnea	
Palpitations	
Chest pain	Supraventricular tachycardia
	Frequent ventricular extrasystoles

Differential Diagnosis:

Myocardial infarction
Pericarditis
Mediastinitis
Angina pectoris
Idiopathic hypertrophic subaortic stenosis (IHSS)
Mitral valve prolapse
Aortic aneurysm
Pleuritis
Pneumonia

Neoplasm (pulmonary, cardiac, chest)
Esophageal lesion
Congestive heart failure
Primary tachyarrhythmia
Hypoxia
Electrolyte disturbances
Collagen vascular disease
Thyrotoxicosis
Pheochromocytoma
Drug toxicity (especially cocaine, alcohol,
    catecholamines, arsenic, methyldopa, and
    certain chemotherapeutic agents
    [cyclophosphamide, daunorubicin, adriamycin])
Arachnid poisoning
Sarcoid
Giant cell myocarditis
Kawasaki's disease

Suggested Workup:

- Physical findings:
    - Tachycardia out of proportion to any fever
      present
    - Unexplained ventricular and
      supraventricular cardiac arrhythmias
- Electrocardiogram (ECG):
    - Nonspecific ST-segment and T-wave
      abnormalities
    - Usually, sequential ST-segment elevations
      and T-wave inversions without
      development of Q waves or R-wave
      depression
    - Atrioventricular or intraventricular
      conduction disturbances
- Serum cardiac enzymes:
    - Creatine kinase-myoglobulin (CK-MB) is
      frequently elevated
    - Troponin T is elevated

- Serology shows positive titers of a variety of heart-reactive antibodies (of more prognostic than diagnostic value)
- Echocardiography:
  - Local thickening of the myocardium
  - Regional wall motion abnormalities
  - Ventricular dilatation
- Imaging studies:
  - ^{111}In-antimyosin antibody imaging: detects myocardial necrosis; correlates very well with results seen with endomyocardial biopsy (high sensitivity), but specificity may be as low as 40%
  - MRI: detects focal myocardial edema and inflammation
- Endomyocardial biopsy—the "gold standard" for the diagnosis of myocarditis
  - Variability still persists in confirming the clinical diagnosis of myocarditis due to sampling error, variability in observer histopathologic criteria for diagnosis, and timing of biopsy with respect to onset of disease
  - Proof of causation requires isolating virus from, or demonstrating viral proteins or nucleic acids in the myocardial tissue sampled; most commonly:
    —Coxsackie A or B virus
    —Echovirus
    —Poliovirus
    —Mumps virus
    —Rubeola virus
    —Epstein-Barr virus (EBV)
    —Influenza virus
    —Rubella virus
    —Adenovirus
    —Varicella-zoster virus (VZV)
    —Cytomegalovirus (CMV)
    —Vaccinia virus

Definitive Diagnosis:

Acute viral myocarditis   ICD-9-CM 422.91
Coxsackievirus myocarditis   ICD-9-CM 074.23

Suggested Treatment:

- Supportive care is appropriate
  - Bed rest
  - Adequate oxygenation
  - Treatment of fluid overload
  - Monitoring and treatment of ventricular arrhythmias
- Pharmacologic therapy:
  - Glucocorticoids have generally caused rapid clinical deterioration and are NOT recommended
  - Immunosuppressive agents (e.g., cyclosporine) have resulted in mixed patient responses and are currently NOT recommended unless the patient is enrolled in a controlled clinical trial
  - Antiviral agents are EXPERIMENTAL and UNPROVED

Follow-Up:

- Bed rest is recommended; patients can be monitored carefully as outpatients if they are hemodynamically stable and do not develop supraventricular or ventricular arrhythmias
- **Watch for:** signs and symptoms of
  - Fluid overload
  - Ventricular arrhythmias
  - Dilated cardiomyopathy

PERICARDITIS

Presenting Symptoms:

SUBJECTIVE	OBJECTIVE
Retrosternal or precordial, sharp or	Three-component pericardial friction

dull chest pain,
radiating to shoulder
and neck and
aggravated by deep
breathing, cough,
swallowing, or lying
supine
Fever
Prodromal flu-like
illness
Dyspnea (most
common in bacterial
pericarditis)
Weight loss, night
sweats, cough
(tuberculous
pericarditis)

rub, with ventricular
systolic component
loudest and easiest
to appreciate
—Often evanescent
—Usually high-
pitched, scratching
or grating
Jugular venous
distension may be
present if there is a
significant
pericardial effusion
Acute cardiac
tamponade
Pulsus paradoxus
greater than
10 mm Hg
Prominent x descent
and loss of y descent
in jugular venous
pressure may be
present
Clear lung fields
(differentiates from
cardiogenic shock)
Tachypnea
Tachycardia

Differential Diagnosis:

Acute myocardial infarction
Acute cardiogenic shock
Pneumonia with pleurisy
Pulmonary emboli
Dissecting aortic aneurysm
Pneumothorax
Mediastinal emphysema

Cholecystitis
Pancreatitis
Uremia
Neoplasm (breast, lung, lymphoma,
  mesothelioma)
Postirradiation chest injury
Chest trauma (blunt or penetrating)
Dressler's syndrome
Postpericardiotomy syndrome
Sarcoidosis
Collagen vascular disease
Myxedema
Inflammatory bowel disease
Drug-induced (e.g., procainamide, hydralazine)

Suggested Workup:

- Laboratory:
  - Leukocytosis
  - Elevated ESR
  - Elevated serum CK-MB, lactate
    dehydrogenase (LDH), and aspartate
    aminotransferase (AST)
  - Collagen vascular profile (antinuclear
    antibody [ANA], RF)
  - Purified protein derivative (PPD) skin test
- Serology: acute and convalescent sera for
  common viral antibodies
- ECG:
  - Abnormal in 90% of patients
  - ST-segment elevation without change in
    QRS morphology (early changes)
  - ST-segment normalization with T-wave
    flattening and PR segment depression (later
    changes)
  - Reduced QRS voltage and electrical
    alternans in the presence of pericardial
    effusion

- Sinus tachycardia generally present, but presence of other cardiac arrhythmias generally suggest underlying heart disease
- Differentiate from acute myocardial infarction: T-wave inversions do not occur until AFTER ST segment has normalized
- Echocardiogram:
  - Can be used to detect presence of and quantify pericardial effusion
  - Can be used to monitor hemodynamic compromise
- Chest radiograph:
  - "Water bottle" silhouette of heart in pericardial effusion
  - Pleural effusion can be detected
- CT/MRI of chest:
  - CT can be used to detect pericardial thickening and may be able to differentiate transudative from high-density exudative pericardial effusions
  - MRI can be used in the same way as CT
- Pericardiocentesis and/or pericardial biopsy add little diagnostically and carry a poor risk/benefit ratio, but may be indicated for patients where:
  - Purulent pericarditis is suspected
  - Pericardial effusion has persisted for more than 3 weeks
  - Cardiac tamponade or significant hemodynamic compromise appears imminent

Definitive Diagnosis:

Viral pericarditis	ICD-9-CM 420.91
Acute suppurative pericarditis	ICD-9-CM 420.99
Tuberculous pericarditis	ICD-9-CM 017.9
Idiopathic pericarditis	ICD-9-CM 420.91

Suggested Treatment:

- Viral or idiopathic pericarditis:
  - Bed rest
  - Ibuprofen 400 to 600 mg orally every 6 hours for 2 weeks, or
    - Indomethacin 25 to 50 mg orally every 6 to 8 hours for 2 weeks, or
    - Aspirin 650 mg orally every 4 hours for 2 weeks
  - Careful monitoring for hemodynamic compromise
  - Glucocorticosteroids are NOT recommended during active disease because they are known to enhance myocardial injury during active virus replication
- Purulent (bacterial) pericarditis:
  - Pericardiocentesis
  - Cefotaxime 2 to 12 g/day IV/ intramuscularly given every 6 hours, or
    - Ceftriaxone 1 to 2 g/day IV/ intramuscularly every 24 hours for 2 weeks
  - For less severe infections:
  - —Clarithromycin 500 mg orally every 12 hours, or
    - Azithromycin 500 mg orally once, then 250 mg orally every 24 hours for 4 days , or
    - Ciprofloxacin 500 to 750 mg orally every 12 hours, or
    - Ofloxacin 200 to 400 mg orally every 12 hours, or
    - Norfloxacin 400 mg orally every 12 hours
  - —All (except azithromycin) for 2 weeks

- Tuberculous pericarditis:
  - Isoniazid (INH) 300 mg orally once
    daily, and
      Rifampin 600 mg orally once daily, and
      Pyrazinamide 25 mg/kg/day orally
        given daily or twice a day,
      and (some studies suggest adding)
      Ethambutol 15 mg/kg/day orally for 6
        to 9 months
  - Prednisone 40 to 60 mg/day orally for 3 to
    5 days, then taper over 3 to 4 weeks
  - Pericardiocentesis or pericardiectomy is
    recommended for patients with
    hemodynamic compromise or progressive
    pericardial thickening from recurrent
    effusion and inflammation

Follow-Up:

- Intensive care unit (ICU) care for patients with
  constrictive pericarditis, impending cardiac
  tamponade, or hemodynamic compromise
- Outpatient care for those with viral/idiopathic
  disease and no hemodynamic impairment;
  follow closely and see in office after 2 weeks
  to re-evaluate cardiac status and
  symptomatology
- Repeat chest radiograph and ECG after 2 to 4
  weeks
- **Watch for:** signs and symptoms of
  - Hemodynamic compromise
  - Pericardial tamponade
  - Noncompressive pericardial
    effusion
  - Recurrent disease
  - Chronic, constrictive pericarditis
  - Right-sided heart failure

MEDIASTINITIS

Presenting Symptoms:

SUBJECTIVE

Chest pain: may be
—Cervical or
  substernal (anterior
  mediastinitis)
—Epigastric with
  radiation to
  intrascapular region
  (posterior
  mediastinitis)
Respiratory distress
Dysphagia
Fever

OBJECTIVE

Crepitus and/or
  edema of the chest
  or neck
Hamman's sign: a
  crunching rasping
  sound heard over
  the precordium
  synchronous with
  the cardiac rhythm
  (indicates
  pneumomediastinum)
Distant, dull heart
  sounds
Signs of bacteremia
  and sepsis (late in
  disease)
Interrupted, staccato
  type of inspiration
  (especially in
  children)

Differential Diagnosis:

Thymoma
Substernal thyroid
Neoplasm (germinal cell or mesenchymal)
Lymphoma
Aortic aneurysm
Parathyroid tumor
Hematoma
Sarcoidosis
Bronchogenic cyst
Vascular anomaly

Lymph node hyperplasia
Esophageal lesion
Thoracic spine lesion
Pancreatic pseudocyst
Hernia of Morgagni
Bronchogenic or tracheal tumors
Neurogenic tumors
Anterior meningocele (infant)

Suggested Workup:

- Laboratory: leukocytosis with left shift
- Microbiology:
  - Send material collected by transtracheal or transthoracic drainage, or collected on epicardial pacing wires for Gram stain and culture and sensitivity testing
  - Blood culture and sensitivity testing
- Chest radiograph (posterior to anterior [PA] and lateral):
  - Mediastinal widening
  - Air-fluid levels
  - Subcutaneous or mediastinal emphysema (especially on lateral views)
  - Pleural effusion
  - Pneumoperitoneum
- Contrast esophagography with water-soluble contrast agent:
  - May be used to demonstrate esophageal perforation
  - Avoid barium contrast material unless no extravasation is seen with water-soluble material
- Imaging studies:
  - CT scan of chest is helpful in making diagnosis when clinical signs and radiograph have not established diagnosis

- Technetium 99m- or ^{111}In-labeled WBC scan may be useful where CT scan is not available
- MRI imaging has not been well established in diagnosing mediastinitis

Definitive Diagnosis:

Acute mediastinitis   ICD-9-CM 519.2

Suggested Treatment:

- Mediastinitis secondary to extension from infection of head (odontogenic) or neck (pharyngeal) or from esophageal perforation (polymicrobic):
  - PCN G 1 to 2 g/day orally given every 6 hours
    (Penicillin allergy: Clindamycin 300 mg orally every 8 hours), and
    Metronidazole 500 mg orally every 12 hours
  - If penicillinase-producing *Staphylococcus* or penicillin-resistant anaerobes are suspected, may substitute for PCN G:
    Ampicillin + sulbactam 1 g ampicillin IV/intramuscularly every 6 hours
    (Penicillin allergy: Ceftriaxone 1 to 2 g IV/intramuscularly every 24 hours, or
    Cefotaxime 0.5 g IV/intramuscularly every 6 hours, or
    Clindamycin 300 mg orally every 8 hours)
  - If Gram-negative enteric bacilli are implicated, can add: Imipenem 0.5 to 1.0 g IV every 6 hours
  - Duration of therapy may be weeks or months and is determined by patient's clinical response
  - Surgical intervention needed for repair of esophageal perforation
  - Transthoracic drainage may be necessary

- Mediastinitis related to cardiothoracic surgery (primarily Gram-positive cocci and some Gram-negative aerobic bacilli):
  - Aggressive surgical drainage and debridement with subsequent irrigation of mediastinum with antibiotic solutions through drainage tubes (NOTE: this procedure has been associated with a variety of complications, including emergence of resistant organisms, pericardial and tissue toxicity, and systemic absorption and toxicity; this technique must be used with great CAUTION)
  - Percutaneous catheter drainage has been used in a small number of patients with some success, but remains EXPERIMENTAL
  - Nafcillin 1 to 2 g IV every 6 hours
    —(Penicillin allergy: Vancomycin 1 g IV every 12 hours), and
      Cefazolin 1 g IV every 8 hours, or
      Cefotaxime 2 g IV every 6 hours, or
      Ceftriaxone 2 g IV every 24 hours, or
- Ceftazidime 1 to 2 g IV every 8 hours, or
  - Piperacillin + tazobactam 3 g piperacillin IV every 6 hours
    —and (especially if *Pseudomonas* or heavy aerobic Gram-negative burden is suspected) Gentamicin 3 to 5 mg/kg/day IV given every 8 hours

Follow-Up:

- Because surgical repair is commonly required in patients with mediastinitis, in-hospital care is generally required
- Follow carefully serum BUN, WBC count, blood cultures, and chest radiograph

- **Watch for:** signs and symptoms of
  - Extension of infection into contiguous areas
    - —Pericardial space → pericardial effusion and tamponade
    - —Pleural space
    - —Peritoneum → peritonitis
  - Sternal osteomyelitis
  - Superior vena cava obstruction
  - Inferior vena cava obstruction
  - Esophageal obstruction
  - Esophagobronchial obstruction or fistula
  - Tracheobronchial obstruction or fistula
  - Pulmonary venous or arterial obstruction
  - Pulmonary hypertension
  - Pulmonary infarction
  - Cor pulmonale
  - Thoracic duct obstruction
  - Constrictive pericarditis
  - Coronary artery stenosis
  - Mediastinal nerve entrapment
  - Recurrent laryngeal nerve palsy
  - Sclerosing or granulomatous (chronic) mediastinitis

Gastrointestinal, Intra-abdominal, and Peritoneal Infections   6

INFECTIONS COVERED

ESOPHAGITIS

Presenting Symptoms:

SUBJECTIVE	OBJECTIVE
Difficulty in swallowing	Elicit history of odynophagia that is worse on swallowing fruit juice or acid liquids
Pain on swallowing	Elicit history of odynophagia and dysphagia that is worse on ingesting large, firm objects (e.g., meat) rather than liquids
—Substernal	
—Anterior cervical	
—Epigastric	
Dull sense of obstruction low in throat or in substernal area on swallowing	Elicit history of risk factors for esophagitis:
	—Human immunodeficiency virus (HIV) infection/acquired immunodeficiency syndrome (AIDS)
	—Diabetes mellitus
	—Chronic antibiotic therapy
	—Immunosuppressive therapy
	–Corticosteroids
	–Antineoplastic agents
	–Post-transplant drug therapy
	—Oropharyngeal herpes simplex infections

Differential Diagnosis:

Peptic esophagitis (regurgitant; reflux)
Mucositis, especially caused by
—Antineoplastic drugs (common with
  methotrexate or 5-fluorouracil)
—Antimicrobial agents (e.g., doxycycline,
  zidovudine)
Aphthous ulcers
Esophageal neoplasm
Systemic sclerosis/scleroderma
Barrett's esophagus
Achalasia
Neurologically disordered esophageal motility
Ingestion of corrosive or chemical substances
Postsclerotherapy for esophageal varices

Suggested Workup:

- Barium contrast esophagram:
  - Generally not diagnostic
  - May show irregular plaques consistent
    with *Candida* esophagitis
  - May be normal
- Endoscopy with brushings and/or biopsy:
  - Gold standard diagnostic tool
  - Permits classification of esophagitis into
    severity stage
  - Brushings:
    —Brush or smears or brushing sent for
      —Wet mount (*Candida*)
      —Calcifluor white stain (*Candida*)
      —Gram stain (*Candida*)
      —Direct or immunochemical stain
        (herpes simplex virus [HSV],
        cytomegalovirus [CMV])
  - Biopsy: Sample lesions and edges of ulcers
    and send for
      —Fungal, HSV, and CMV culture
      —Histopathology

- *Candida:*
  - —Typical white plaques in distal third of esophagus
  - —Demonstrate pseudohyphae and yeasts in biopsies or smears of brushings
- Herpes simplex:
  - —Discrete ulcerations of mucosa in distal third of esophagus
  - —Culture brushings or biopsies
  - —Direct fluorescent antibody staining for HSV-1
  - —Biopsy shows characteristic pathology (Cowdry type A inclusions)
- CMV:
  - —Extensive, large shallow ulcers of distal esophagus
  - —Biopsy shows characteristic pathology (large cells with dense intranuclear inclusions and small intracytoplasmic inclusions)
  - —Immunohistochemical stains and direct fluorescent stains for CMV

Definitive Diagnosis:

Acute esophagitis   ICD-9-CM 530.10
Candidal esophagitis   ICD-9-CM 112.84

Suggested Treatment:

- Fungal esophagitis:
  - Mild to moderate nondisseminated disease:
  - Nystatin suspension (100,000 units (U)/mL) 5 mL orally 4 times a day, or
    - Clotrimazole troche 10 mg orally 5 times a day, or
    - Ketoconazole 400 mg orally once a day (NOTE: cannot be given if gastric acid is to be suppressed), or

  Itraconazole 200 mg orally once a day, or
  Fluconazole 100 to 200 mg orally once
    a day
- Moderate to severe nondisseminated
  disease in afebrile, non-neutropenic patient:
  —Fluconazole 100 to 200 mg intravenously
    (IV) once a day, or
  —Amphotericin B 0.3 to 0.5 mg/kg/day IV
- Febrile patient who is neutropenic and/or
  has disseminated disease:
  Amphotericin B 0.5 to 1.0 mg/kg/day IV
- Herpes simplex esophagitis:
  - Acyclovir 15 mg/kg/day IV given every 8
    hours; if no clinical improvement, change to
  - Foscarnet 40 mg/kg IV every 8 hours
- CMV esophagitis:
  - Ganciclovir 5 mg/kg IV every 12 hours for
    14 to 21 days, then 5 mg/kg/day IV or
    1000 mg orally 3 times a day, or
  - Foscarnet 60 mg/kg IV given every 8 hours
- Empiric therapy where endoscopy is not
  available or contraindicated:
  - Clotrimazole or Ketoconazole → failure, go to
  - Fluconazole → failure, go to
  - Acyclovir → failure, go to
  - Ganciclovir if CMV is suspected; otherwise,
    go to Foscarnet

Follow-Up:

- Follow symptomatically
- In-patient care required in leukopenic patients
  or those with profound immunosuppression
- Treat underlying cause of immunosuppression
- Consider repeat endoscopy 1 to 2 weeks after
  clinical resolution
- Consider long-term prophylaxis for recurrent
  Candida esophagitis after resolution of acute
  infection

- **Watch for:** signs and symptoms of
  - Disseminated disease
  - Esophageal ulceration and perforation
  - Esophagopulmonary fistula
  - Relapse

PEPTIC ULCER DISEASE (*HELICOBACTER PYLORI* INFECTION)

Presenting Symptoms:

SUBJECTIVE

Epigastric pain, usually 1 to 3 hours after meals, relieved by food or antacids (duodenal ulcer)

Nocturnal epigastric pain

"Heartburn"

Dyspeptic complaints

—Belching

—Bloating

—Abdominal distention

—Food intolerance

Anorexia, weight loss

Early satiety

Nausea, vomiting

Hematemesis

Blood on stool

OBJECTIVE

Elicit history of:

—Cigarette smoking

—Nonsteroidal anti-inflammatory drug (NSAID) use

—Family history of peptic ulcer disease

—Corticosteroid use

Abdominal examination generally benign

Melena or heme-positive stool

Differential Diagnosis:

Nonulcer dyspepsia
Gastric carcinoma
Gastritis without ulcer
Gastroesophageal reflux
Gastroduodenal Crohn's disease
Pancreatitis

Variant angina pectoris
Cholelithiasis
Atrophic gastritis
Gastric lymphoma
Zollinger-Ellison syndrome
Gastric outlet obstruction
Pyloric stenosis

Suggested Workup:

- Laboratory:
  - Complete blood count (CBC) may show lowered hemoglobin (Hb)/hematocrit (HCT)
  - Fecal occult blood may be positive
  - Serum gastrin to rule out Zollinger-Ellison syndrome
- Imaging studies:
  - Barium swallow may reveal ulcer crater (accuracy 70% to 90%)
  - Barium enema indicated in the presence of fecal occult blood to rule out colonic involvement
- Urea breath test:
  - Commercially available, noninvasive test for *H. pylori* (90% sensitivity and specificity)
  - Drawback is exposure of patient to small doses of radioactivity
- Upper endoscopy with biopsy of lesion:
  - Cytology
  - Gram stain
  - Hematoxylin and eosin stain
  - Warthin-Starry silver stain
  - Rapid urease test (CLOtest) for urease activity in biopsy specimen is a rapid, commercially available alternative to waiting for cytology and microbiology results

- Serology:
  - Enzyme-linked immunosorbent assay (ELISA) tests for immunoglobulin (Ig)A and IgG anti-*H. pylori* antibodies (95% sensitivity; 75% specificity)
- Proposed algorithm for evaluation of the patient with symptoms of dyspepsia (Figure 6.1)

Definitive Diagnosis:

Duodenal ulcer   ICD-9-CM 532.9
Gastric ulcer   ICD-9-CM 531.9

Suggested Treatment:

- Classic triple therapy:
  - ℞ Bismuth subsalicylate (™Pepto-Bismol) 2 tablets orally 4 times a day, and
    Metronidazole 250 mg 3 or 4 times a day, or
    Tinidazole 250 mg orally 3 times a day, and
    Amoxicillin 500 mg or Tetracycline 500 mg orally 4 times a day for 14 days
  - Ninety to 95% eradication of *H. pylori*
  - Inexpensive, but complex regimen requiring up to 14 pills per day
  - Poor compliance, leading to treatment failures
  - Ranitidine 300 mg orally once a day or Omeprazole 20 mg orally twice a day may be given with antibiotics for 2 weeks, then continued for another 4 to 6 weeks alone for relief of an acute, highly symptomatic ulcer
- Protein pump inhibitor (PPI) dual therapy:
  - Omeprazole 20 to 40 mg orally twice a day, or

Patient with symptoms of dyspepsia:

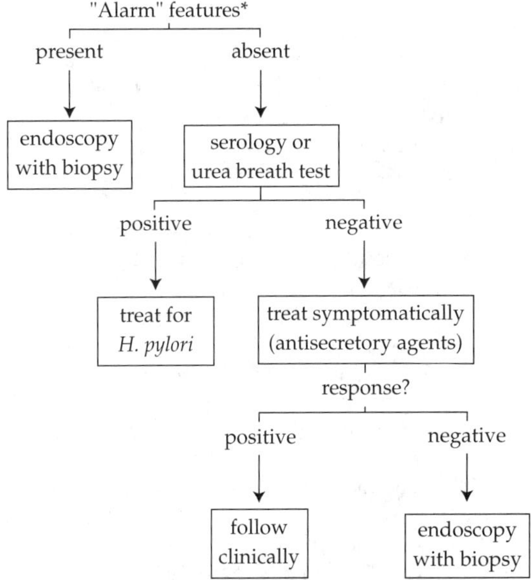

Fig. 6.1 Proposed Algorithm for Evaluation of the Patient with Dyspepsia

*** "Alarm" features include: advanced age, long history of symptoms, unintended weight loss, persistent anorexia, long history of use of nonsteroidal anti-inflammatory drugs (NSAIDs), gastrointestinal bleeding, anemia, persistent vomiting, barium swallow consistent with malignancy.**

Lansoprazole 30 mg orally once a
day, and
Clarithromycin 500 mg orally 3 times a
day, or
Amoxicillin 500 mg orally 4 times a day
or 1 g orally twice a day for 14 days
- Sixty to 80% eradication of *H. pylori*
- Simpler, better tolerated, but more
expensive regimen
- PPI triple therapy:
  - Omeprazole 20 mg orally twice a day, or
Lansoprazole 30 mg orally once a
day, and
Clarithromycin 500 mg orally twice a
day, and
Metronidazole 500 mg orally twice a
day, or
Amoxicillin 1 g orally twice a day for
7 days
  - Results in greater than 90% eradication of
H. pylori
- New combinations:
  - Clarithromycin 500 mg orally 3 times a
day, and
Ranitidine-bismuth citrate complex
400 mg orally 2 times a day for
14 days, then
Ranitidine-bismuth citrate complex alone
400 mg orally 2 times a day for
14 days
—Eighty-five to 90% eradication of *H. pylori*
—Simpler, well-tolerated regimen
  - Omeprazole 20 mg orally every other
day, and
Tinidazole 500 mg orally twice a
day, and
Clarithromycin 250 mg orally 3 times a
day for 7 days

  —THIS IS AN EXPERIMENTAL
    PROTOCOL tested in a small number of
    patients
  —Complete (100%) eradication of *H. pylori*
- Omeprazole 40 mg orally in the morning, and
    Clarithromycin 500 mg orally 3 times a
      day for 14 days, then
    Omeprazole 20 mg orally in the morning
      for 14 days

Follow-Up:

- Recheck patient 4 to 6 weeks after treatment
  by urea breath test or re-endoscopy with
  biopsy to confirm eradication of *H. pylori* in
  patients with "alarm" features or acute gastric
  ulcer
- Monitor clinical response in patients with no
  "alarm" features and duodenal ulcer; no need
  for retesting unless poor clinical response
  noted
- Continue H2 blocker or PPI therapy on
  maintenance doses (e.g., ranitidine 150 to
  300 mg orally each night at bedtime) in
  patients with bleeding ulcers even if *H. pylori*
  has been eradicated (NOTE: there is
  controversy as to how long maintenance
  therapy should be continued and even
  whether it is necessary at all)
- **Watch for:** signs and symptoms of
    - Hemorrhage (25% of cases)
    - Perforation of viscus (less than
      5% of cases)
    - Gastric outlet obstruction (5% of
      cases)
    - Reinfection with *H. pylori*
    - Development of atrophic
      gastritis and gastric malignancy

PSEUDOMEMBRANOUS COLITIS

Presenting Symptoms:

SUBJECTIVE

Profuse watery and/or
  bloody diarrhea
—Foul-smelling
—Mucoid green
Cramping abdominal
  pain
Fever

OBJECTIVE

Elicit history of
  antibiotic use within
  4 weeks (average 4
  to 9 days) of onset of
  symptoms,
  particularly:
—Clindamycin
—Lincomycin
—Ampicillin
—Cephalosporins
—Some beta-lactams
Elicit history of cancer
  chemotherapy,
  particularly:
—5-Fluorouracil
—Methotrexate
Elicit history of
  treatment for
  arthritic conditions,
  particularly:
—Gold compounds
—Certain NSAIDs
Lower abdominal
  tenderness
High fevers (102° to
  105°F)

Differential Diagnosis:

Inflammatory bowel disease (especially Crohn's
  disease)
Idiopathic ulcerative colitis
Inflammatory enteritis (especially *Salmonella,
  Shigella, Edwardsiella,* invasive *Escherichia coli,
  Entamoeba histolytica, Staphylococcus aureus,
  Campylobacter, Yersinia,* and *Strongyloides*)
Toxic megacolon

Peritonitis
Colonic perforation
Ischemic colitis
Typhlitis

Suggested Workup:

- Laboratory:
  - Stool for fecal leukocytes
  - Stool for detection of *Clostridium difficile* toxins A & B
    —ELISA tests are now commercially available
  - Microbiology: Stool culture for *C. difficile* using selective medium containing cycloserine, cefoxitin, and fructose in agar (CCFA)
- Colonoscopy:
  - Detects lesions in rectum, colon, and distal ileum
  - Colitis and pseudomembranous lesions are typical gross findings
  - Biopsy needed when gross findings are not definitive
    —Microscopic pseudomembranes can be detected
- Imaging studies (may be helpful in cases where colonoscopy is contraindicated):
  - Computed tomography (CT) of the abdomen
  - Air-contrast barium enema (contraindicated in severe colitis because of fear of precipitating toxic megacolon, perforation, or other complications)

Definitive Diagnosis:

Pseudomembranous colitis   ICD-9-CM 008.45
  (*C. difficile*)

Suggested Treatment:

- Mild to moderate cases:
  - Metronidazole 250 to 500 mg orally 4 times a day or 500 to 750 mg orally 3 times a day for 7 to 10 days, or

> Bacitracin 25,000 U (500 mg) orally
> 4 times a day for 7 to 10 days

- Severe or resistant cases:
  - Vancomycin 125 to 500 mg orally 4 times a day for 5 to 14 days (dose and length of therapy should be based on patient response)
  - Where oral therapy is not possible:
    —Vancomycin 500 mg per nasogastric (NG) tube 4 times a day, or
    —Vancomycin 200 to 500 mg/L solution infused by enema into the colonic lumen
  - For patients with adynamic ileus:
    —Vancomycin 500 to 1000 mg IV every 12 hours, and
    —Metronidazole 500 mg IV every 6 to 8 hours, and
    —Vancomycin 200 to 500 mg/L solution infused by enema into the colonic lumen, an ileostomy, or colostomy
- Symptomatic relief:
  - Cholestyramine 4 g orally 3 or 4 times a day
  - Reserved for MILD cases only
  - NOT TO BE USED with Vancomycin (it will bind to the antibiotic and reduce its action)
- Antidiarrheal agents: Opiates and antiperistaltic agents should be AVOIDED: may result in toxic megacolon
- Surgery:
  - Diversion of fecal stream or resection of diseased bowel are rarely performed except in life-threatening situations as with toxic megacolon or cecal perforation
  - Colostomy or ileostomy may be needed to facilitate instillation of vancomycin or metronidazole into the colonic lumen of patients with ileus

Follow-Up:

- Careful monitoring during acute infection (outpatient for mild cases; inpatient for fulminant cases)
- Prevention of recurrence
  - Avoid prolonged antibiotic usage
  - Supplement patient's diet with organisms that compete with *C. difficile* (e.g., *Lactobacillus*)
  - Gamma-globulin 400 mg/kg IV given every 3 weeks (proven in pediatric cases only)
  - Lyophilized preparation of *Saccharomyces boulardii:* 500 mg orally twice a day for 30 days (EXPERIMENTAL THERAPY)
- **Watch for:** signs and symptoms of
  - Dehydration
  - Reactive arthritis
  - Reiter's syndrome
  - Hypoalbuminemia
  - Edema
  - Shock
  - Intestinal perforation
  - Toxic megacolon
  - Recurrence
  - Death (10% to 30% of cases)

INFLAMMATORY ENTERITIDES AND ACUTE DIARRHEA

Presenting Symptoms:

SUBJECTIVE	OBJECTIVE
Bacillary Dysentery (Shigellosis and Enteroinvasive **E. coli** *[EHEC])*	
Acute bloody diarrhea	Diffuse abdominal
High fever	tenderness
Abdominal pain	High fever
Malaise	Meningismus

Headache   Conjunctivitis

Arthralgias   Arthritis similar to

Conjunctivitis   Reiter's syndrome

Elicit history of symptom onset 3 to 4 days after suspect meal

Campylobacter *Enteritis*

Severe abdominal pain   Diffuse abdominal

High fever   tenderness

Diarrhea with blood and pus   High fever

Amebic Dysentery **(E. histolytica)**

Severe abdominal pain   Diffuse abdominal

Bloody diarrhea   tenderness that may

Fever   localize to the right

Rectal pain   upper quadrant

Nausea and vomiting   Fever

May see systemic symptoms

Elicit history of risk factors

—Low socioeconomic status

—Institutional living

—Male homosexuality

—Travel to endemic areas (Mexico, India, South Africa)

Schistosomiasis

Acute bloody diarrhea   Diffuse abdominal pain

Abdominal pain   Fever

Weight loss   Rectal polyps

Fever

Salmonellosis

Fever   Diffuse abdominal pain

Cramping abdominal
pain
Diarrhea with blood
and pus
Onset 8 to 48 hours
after suspect meal
Nausea and vomiting

Fever
Elicit history of suspect
meal within 48 hours
of onset of
symptoms

Differential Diagnosis:

Pseudomembranous colitis
Necrotizing enterocolitis
Inflammatory bowel disease
Hepatitis
Hepatic abscess
Diverticulitis
Zollinger-Ellison syndrome
Ischemic bowel
Gastrinoma
Gastric or intestinal malignancy
Viral enteritis

Suggested Workup:

See Figure 6.2

Definitive Diagnosis:

Bacterial enteritis   ICD-9-CM 008.5
Amebic enteritis   ICD-9-CM 006.9
Viral enteritis   ICD-9-CM 008.8
Bacillary dysentery   ICD-9-CM 004.9
Amebic dysentery   ICD-9-CM 006.9
Schistosomiasis   ICD-9-CM 120.9
Salmonellosis   ICD-9-CM 003.0

Suggested Treatment:

- Empiric antibiotic therapy for presumptive
  inflammatory enteritis should be initiated
  when diagnosis is suspected, before the results
  of the laboratory tests are obtained; therapy

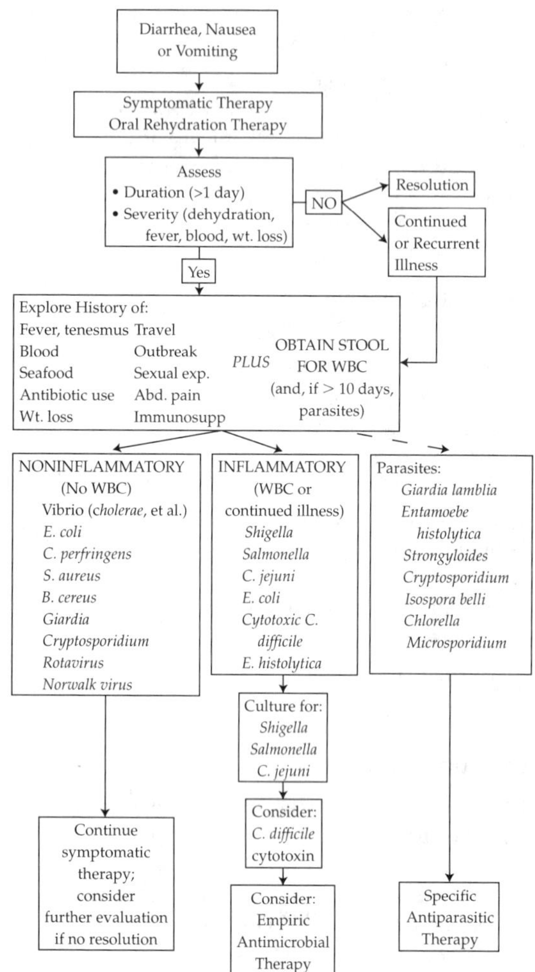

Fig. 6.2 Suggested Workup for Inflammatory Enteritides and Acute Diarrhea

Wt. loss = weight loss; Sexual exp. = sexual exposure;
Abd. pain = abdominal pain; Immunospp = immunosuppression;
WBC = white blood cells.

may be modified as laboratory results become available:
- Bacterial: Ciprofloxacin 500 mg orally twice a day for 10 days, or
    Trimethoprim-sulfamethoxazole (TMP-SMX) DS 1 tablet orally twice a day for 5 days
- Amebic: Metronidazole 500 to 750 mg orally 3 times a day for 10 days
- Schistosomal: Praziquantel 20 mg/kg orally every 4 to 6 hours for 3 doses, all in 1 day
- Supportive care:
  - Replacement of lost fluids and electrolytes
  - Dietary management

Follow-Up:

- Outpatient care except for dehydration
- Strict attention to fluids, nutrition, and electrolyte management
- **Watch for:** signs and symptoms of
    - Dehydration
    - Sepsis
    - Shock
    - Anemia
    - Abscess formation (intestinal, hepatic)
    - Intestinal perforation
    - Intestinal obstruction
    - Toxic megacolon
    - Salmonella osteomyelitis and endarteritis (especially in the elderly)

ENTERIC FEVER (TYPHOID FEVER)

Presenting Symptoms:

SUBJECTIVE	OBJECTIVE
Fever, initially remittent, then rising	Elicit history of initially intermittent, then

in a stepwise fashion
to sustained levels
Headache
Altered bowel habits
ranging from
constipation to
diarrhea
Dry cough
Conjunctivitis
Nausea and vomiting
Abdominal cramps
Rash
Malaise
Sore throat
Anorexia
Myalgias

sustained fever
Bradycardia
Lethargy/confusion
Conjunctivitis (45%)
Abdominal tenderness,
diffuse or localized,
usually in right
lower quadrant
Splenomegaly
Hepatomegaly
Lymphadenopathy rare
Rales or rhonchi may
be heard (highly
variable finding)
Rose spots (50% of
patients)
—Transient,
erythematous
maculopapular
eruption on anterior
thorax or upper
abdomen
Meningismus (up to
10% of patients)
Elicit history of travel
to endemic area
(Mexico, India,
Pakistan) or contact
with known typhoid
case 2 to 8 weeks
before appearance of
symptoms

Differential Diagnosis:

Septicemic plague (*Yersinia pestis*)
Intestinal anthrax
Acute bartonellosis
Leptospirosis

Relapsing fever (*Borrelia* spp.)
Intestinal tuberculosis
Abdominal actinomycosis
Intra-abdominal abscess
Rat bite fever
Bacterial or atypical pneumonia
Hepatitis
Infectious mononucleosis
Rickettsial infections
   Scrub and endemic typhus
   Rocky Mountain spotted fever
   Q fever
   Brill-Zinsser disease
Mycotic infections
Parasitic infections
Abdominal and hematologic malignancies
Sarcoidosis
Inflammatory bowel disease
Acute or subacute appendicitis
Malaria
Subacute bacterial endocarditis

Suggested Workup:

- Laboratory:
  - CBC: leukopenia (up to 50% of patients) depressed eosinophils (up to 70% of patients)
  - Liver function tests (LFTs):
    —Mildly elevated bilirubin
    —Elevated alkaline phosphatase
    —Elevated transaminase levels
  - Urinalysis:
    —Proteinuria
    —Pyuria
    —Red blood cell casts
  - Positive fecal leukocytes (usually mononuclear cells)

- Microbiology:
  —Blood cultures
  —Urine cultures
  —Stool cultures
    –Look for *Salmonella typhi* or another *Salmonella* spp.
    –Seventy-three to 97% positive blood cultures for *S. typhi* if multiple cultures are obtained
    –Fifty percent or less positive stool cultures
    –Forty percent or less positive urine cultures
  —Bone marrow aspirate cultures may be performed if blood cultures are negative and clinical suspicion is high
    –Eighty to 95% positive even in patients who have been taking antibiotics for several days
- Serology:
  - Counter-Immunoelectrophoresis (CIE) testing of serum for circulating anti-*S. typhi* antibody
  - Widal reaction testing (test for agglutinating antibodies to the O and H antigens of *S. typhi*)
    —High degree of cross-reactivity with a variety of non-*S. typhi* antigens
    —Highly variable test results with widely varying sensitivity and specificity
    —Should be used primarily in areas for which data on Widal titer results in control groups of patients without enteric fever are available
- Biopsy rose spots: *S. typhi* often isolated
- Newer Tests:
  - Determination of *S. typhi* antigen in urine, serum, feces
    —Low specificity
    —Not widely available commercially

- Polymerase chain reaction (PCR) testing of blood and stool for *S. typhi:* not widely available commercially

Definitive Diagnosis:

Typhoid fever   ICD-9-CM 002.0

Suggested Treatment:

- Empiric antimicrobial therapy should be started immediately after specimens of blood, stool, urine (and possibly, bone marrow) for culture are drawn, but before diagnosis is documented by culture:
  - Standard therapy:
    —Chloramphenicol 50 mg/kg/day orally given every 6 hours for 2 weeks (adults or children), or
    —Ampicillin 500 mg orally every 6 hours (adults) or 100 mg/kg/day orally given 4 times a day for 2 weeks, or
    —TMP-SMX DS 1 tablet orally twice a day for 2 weeks
    —Multiple-drug-resistant isolates unresponsive to these antibiotics are now becoming increasingly prevalent
  - For multi-drug resistant infections:
    —Ceftriaxone 1 to 2 g IV given once a day (adults) or 75 mg/kg/day IV (children) for 2 weeks, or
    —Cefoperazone 2 to 4 g IV every 6 to 12 hours for 2 weeks, or
    —Ciprofloxacin 500 mg orally twice a day or 200 to 400 mg IV every 12 hours for 2 weeks (adults only), or
    —Cefixime 5 mg/kg orally twice a day for 2 weeks (children only)
- Carrier state (patient who excretes *S. typhi* in the stool 1 year after his or her initial illness; usually 3% to 5% of patients):

- Ampicillin or amoxicillin 4 to 5 g/day orally given every 6 hours, and
- Probenecid 500 mg orally 4 times a day for 6 weeks, or
- TMP-SMX DS 1 tablet orally twice a day for 6 weeks, or
- Ciprofloxacin 500 mg orally twice a day for 4 to 6 weeks

Follow-Up:

- Inpatient care for acutely ill
- Outpatient care for carrier or less ill patient
- Fluid and electrolyte support
- Strict isolation of patient's linen, stool, and urine
- Serial abdominal radiographs prudent to monitor for evidence of intestinal perforation
- Consider vaccination of family members and close contacts
- **Watch for:** signs and symptoms of
    - Intestinal hemorrhage
    - Intestinal perforation
    - Metastatic infection
        —Endovascular (especially in the elderly patient)
        —Osteomyelitis (especially in immunocompromised patients)
    - Chronic carrier state
    - Relapse of infection
        —May consider cholecystectomy in patients with relapse or chronic carrier state because seeding of biliary tract contributes significantly to these conditions

FOODBORNE INFECTIONS

Presenting Symptoms:

SUBJECTIVE

S. aureus, Bacillus cereus
Nausea, vomiting, and diarrhea within 1 to 8 hours after a meal
Fever uncommon
Illness usually lasts less than 12 hours
Clostridium perfringens; B. cereus
Abdominal cramps and diarrhea within 8 to 16 hours after a meal
Occasional nausea
Fever and vomiting are uncommon
Campylobacter jejuni; Vibrio parahaemolyticus; **invasive** *E. coli; Salmonella; Shigella*
Fever, abdominal cramps, and diarrhea within 16 to 48 hours after a meal
Vomiting is common
Resolution of illness is within 2 to 7 days
Diarrhea is frequently bloody
Enterotoxigenic *E. coli; V. parahaemolyticus; Vibrio cholerae; C.*

OBJECTIVE

Physical findings are of little help in diagnosing or distinguishing between any of the foodborne infections
Suspicion is aroused based on epidemiologic findings:
—Multiple persons become ill after eating the same meal
—Timing and type of clinical presentation as outlined under Subjective Symptoms are the most important clues in establishing diagnosis
Elicit history for appropriate risk factors:
—*S. aureus:* egg salad, cream pastries, poultry, ham
—*B. cereus:* cereals, fried rice, dried foods, meats, vegetables, sauces
—*C. perfringens:* meats, gravies, dried foods,

jejuni; Salmonella; Shigella

Abdominal cramps and watery diarrhea within 16 to 72 hours after a meal

Illness usually resolves within 96 hours, but can last up to 7 days

Vomiting and muscular cramps seen in cholera

Yersinia enterocolitica

Fever and abdominal cramps within 16 to 48 hours after a meal

Mesenteric adenitis is common

Verotoxigenic E. coli

Bloody diarrhea without fever within 72 to 120 hours after a meal

Severe abdominal cramps are common

Uncomplicated illness lasts 1 to 12 days

Complications occur in less than 10% of patients

—Hemolytic uremic syndrome

—Thrombotic thrombocytopenic purpura (TTP)

vegetables, Mexican food

—*C. jejuni:* undercooked poultry, meat, raw dairy

—*Y. enterocolitica:* undercooked pork, meat, dairy

—*E. coli:* raw vegetables, contaminated water

—*V. parahaemolyticus:* raw and cooked seafood

—*Shigella:* raw vegetables, egg salad, contaminated water

—*Salmonella:* undercooked eggs, poultry, dairy, meat

Clostridium botulinum
Nausea, vomiting,
  diarrhea, and
  paralysis within 18
  to 36 hours after
  a meal
Simultaneous
  gastrointestinal (GI)
  symptoms with/just
  prior to onset of
  symmetric
  descending
  weakness/paralysis
  is pathognomonic for
  foodborne botulism

Differential Diagnosis:

Infectious gastroenteritis
Inflammatory bowel disease
Acute appendicitis
Viral hepatitis
Foodborne disease caused by chemicals or toxins
  of nonmicrobial origin
—Heavy metals (copper, zinc, tin, cadmium)
—Histamine fish poisoning (scombroid)
—Ciguatera
—Paralytic shellfish poisoning
—Neurotoxic shellfish poisoning
—Amnesic shellfish poisoning
—Mushroom poisoning
—Monosodium glutamate (MSG) poisoning
  ("Chinese restaurant syndrome")
—Niacin poisoning
—Raw milk ingestion (Brainerd diarrhea)
—Organophosphate poisoning
—Aminoglycoside poisoning
Parasitic infestation

Viral gastroenteritis
Guillain-Barré syndrome
Encephalitis
Tick paralysis
Myasthenia gravis
Basilar artery stroke
Acute or chronic cyanide poisoning
Favism

Recommended Workup:

- Stool culture is most reliable method
  - Laboratory must be notified of diagnostic considerations for most pathogens except *Salmonella* and *Shigella*
  - Fecal leukocytes: if positive, indicates that the organism has invaded the GI tract; suggests: *Salmonella, Shigella, C. jejuni,* invasive *E. coli, V. parahaemolyticus,* or *Y. enterocolitica*
- Blood culture
- Toxin assays of serum, stool, and implicated food
- Epidemiologic investigation
  - Verify a common meal for several ill people
  - Interview people who ate the meal and did or did not become ill
  - Identify foodstuffs consumed by people who did and did not become ill
  - Calculate food-specific attack rates for each food: to be incriminated as the vehicle for transmission, the food must have a significantly higher attack rate for those who ate it than for those who did not, and most of those who became ill must have eaten the food
- Culture suspected food sources (if available)
  - Microbiologic evaluation
  - Other tests if noninfectious etiology is suspected

    —Metallic ion of heavy metals
    —Histamine levels in suspect fish
    —Ciguatoxin in suspect fish
    —Assay for specific toxin suspected
- Electromyogram (EMG) (if botulism is suspected): characteristic pattern to distinguish from Guillain-Barré

Definitive Diagnosis:

Salmonella gastroenteritis	ICD-9-CM 003.0
Shigellosis	ICD-9-CM 004.9
Staphylococcal food poisoning	ICD-9-CM 005.0
Botulism	ICD-9-CM 005.1
Food poisoning, *C. perfringens*	ICD-9-CM 005.2
Food poisoning, *V. parahaemolyticus*	ICD-9-CM 005.4
Food poisoning, *B. cereus*	ICD-9-CM 005.8
Food poisoning, unspecified	ICD-9-CM 005.9
E. coli intestinal infection	ICD-9-CM 008.0

Suggested Treatment:

- Usually self-limited infections requiring only supportive care:
  - Rehydration
    —Oral solutions for most patients
    —Intravenous fluids for more severe dehydration and for the elderly
  - Correct electrolyte imbalances
  - Bland diet during recovery
  - Nothing by mouth if there is excessive vomiting or diarrhea
  - Antiperistaltic agents appear to be of little value and are contraindicated in patients positive for fecal leukocytes
- Specific antimicrobial therapy:
  - Shigellosis:
    Ciprofloxacin 500 mg orally twice a day for 3 to 5 days, or

> TMP-SMX DS 1 tablet orally twice a day
> for 3 to 5 days

- *V. cholera:* Tetracycline 500 mg orally 4 times a day for 2 days
- *C. jejuni:*
  > Erythromycin 250 to 500 mg orally 4
  > times a day for 5 to 7 days, or
  > Ciprofloxacin 500 mg orally 2 times a
  > day for 7 days
- Invasive or enterotoxigenic *E. coli:*
  > TMP-SMX DS 1 tablet orally twice a day
  > for 3 to 5 days, or
  > Ciprofloxacin 500 mg orally twice a day
  > for 3 to 5 days (or 1 g orally once)
- Invasive *Salmonella* or systemic salmonellosis:
  > —Ceftriaxone 3 to 4 g/day IV given for 5
  > to 7 days, or
  > —Ciprofloxacin 400 mg IV twice a day for
  > 7 to 10 days, then
  > —Ciprofloxacin 500 to 750 mg orally twice
  > a day for 3 to 4 weeks
  > —**NOTE:** Antimicrobial therapy for
  > uncomplicated, self-limiting salmonellosis
  > is not indicated, and may prolong
  > bacterial shedding
- *C. botulinum:*
  > —Antitoxin therapy with trivalent A-B-E
  > antitoxin 1 vial IV + 1 vial
  > intramuscularly, repeated in 2 to 4 hours
  > IV as needed in severe or progressive cases
  > —Antitoxin is available from the Centers
  > for Disease Control and Prevention
  > (CDC) at (404) 639-2206 or 639-2888

Follow-Up:

- For most infections, outpatient care is sufficient

- Hospitalization for septicemias, focal infections, severe dehydration, or electrolyte imbalances is required, with meticulous attention to fluid status
- Inpatient care for botulism is mandatory, with maximal monitoring, especially for respiratory failure
  - Meticulous airway management
  - Cardiac monitoring
  - Physical therapy
- NG or intravenous feedings as required
- **Watch for:** signs and symptoms of
    - Cardiovascular collapse
    - Cardiac arrhythmias from electrolyte disturbances
    - Septicemia
    - Metastatic infections
    - Invasion of GI tract by bacteria
    - Hypoglycemia
    - Aspiration pneumonia (especially in botulism patients)
    - Hypoxia and respiratory failure (especially in botulism patients)

TROPICAL SPRUE

Presenting Symptoms:

SUBJECTIVE	OBJECTIVE
Fatigue	Asthenia, pallor
Asthenia	Borborygmi
Anorexia, weight loss	Stomatitis
Chronic diarrhea	Glossitis
Abdominal cramps	Cheilosis
Borborygmus	Hyperkeratosis
Night blindness	Edema
Tongue pain and inflammation	Hyperpigmentation
	Koilonychia

Chapped and
  fissured lips
Rash
Fever

Peripheral neuropathy
Fever may be present
Elicit appropriate
  travel or exposure
  history:
—South Africa
—India
—Haiti
—Caribbean countries

Differential Diagnosis:

Megaloblastic anemia of other causes
Malabsorptive syndrome
Celiac disease
Inflammatory bowel disease
Giardiasis
Cryptosporidiosis
Coccidiosis (*Isospora belli*)
Capillariasis
Gluten enteropathy
Lymphoma
Intestinal tuberculosis
Blind loop syndrome
Pancreatic neoplasm
Whipple's disease
HIV enteropathy
Microsporidia in HIV infection

Suggested Workup:

- Laboratory:
  - CBC: macrocytic anemia
  - Serum vitamin B_{12} level decreased
  - Serum iron decreased
  - Serum calcium decreased
  - Serum folic acid decreased
  - Serum carotene decreased

- • Serum cholesterol decreased
  - • Serum albumin decreased
  - • Serum magnesium decreased
  - • Seventy–two-hour fecal fat analysis: steatorrhea
- • Imaging studies:
  - • Upper GI series with small bowel follow-through:
    - —Flattened mucosal folds
    - —Luminal dilatation
    - —Flocculation of the barium
    - —Abnormally slow transit time
  - • Highly suggestive, but not definitive
- • Upper endoscopy:
  - • Duodenal aspirate for parasites
  - • Biopsy
  - • Quantitative small bowel culture
- • Malabsorption studies:
  - • D-xylose
  - • Fat
  - • Vitamin B_{12}
  - • Malabsorption of two of these nutrients is essential for diagnosis

Definitive Diagnosis:

Tropical sprue   ICD-9-CM 579.1

Suggested Treatment:

- • Antimicrobial therapy:
  - • Tetracycline 250 mg 4 times a day for 1 to 6 months
  - • Duration of therapy varies for travelers to tropics (1 to 2 months) versus residents of tropics (6 months)
- • Folate replacement: Folic acid 5 mg orally once a day for 1 to 6 months, or

- Folic acid 5 mg/iron 500 mg/B_{12} 125 μg combination elixir (Niferex forte) orally once a day for 1 to 6 months

Follow-Up:

- Follow symptomatically
- Monitor fluid status
- Monitor nutritional status
- Recheck CBC periodically
- **Watch for:** signs and symptoms of
  - Complications of malabsorption
    - —Stomatitis
    - —Glossitis
    - —Cheilosis
    - —Night blindness
    - —Peripheral neuropathy
    - —Hyperkeratosis
    - —Hyperpigmentation
    - —Koilonychia
  - Relapse: continue medication for longer period and/or reevaluate diagnosis

WHIPPLE'S DISEASE

Presenting Symptoms:

SUBJECTIVE	OBJECTIVE
Intermittent arthralgias involving multiple joints (may have occurred over a period of years)	Distended abdomen that is tender to palpation
Gradual onset of diarrhea	Tenderness of large joints
Anorexia and weight loss	Evidence of weight loss
Vague abdominal pain	Palpable abdominal lymphadenopathy
	Hyperpigmentation of

Low-grade fever

the skin (50% of
cases)
Hypotension
Low-grade fever, but
may spike to 103°F
Peripheral
lymphadenopathy
Cardiac murmurs (25%
of cases)
Evidence of
malabsorption
Neurologic
abnormalities
—Ophthalmoplegia
—Dementia
—Ataxia
—Myoclonus
—Hyperreflexia
—Paresis
—Hearing loss
—Visual disturbances
—Personality changes
(may be first
presenting signs
without significant
GI signs or
symptoms)
Typical patient is
a middle-aged
white man

Differential Diagnosis:

Iron deficiency anemia of other causes
Malabsorptive syndrome
Celiac disease
Tropical sprue
Inflammatory bowel disease

Giardiasis
Cryptosporidiosis
Coccidiosis
Lymphoma
Pancreatic neoplasm
HIV enteropathy
Histoplasmosis
Mycobacterium avium infection in AIDS

Suggested Workup:

- History and physical provide high index of
  suspicion:
  - A middle-aged white man with a history of
    arthralgias, followed by weight loss,
    diarrhea, and abdominal pain should be
    highly suggestive of Whipple's disease
- Laboratory:
  - Normocytic, normochromic anemia
  - Iron deficiency
  - Normal white blood cell (WBC) count and
    differential
  - Decreased albumin
  - Decreased cholesterol
  - Decreased serum potassium
  - Prolonged prothrombin time
  - Seventy–two-hour fecal fat analysis →
    steatorrhea
- Absorption studies:
  - Decreased D-xylose absorption (93% of
    patients)
  - Decreased vitamin B_{12} absorption (15% of
    patients)
- Upper endoscopy with small bowel biopsy:
  - Definitive diagnostic procedure
  - Finding of periodic acid-Schiff (PAS) stain-
    positive macrophages and the presence of
    characteristic Whipple bacteria (proposed

name is *Tropheryma whippelii*) is pathognomonic

Definitive Diagnosis:

Whipple's disease   ICD-9-CM 040.2

Suggested Treatment:

- Standard antimicrobial therapy: TMP-SMX DS 1 tablet orally twice a day for 1 year
- Seriously ill patients:
  - TMP-SMX DS 1 tablet orally 3 times a day for 2 weeks, then 2 times a day for 1 year
  - Folinic acid 3 mg orally 2 times a week during 2 weeks of therapy with TMP-SMX DS
- Sulfonamide allergy or intolerance:
  - Penicillin (PCN)-V 250 mg orally 4 times a day for 1 year
  - Where cerebral involvement is suspected: PCN-G 20 million U/day IV for 30 days, then oral therapy
  - Penicillin allergy: Chloramphenicol 250 mg orally 4 times a day for 1 year
- Treatment of relapse:
  - Repeat TMP-SMX or chloramphenicol therapy for 6 to 12 months, or
  - In noncentral nervous system (CNS) relapse, tetracycline 250 mg orally 4 times a day for 6 to 12 months
- Dietary supplements: Consider supplements of
  - Folate
  - Vitamin B_{12}
  - Vitamin K
  - Iron

Follow-Up:

- Careful clinical follow-up monthly for 6 months, then annually thereafter, even after treatment is completed

- If relapse is suspected, intestinal biopsy should be repeated and/or empirical trial of antibiotics should be instituted
- **Watch for:** signs and symptoms of
    - CNS involvement
    - Complications of malabsorption
    - Malnutrition
    - Relapse

ACUTE VIRAL HEPATITIS (HEPATITIS A, B, C, D, AND E ARE DENOTED AS HAV, HBV, HCV, HDV, AND HEV, RESPECTIVELY)

Presenting Symptoms:

SUBJECTIVE	OBJECTIVE
Pre-icteric phase (3 to 10 days):	**Acute disease:**
Fever (unusual with HBV, HCV)	Icterus (best observed in sclera and sublingual area)
Malaise	Abdominal palpation reveals slightly enlarged and tender liver
Nausea, vomiting	
Anorexia	
Dull, right upper quadrant abdominal pain	Borderline splenomegaly
Headache	Modest lymphadenopathy
Flu-like symptoms	
Urticarial rash	Vascular spiders
Polyarticular, migratory arthralgic symptoms	Urticarial rash
	Red, warm, tender joints (5% to 15% of cases)
Icteric phase:	
Jaundice	Exacerbation of underlying dermatitis (e.g., acne)
Dark urine	
Light-colored stools	
Pruritus	

Fulminant disease with liver failure (usually HBV):
Encephalopathy manifested by
—Lethargy
—Somnolence
—Change in personality
—Stupor
—Coma

Fulminant disease:
Encephalopathy
—Lethargy
—Somnolence
—Confusion
—Asterixis
—Stupor
—Coma
—Fetor hepaticus
—Decerebrate posturing
Ascites

Differential Diagnosis:

Infectious mononucleosis (Epstein-Barr virus [EBV] infection)
Hepatic malignancy
Drug- or chemical-induced hepatitis
Ischemic hepatitis
Alcoholic hepatitis
Chronic active hepatitis
Cytomegalovirus (CMV) infection
Wilson's disease
Serum sickness
Pneumococcal pneumonia
Leptospirosis
Miliary tuberculosis
Q fever
Syphilis
Anoxic liver injury
Sickle cell crisis

Suggested Workup:

- Serology: See Figure 6.3
- Laboratory:
  - LFTs
    —Aspartate aminotransferase (AST)/alanine aminotransferase (ALT) markedly elevated (ALT can be 400 to several thousand U/L)

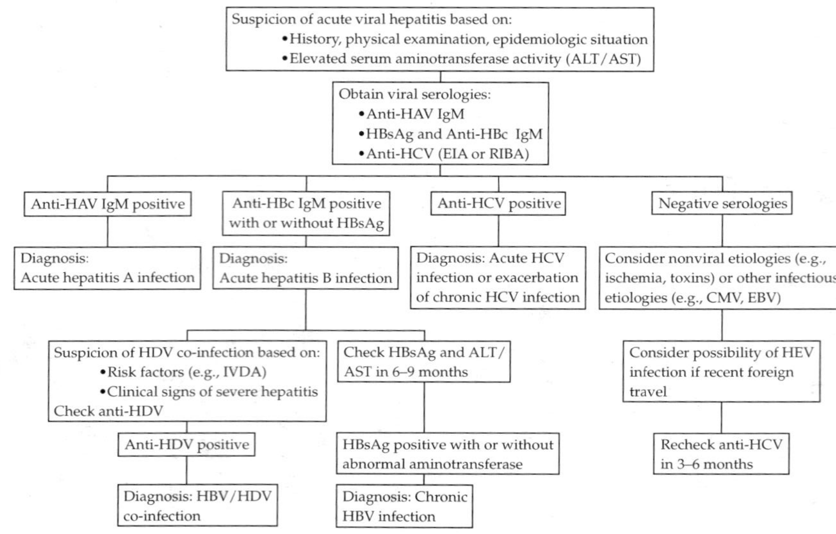

Suspicion of acute viral hepatitis based on:
•History, physical examination, epidemiologic situation
•Elevated serum aminotransferase activity (ALT/AST)
Obtain viral serologies:
•Anti-HAV IgM
•HBsAg and Anti-HBc IgM
•Anti-HCV (EIA or RIBA)
Anti-HAV IgM positive
Anti-HBc IgM positive with or without HBsAg
Anti-HCV positive
Negative serologies
Diagnosis: Acute hepatitis A infection
Diagnosis: Acute hepatitis B infection
Diagnosis: Acute HCV infection or exacerbation of chronic HCV infection
Consider nonviral etiologies (e.g., ischemia, toxins) or other infectious etiologies (e.g., CMV, EBV)
Suspicion of HDV co-infection based on:
•Risk factors (e.g., IVDA)
•Clinical signs of severe hepatitis
Check anti-HDV
Check HBsAg and ALT/AST in 6–9 months
Consider possibility of HEV infection if recent foreign travel
Anti-HDV positive
HBsAg positive with or without abnormal aminotransferase
Recheck anti-HCV in 3–6 months
Diagnosis: HBV/HDV co-infection
Diagnosis: Chronic HBV infection

—Bilirubin usually elevated
—Prothrombin time (PT)/partial thromboplastin time (PTT) markedly elevated in more severe cases

- Clues from history, physical examination, and epidemiology:
  - **HAV**
    - —Acute, sudden onset of flu-like symptoms
      - –Fifteen- to 60-day incubation period
      - –Symptoms generally last 2 to 4 weeks
    - —Generally anicteric
    - —Low mortality
    - —No chronic disease or carrier state
    - —Fecal-oral transmission
      - –Contaminated water
      - –Poor sanitary conditions
      - –Ingestion of raw or undercooked shellfish
      - –Travel to endemic areas
    - —Exposure to children in day care centers
    - —Male homosexuality recently found to be a risk factor
    - —Intravenous drug abuse recently found to be a risk factor
  - **HBV**
    - —More insidious onset: 30- to 180-day incubation period

---

Fig. 6.3 Algorithm for the Diagnosis of Acute Viral Hepatitis

ALT = alanine aminotransferase; AST = aspartate aminotransferase; HBsAg = HBV surface antigen; HBc = HBV core antigen; EIA = enzyme immunoassay; RIBA = Recombinant immunoabsorbent assay; CMV = cytomegalovirus; EBV = Epstein-Barr virus; IVDA = intravenous drug abuser.

—Prolonged course: symptoms generally last 4 to 8 weeks
—Higher incidence of serum sickness-like symptoms: fever, rash, and polyarthralgias in the pre-icteric phase
—Parenteral transmission
  –Transfusion of blood or blood products
  –Renal dialysis
  –Exposure to contaminated needles and syringes
    —Oncology ward patients
    —Intravenous drug addicts
—Intimate transmission
  –Maternal-fetal
  –Sexual contact
  –Exposure to body fluids or excreta
—Five to 10% risk of long-term disease or carrier rate (chronically hepatitis B surface antigen [HB_sAg]-positive): must demonstrate anti-hepatitis B core antigen (HB_cAb) IgM in these patients to diagnose acute HBV superimposed on the carrier state

- **HCV**
  —More indolent and prolonged course than HBV
    –Fourteen- to 180-day incubation period
    –Symptoms generally last 8 to 10 weeks
  —Parenteral transmission
    –Accounts for 70% to 95% of post-transfusion hepatitis
    –Intravenous drug abuse with needle sharing
  —Progresses to chronic hepatitis, chronic active disease, fibrosis, and cirrhosis (50% to 85% risk of long-term disease)
    –Often indolent and silent

- –Twenty-five percent progress to cirrhosis
- —May be a risk factor for hepatocellular carcinoma
- **HDV**
  - —Defective delta virus that requires coinfection with HBV (40- to 180-day incubation period)
  - —Most common in persons with multiple parenteral exposures
    - –Intravenous drug addicts
    - –Hemophiliacs
    - –Persons receiving multiple transfusions
  - —Uncommon in homosexuals
  - —Endemic areas are those where HB_sAg carrier rate is high
  - —Two to 70% risk of long-term disease
- **HEV**
  - —Acute, self-limited disease
    - –Fifteen- to 60-day incubation period
    - –No risk of chronic, long-term disease
  - —Often cholestatic with prolonged jaundice
  - —Associated with lower serum AST/ALT levels but higher serum alkaline phosphatase levels than other forms of hepatitis
  - —Fecal-oral transmission, usually linked to fecal contamination of the water supply
  - —May present as fulminant disease in pregnant women
- Liver biopsy:
  - May be necessary in clinically persistent disease and to exclude other diseases
  - Determines type and extent of liver injury
  - Indicated if interferon (IFN) therapy is contemplated

Definitive Diagnosis:

Hepatitis type A	ICD-9-CM 070.1
Hepatitis type A with coma	ICD-9-CM 070.0
Hepatitis type B	ICD-9-CM 070.30
Hepatitis type B with coma	ICD-9-CM 070.20
Hepatitis type C	ICD-9-CM 070.51
Hepatitis type C with coma	ICD-9-CM 070.41
Hepatitis type D	ICD-9-CM 070.52
Hepatitis type E	ICD-9-CM 070.53

Suggested Treatment:

- Interferon:
    - —IFN-α_{2b} recombinant may help to induce remission in 25% to 50% of HBV and 40% of HCV patients and to decrease abnormal LFTs in chronic HBV and HCV infections
    - —For HBV: 5 million international units (IU) intramuscularly/subcutaneously once a day or 10 million IU intramuscularly/ subcutaneously 3 times a week for 16 weeks
    - —For HCV: 3 million IU intramuscularly/ subcutaneously 3 times a week for 24 weeks
- Corticosteroids:
    - Not indicated for a typical uncomplicated case of viral hepatitis
    - May be helpful in
        - —Prolonged cholestasis following HAV
        - —Fulminant hepatic failure
- General management:
    - Outpatient care is generally adequate, except for patients:
        - —In danger of dehydration
        - —With prolonged PT
        - —With rising bilirubin levels greater than 15 to 20 mg/dL
        - —With clinical evidence of hepatic failure

- Segregation necessary only for
  —Food handlers with HAV
  —Health care workers with HBV or HCV
- Bedrest while patient is symptomatic
- Avoidance of alcohol and unnecessary drugs
- Low fat, high carbohydrate diet
- Correct laboratory abnormalities
  —Coagulation defects
  —Abnormal fluid and electrolyte concentrations
  —Acid-base imbalance
  —Hypoglycemia
  —Renal impairment
- Fulminant hepatitis
  —Bedrest
  —Low-protein diet (less than 20 to 30 g/day)
  —Bowel-cleansing enemas
  —Neomycin 1 to 1.5 g orally every 6 hours, or lactulose 30 to 60 mL orally every 2 to 6 hours until loose stools are achieved
  —Correct coagulation defects with fresh frozen plasma (FFP)
  —Cimetidine 300 to 500 mg IV every 6 hours to prevent GI bleeding
  —Consider liver transplant

Follow-Up:

- Outpatient care is usual
- Monitor serum AST/ALT periodically
- Monitor biochemical markers
- Serology to monitor convalescence (as per algorithm above)
- Monitor CBC and platelets if patient is receiving IFN

- Patient education regarding prevention and avoidance
  - Proper disposal of needles
  - Good sanitation
  - Consider HAV and/or HBV vaccine for
    - —Travelers to endemic areas
    - —Close contacts of patients
    - —Staff at institutions where case has occurred
- **Watch for:** signs and symptoms of
    - Acute or subacute hepatic necrosis
    - Chronic or chronic active hepatitis
    - Cirrhosis
    - Liver failure
    - Hepatocellular carcinoma
    - Immune complex nephritis
    - Anemia
    - HBV cardiomyopathy
    - HCV mixed cryoglobulinemia
    - HCV-induced porphyria cutanea tarda

CHRONIC HEPATITIS (HEPATITIS B, C, AND D ARE DENOTED HBV, HCV, AND HDV, RESPECTIVELY)

Presenting Symptoms:

SUBJECTIVE	OBJECTIVE
Wide range of patient symptoms	Wide range of physical findings
—Asymptomatic	None, with only abnormal LFTs to suggest diagnosis
—Mild nonspecific symptoms	
—Severe, fulminant symptoms	Fulminant hepatic failure

Extrahepatic symptoms not uncommon
—Migratory, nondeforming polyarthritis
—Polyarteritis nodosa
—Glomerulonephritis
—Essential mixed cryoglobulinemia
—Porphyria cutanea tarda

Elicit history of risk factor
—Acute viral hepatitis
—Intravenous drug abuse
—Multiple transfusions of blood or blood products
—HIV infection

Differential Diagnosis:

Polyarteritis nodosa
Glomerulonephritis
Essential mixed cryoglobulinemia
Porphyria cutanea tarda
α_1-antitrypsin deficiency
Wilson's disease
Primary biliary cirrhosis
Primary sclerosing cholangitis
Inflammatory bowel disease
AIDS cholangiopathy
Granulomatous hepatitis
Systemic lupus erythematosus
Graft-versus-host disease
Drug-induced hepatitis
Alcoholic hepatitis
Hemochromatosis

Suggested Workup:

- History and/or epidemiology may be helpful
  - History of acute viral hepatitis (especially HBV, HCV, or HDV)
  - Presence of tattoos
  - Scars of acupuncture or intravenous drug use
  - History of major surgery and/or transfusion of blood or blood products
- Serology:
  - **Chronic HBV**
    - —HB_sAg-positive
    - —Anti- HB_cAb-positive
    - —Hepatitis B e antigen (HB_eAg)-positive and anti-HB_e antibody (HB_eAb)-negative patients are in the viral replicative stage (antigen-negative and antibody-positive patients are in the nonreplicative stage)
    - —Serum HBV DNA-positive in patients in the replicative stage
  - **Chronic HCV**
    - —Anti-HCV antibody-positive
    - —Serum HCV RNA-positive by PCR technique
  - **Chronic HDV**
    - —HDV antigen-positive
    - —Anti-HDV antibody-positive
    - —Serum HDV RNA-positive
- Laboratory:
  - LFTs:
    - —Elevated serum ALT
    - —Serum bilirubin may be elevated
- Liver biopsy:
  - Helps distinguish between a viral carrier state and true chronic hepatitis
  - Chronic necroinflammatory changes seen in true chronic disease

Definitive Diagnosis:

Chronic hepatitis type B	ICD-9-CM 070.32
Chronic hepatitis type C	ICD-9-CM 070.54
Chronic hepatitis type D	ICD-9-CM 070.33

Suggested Treatment:

- HBV: IFN-α_{2b} recombinant 5 million IU intramuscularly/subcutaneously once a day or 10 million IU intramuscularly/subcutaneously 3 times a week for 16 weeks
- HCV:
    - IFN-α_{2b} 3 million IU subcutaneously 3 times a week for 6 months
    - Only 10% to 25% of patients show sustained response
- Orthotopic liver transplantation: Option for patients who do not respond to treatment

Follow-Up:

- Monitor LFTs and serology periodically
- Repeat liver biopsy after treatment to gauge response
- **Watch for:** signs and symptoms of
    - Liver failure
    - Cirrhosis
    - Granulomatous hepatitis
    - Autoimmune hepatitis
    - Immune cholangiopathy
    - Hepatocellular carcinoma

PERITONITIS

Presenting Symptoms:

SUBJECTIVE	OBJECTIVE
Acute abdominal pain, often exacerbated by motion	Diffuse abdominal tenderness on palpation with
Fever	guarding

Nausea, vomiting
Constipation/diarrhea
Dyspnea
Abdominal distention

Rebound tenderness
General abdominal
  rigidity
Hypoactive/absent
  bowel sounds
Abdominal hyper-
  resonance to
  percussion
Facies hippocratica
Ascites may be
  present
Paralytic ileus
Tachycardia and
  tachypnea
Hypotension
Cutaneous
  vasoconstriction
Respiratory splinting
Elicit possible risk
  factors:
—**Primary peritonitis:**
  none
—**Secondary
  peritonitis:**
  –Peptic ulcer disease
  –Abdominal trauma
  –Colitis
  –Diverticulitis
  –Appendicitis
  –Pancreatitis
  –Acute cholecystitis
  –Postabdominal or
    pelvic surgery
  –Puerperal sepsis
  –Suppurative
    prostatitis
  –Peritoneal dialysis

–Peritoneal shunts
–Advanced liver
 disease
–Renal abscess
–Intestinal neoplasm

Differential Diagnosis:

Subdiaphragmantic abscess
Peritoneal abscess
Subhepatic abscess
Pelvic abscess
Pelvic inflammatory disease
Volvulus
Intussusception
Acute appendicitis
Gangrene of the bowel
Inflammatory bowel disease
End-stage liver disease
Mesenteric adenitis
Pancreatitis
Chemical peritonitis
Bowel obstruction with strangulation
Pneumonia
Sickle cell anemia
Diabetic ketoacidosis
Tabes dorsalis
Porphyria
Familial Mediterranean fever
Plumbism
Systemic lupus erythematosus
Uremia

Suggested Workup:

- Laboratory:
  - CBC:
    - Elevated WBCs 17,000 to 25,000/mm^3 not
      unusual, with marked shift to the left

—Hemoconcentration with elevated red blood cells (RBCs) and HCT
- Elevated blood urea nitrogen (BUN)
- Elevated amylase (very high levels more consistent with acute pancreatitis)
- Metabolic and respiratory acidosis
- Blood cultures positive for infecting organism(s)
- Hyperglycemia and glycosuria more consistent with diabetic acidosis and acute pancreatitis
- Hematuria and pyuria more consistent with appendicitis or other intra-abdominal infection adjacent to urinary tract
- Hyponatremia in the absence of large volume nonisotonic fluid replacement more consistent with porphyria
- Imaging studies:
  - Supine, upright, and lateral decubitus radiographs of the abdomen
    —Free air in peritoneal cavity
    —Small and large bowel dilatation
    —Intestinal wall edema
    —Features of mechanical intestinal obstruction
    —Trapped gas with an air-fluid level seen if there is intra-abdominal abscess
  - Upright chest radiograph
    —Elevated diaphragm
    —Trapped air beneath the diaphragm
    —Calcification of gall bladder or other organ
- Abdominal CT or ultrasound can be used to detect ascites or abscess
- Paracentesis: Needle aspiration of peritoneal cavity or peritoneal lavage with Ringer's lactate solution (may need ultrasound or CT guidance)

- Examine peritoneal fluid grossly for:
  —Blood
  —Pus
  —Bile
- Laboratory analysis
  —Amylase
  —Microbiologic analysis
  —Gram stain and culture
- Exploratory laparotomy is reserved for patients in whom diagnosis is still uncertain after all other tests have been completed, or for those who do not respond clinically to therapy for acute peritonitis

Definitive Diagnosis:

Acute generalized peritonitis   ICD-9-CM 567.2
Acute primary peritonitis,   ICD-9-CM 567.9
  localized

Suggested Treatment:

- Empiric antibiotic therapy should be started immediately after blood and peritoneal fluid cultures are obtained; the regimen can be modified after the results of culture and antibiotic sensitivity testing are known
  - Variables that must be considered in selecting a therapeutic option include:
    —Nature of patient involved (i.e., age, presence of renal disease, types and severity of underlying illnesses)
    —Community versus hospital acquired infection
    —Pathogens isolated
    —Adverse drug reactions encountered
    —Severity of infection
    —Cost of drugs
- Spontaneous or primary peritonitis (usually monomicrobial): 14 days of

- Aztreonam 1 g IV every 8 hours, and
    Ampicillin 1 to 2 g IV every 6 hours, or
- Cefotaxime 1.5 to 2.0 g IV every 6
  hours, and
    Ampicillin 2 g IV every 6 hours, or
- Ticarcillin-clavulanate 3 g IV every 6
  hours, or
- Gentamicin 1.7 mg/kg IV every 8
  hours, and
    Cefoxitin 2 g IV every 6 hours, or
    Cefotaxime 1.5 to 2.0 g IV every 6
      hours, or
    Piperacillin 4 to 5 g IV every 6 hours
- Penicillin allergy: can substitute
  Vancomycin 1 g IV every 12 hours
- Secondary peritonitis from an enteric source
  (usually polymicrobial): treatment should be
  continued until patient's clinical status
  resolves and cultures become negative; 5 to 14
  days of:
    - Clindamycin 600 to 900 mg IV every 6 to 8
      hours, or
        Metronidazole 750 to 1000 mg IV every
          12 hours, and
        Gentamicin 3 to 5 mg/kg/day IV given
          every 8 hours, or
        Cefotaxime 1.5 to 2.0 g IV every 6
          hours, or
        Ceftriaxone 1 g IV every 12 hours
        (best for young patient, with no
          hypotension or renal failure), or
    - Clindamycin 600 to 900 mg IV every 6 to 8
      hours, and
        Aztreonam 1.0 to 1.5 g IV every 6
          hours, or
    - Cefotaxime 1 to 2 g IV every 4 to 8
      hours, or
        Ceftriaxone 1 to 2 g IV every 24 hours, or

Cefoxitin 1.5 to 2.0 g IV every 6 hours, or
Cefotetan 1.5 to 2.0 g IV every 12
hours, or
Cefmetazole 1.5 to 2.0 g IV every 6 to 8
hours
(best for community-acquired infections
of mild to moderate severity), or

- Ampicillin 1 to 2 g IV every 6
hours, and
Gentamicin 1.7 mg/kg IV every 8
hours, and
Metronidazole 500 mg IV every 6 to 8
hours, or
Clindamycin 600 to 900 mg IV every 8
hours
(best where a strong anaerobic
component to the infection is
suspected), or

- Imipenem 0.5 to 1.0 g IV every 6 to 8
hours, or
Meropenem 1.0 g IV every 8 hours
(best where mixed aerobic and anaerobic
infection with beta–lactamase-
producing bacteria is suspected and/or
aminoglycosides are contraindicated)

- Peritonitis during peritoneal dialysis:
  - Dialysate shows bacteria:
    —Vancomycin 30 to 50 mg/L dialysate or
    2 g in one 6-hour exchange every 7 days
    plus 1 g intravenous load, and
    Gentamicin 6 to 8 mg/L dialysate, or
    Ceftazidime 20 mg/L dialysate for 1 to
    4 days
  - Dialysate shows fungi:
    —Amphotericin B 1 g intraperitoneal (ip)
    per day, and
    Fluconazole 150 mg ip every other day
    (qod), or

—If dialysis catheter is removed; this is
necessary in 10% to 20% of patients:
Amphotericin B 30 mg IV/day

Follow-Up:

- Follow as inpatient carefully with close
  monitoring of clinical status, CBC, and repeat
  cultures of blood and peritoneal fluid
- Treat underlying condition(s) in secondary
  peritonitis, including by surgery if necessary
- Monitor fluid status; intravenous hydration as
  necessary
- Monitor nutritional status; total parenteral
  nutrition (TPN) if necessary
- Nasogastric decompression for ileus
- **Watch for:** signs and symptoms of
    - Hypovolemia and shock
    - Septicemia
    - Acute renal failure
    - Acute respiratory insufficiency
    - Liver failure
    - Abscess formation requiring
      surgical drainage
    - Bowel perforation

INTRAPERITONEAL ABSCESS

Presenting Symptoms:

SUBJECTIVE	OBJECTIVE
Acute onset abdominal pain	History of risk factor(s) for intraperitoneal abscess:
High intermittent fever	—Primary or secondary peritonitis
Shaking chills	—Appendicitis
	—Diverticulitis
	—Biliary tract lesions

—Pancreatitis
—Perforated peptic ulcer
—Inflammatory bowel disease
—Abdominal trauma
—Abdominal surgery
Physical signs vary with location of abscess:
—Subphrenic abscess causes costal tenderness and pleural or pulmonary involvement
—Subhepatic abscess causes upper abdominal or subcostal symptoms and few pulmonary changes

Differential Diagnosis:

Peritonitis
Perforated peptic ulcer
Appendicitis
Cholangitis
Cholecystitis
Inflammatory bowel disease
Diverticulitis
Regional enteritis
Pneumonia
Hepatitis
Pelvic inflammatory disease
Intestinal obstruction
Intestinal ischemia

Suggested Workup:

- Laboratory:
  - CBC: leukocytosis with left shift
  - Blood cultures positive in less than 25% of cases
- Imaging studies:
  - Abdominal radiograph can suggest the location of peritoneal abscesses in up to 50% of cases
  - Gallium (^{67}Ga-) and indium (^{111}In)-tagged leukocyte scans can detect intra-abdominal abscesses as "hot" spots (In scan is as sensitive as Ga scan but more specific because In is not secreted into the bowel)
  - Ultrasound of the abdomen can delineate an abdominal mass according to its:
    —Size
    —Shape
    —Consistency
    —Anatomic relationships
  - CT of the abdomen with contrast (oral, rectal, and intravenous) is the test of choice in diagnosing an intra-abdominal abscess
- Invasive techniques:
  - Percutaneous catheter drainage of abscess under ultrasound or CT guidance, or
  - Surgical drainage (the conventional intervention): drainage material should be sent for Gram stain and culture and antibiotic sensitivity testing

Definitive Diagnosis:

Peritoneal abscess   ICD-9-CM 567.2

Suggested Treatment:

- Empiric antimicrobial therapy should be instituted immediately after blood cultures are drawn and before abscess drainage material is collected; coverage may be modified once results of culture and sensitivity testing are known:

- Clindamycin 600 to 900 mg IV every 6 to 8 hours, or
    - Metronidazole 750 to 1000 mg IV every 12 hours, and
    - Gentamicin 3 to 5 mg/kg/day IV given every 8 hours, or
    - Cefotaxime 1.5 to 2.0 g IV every 6 hours, or
    - Ceftriaxone 1 g IV every 12 hours (best for young patient, with no hypotension or renal failure), or
- Clindamycin 600 to 900 mg IV every 6 to 8 hours, and
    - Aztreonam 1.0 to 1.5 g IV every 6 hours, or
- Cefotaxime 1 to 2 g IV every 4 to 8 hours, or
    - Ceftriaxone 1 to 2 g IV every 24 hours, or
    - Cefoxitin 1.5 to 2.0 g IV every 6 hours, or
    - Cefotetan 1.5 to 2.0 g IV every 12 hours, or
    - Cefmetazole 1.5 to 2.0 g IV every 6 to 8 hours
    (best for infections of relatively mild to moderate severity), or
- Ampicillin 1 to 2 g IV every 6 hours, and
    - Gentamicin 1.7 mg/kg IV every 8 hours, and
    - Metronidazole 500 mg IV every 6 to 8 hours or
    - Clindamycin 600 to 900 mg IV every 8 hours

> (best where a strong anaerobic component to the infection is suspected), or

- Imipenem 0.5 to 1.0 g IV every 6 to 8 hours, or Meropenem 1.0 g IV every 8 hours
  (best where mixed aerobic and anaerobic infection with beta—lactamase-producing bacteria is suspected and/or aminoglycosides are contraindicated)
- Surgical drainage is indicated in virtually all intraperitoneal abscesses:
  - Conventional therapy is surgical drainage
  - An alternative to surgery is percutaneous catheter drainage under ultrasound or CT guidance; possible only where:
    - Abscess can be safely approached via a percutaneous route
    - Abscess is unilocular
    - Abscess is not vascular
    - Dependent catheter drainage is possible

Follow-Up:

- Inpatient care with close clinical monitoring
- Repeat blood cultures and culture of abscess drainage fluid during therapy when clinically indicated
- **Watch for:** signs and symptoms of
  - Septicemia
  - Hemorrhage
  - Peritoneal spillage and generalized peritonitis
  - Fistula formation

SUBPHRENIC ABSCESS

Presenting Symptoms:

SUBJECTIVE	OBJECTIVE
High spiking fever	Abdominal tenderness
Chills and sweating	on palpation

Abdominal pain
Chest pain
Nausea
Shortness of breath
Shoulder pain
Intractable hiccups

Evidence of ileus
Erythema of anterior
    abdominal wall
Tachycardia
Evidence of pleural
    effusion
Elevated
    hemidiaphragm
    (usually right) on
    percussion
Tenderness when
    compressing lower
    costal margin
Basilar rales
High, spiking fevers
Elicit history of recent
    abdominal surgery
    (50% of cases) or
    trauma

Differential Diagnosis:

Other intra-abdominal abscess
Peritonitis
Empyema

Suggested Workup:

- Laboratory:
    - CBC: elevated WBC
    - Blood cultures can identify infecting
      organism
- Radiograph of chest and abdomen:
    - Elevation of right hemidiaphragm
    - Fluid in right costophrenic sulcus
    - Air-fluid level in subphrenic space
- CT scan of chest and abdomen
    - May be used to visualize collection of pus
      under diaphragm

- May be used to direct transabdominal needle aspiration; collected material should be sent for Gram stain and culture
- Abdominal ultrasound
  - May be used to visualize collection of pus under diaphragm
  - May be used to direct transabdominal needle aspiration; collected material should be sent for Gram stain and culture
- Ga scan for those patients where CT/ultrasound fail to detect nidus of infection

Definitive Diagnosis:

Subphrenic abscess, ICD-9-CM 998.5
  postoperative

Suggested Treatment:

- Adequate percutaneous or surgical drainage of abscess
- Antimicrobial therapy:
  - Gentamicin or tobramycin 3 to 5 mg/kg/day IV given every 8 hours, and
    Clindamycin 600 mg IV every 6 hours, or
    Metronidazole 15 mg/kg intravenous loading dose, followed by 7.5 mg/kg IV every 6 hours, or
  - Cefoxitin 2 g IV every 4 to 6 hours, or
    Cefoperazone 1 to 2 g IV every 12 hours, or
    Cefotaxime 1 g IV every 6 to 8 hours

Follow-Up:

- Careful in-hospital monitoring with surgical consultation
- Frequent evaluation in office for at least 4 to 6 weeks after discharge
- Periodic CBCs during 6 week post-hospital period

- Repeat chest radiographs until normal
- **Watch for:** signs and symptoms of
    - Multisystem organ failure
    - Recurrent abscess
    - Hemorrhage
    - Bowel obstruction
    - Wound dehiscence
    - Sepsis
    - Pneumonia
    - Pleural effusion
    - Suppurative pylephlebitis
    - Peritonitis
    - Fistula formation

PANCREATIC ABSCESS

Presenting Symptoms:

SUBJECTIVE
Abdominal pain
  radiating to the back
Nausea and vomiting
Fever
Abdominal distention

OBJECTIVE
History of pancreatitis,
  usually 1 to 3 weeks
  into clinical course
Generalized abdominal
  tenderness
Abdominal mass may
  be felt in some cases
Jaundice

Differential Diagnosis:

Worsening acute pancreatitis
Complication of endoscopic retrograde
  cholangiopancreatography (ERCP)
Acute peritonitis
Perforating peptic ulcer
Pancreatic pseudocyst
Biliary tract disease
Intestinal obstruction
Intestinal ischemia/infarction

Ruptured ectopic pregnancy
Aortic aneurysm
Pancreatic neoplasm
Other peritoneal/retroperitoneal abscess

Suggested Workup:

- Laboratory:
    - Elevated serum amylase
    - CBC: leukocytosis
- Imaging studies:
    - Abdominal radiograph
      —Diaphragmatic elevation
      —Pleural effusion
      —Retrogastric mass
      —Forward displacement of gastric air
        shadow (lateral view)
      —Widening of gastrocolic omentum
    - Upper GI series with barium
      —Visceral displacement on the posterior
        gastric wall
    - CT scan of abdomen
      —Demonstrate pancreatic gas collections
      —Difficult to discern abscess from
        pancreatic pseudocyst
    - Ga/In scans not helpful in making
      diagnosis
- Invasive techniques: Fine needle aspiration
  under ultrasound or CT guidance can
  distinguish between abscess and uninfected
  pancreatic pseudocyst
    - May also be used for percutaneous
      drainage
    - Material collected should be sent for Gram
      stain and culture and antibiotic sensitivity
      testing
    - May be sufficient treatment until patient is
      stabilized for definitive surgical drainage

Definitive Diagnosis:

Pancreatic abscess   ICD-9-CM 577.0

Suggested Treatment:

- Antimicrobial therapy should be initiated immediately on an empiric basis and adjusted according to results of sensitivity testing:
  - Clindamycin 600 to 900 mg IV every 6 to 8 hours, or
      Metronidazole 750 to 1000 mg IV every 12 hours, and
      Gentamicin 1.7 mg/kg IV every 8 hours, or
      Cefotaxime 1.5 to 2.0 g IV every 6 hours, or
      Ceftriaxone 1 g IV every 12 hours, or
  - Clindamycin 600 to 900 mg IV every 6 to 8 hours, and
      Aztreonam 1.0 to 1.5 g IV every 6 hours, or
  - Ampicillin 1 to 2 g IV every 6 hours (Penicillin allergy: Vancomycin 1 g IV every 12 hours), and
      Gentamicin 1.7 mg/kg IV every 8 hours, and
      Metronidazole 500 mg IV every 6 to 8 hours, or
      Clindamycin 600 to 900 mg IV every 8 hours, or
  - Imipenem 0.5 to 1.0 g IV every 6 to 8 hours, or Meropenem 1.0 g IV every 8 hours
  - Antibiotics should be continued for 10 to 14 days
- Surgical drainage should be considered early
  - Percutaneous appears inadequate for the majority of patients; may be used until patient is stabilized for optimal surgical debridement and drainage
  - Retroperitoneal laparoscopy may be useful

- Routine therapy for underlying pancreatitis should also be instituted
  - Pain control
  - Appropriate fluid measures
  - NG tube
  - Monitor renal function
  - Monitor serum calcium (Ca) levels
  - Monitor pancreatic endocrine function (diabetes mellitus)

Follow-Up:

- Follow closely in hospital or intensive care unit (ICU)
- Prompt reoperation should be considered for persistent infection
- Repeat CT or ultrasound to follow resolution of abscess to correlate with clinical status
- **Watch for:** signs and symptoms of
  - Pancreatic necrosis
  - Biliary tract disease
  - Septicemia
  - Pleuropulmonary complications
  - Hepatic failure
  - Renal failure
  - Spread of infection in the retroperitoneum
  - Fistula formation between abscess cavity and stomach, duodenum, or transverse colon

HEPATIC ABSCESS

Presenting Symptoms:

SUBJECTIVE	OBJECTIVE
Fever and chills for several days or weeks	Right upper quadrant pain on palpation Tender hepatomegaly

<table>
<tr><td valign="top">

Dull right upper quadrant pain with radiation to right shoulder
Cough
Pleuritic chest pain

</td><td valign="top">

Pleural friction rub
Spiking fevers
History of risk factor:
—Biliary calculus, stricture, or malignancy
—Ascending cholangitis
—Appendicitis
—Diverticulitis
—Inflammatory bowel disease
—Gallbladder disease
—Infection with access to hepatic artery
—Penetrating trauma to liver

</td></tr>
</table>

Differential Diagnosis:

Acute viral hepatitis
Hepatic neoplasm
Ascending cholangitis
Biliary calculus
Cholelithiasis
Cholecystitis
Appendicitis
Diverticulitis
Inflammatory bowel disease (Crohn's disease, ulcerative colitis)
Amebic abscess

Suggested Workup:

- Laboratory:
  - Elevated serum alkaline phosphatase
  - Blood cultures positive in 50% of patients (especially for *Streptococcus viridans*)

- Serology for ameba:
  - —Positive in patients with amebic abscess
  - —Negative in patients with pyogenic abscess
- Imaging studies:
  - Abdominal and chest radiographs
    - —Elevation and limitation of motion of right hemidiaphragm
    - —Basilar atelectasis
    - —Right pleural effusion
    - —Gas within an abscess cavity
  - CT/magnetic resonance imaging (MRI) of abdomen
    - —Sensitive techniques for detecting hepatic abscess
  - Technetium-99m (^{99m}Tc) sulfur colloid liver scan can detect 85% of lesions greater than 2 cm in diameter
  - ^{67}Ga leukocyte scan can differentiate between pyogenic and amebic abscess: amebic abscesses will show decreased central Ga concentration and pyogenic abscesses will show increased central Ga uptake
  - Abdominal ultrasound: abscesses visualized as echo-free lesions to highly echogenic masses within the liver
- Invasive studies:
  - CT or ultrasound-guided percutaneous aspiration
    - —Send for Gram stain and culture and antibiotic sensitivity testing (aerobic and anaerobic)
    - —Brownish, non–foul-smelling sterile fluid is indicative of amebic abscess

Definitive Diagnosis:

Hepatic abscess, pyogenic   ICD-9-CM 572.0
Hepatic abscess, amebic   ICD-9-CM 006.3

Suggested Treatment:

- Antimicrobial therapy should be initiated on an empiric basis as soon as the diagnosis is suspected, and adjusted according to results of sensitivity testing:
  - Clindamycin 600 to 900 mg IV every 6 to 8 hours, or
    - Metronidazole 750 to 1000 mg IV every 12 hours, and
    - Gentamicin 1.7 mg/kg IV every 8 hours, or
    - Cefotaxime 1.5 to 2.0 g IV every 6 hours, or
    - Ceftriaxone 1 g IV every 12 hours, or
  - Clindamycin 600 to 900 mg IV every 6 to 8 hours, and
    - Aztreonam 1.0 to 1.5 g IV every 6 hours, or
  - Ampicillin 1 to 2 g IV every 6 hours
    - (Penicillin allergy: Vancomycin 1 g IV every 12 hours), and
    - Gentamicin 1.7 mg/kg IV every 8 hours, and
    - Metronidazole 500 mg IV every 6 to 8 hours, or
    - Clindamycin 600 to 900 mg IV every 8 hours, or
  - Imipenem 0.5 to 1.0 g IV given every 6 to 8 hours, or
    - Meropenem 1.0 g IV every 8 hours
  - Antibiotics should be continued for 10 to 14 days
- Amebic abscess: Metronidazole 15 mg/kg intravenous loading dose, then 6 hours later 7.5 mg/kg IV every 6 hours
- Drainage of abscess through percutaneous catheters placed by CT or ultrasound guidance:
  - Generally recommended for pyogenic and amebic abscesses

- Repeated aspiration recommended for expanding abscesses or where greater than 250 mL is obtained on initial aspiration

Follow-Up:

- Follow closely in hospital or ICU
- Repeat CT or ultrasound to correlate with clinical resolution
- **Watch for:** signs and symptoms of
  - Relapses (may require up to 4 months of antibiotic therapy)
  - Contiguous spread of infection
  - Hematogenous spread of infection and sepsis
  - Liver failure
  - Renal failure

ACUTE CHOLECYSTITIS

Presenting Symptoms:

SUBJECTIVE	OBJECTIVE
Asymptomatic (5% to 10%)	Abdominal tenderness in right upper quadrant
Sudden onset, sharp abdominal pain	Signs of peritoneal irritation may be present
—Epigastric	
—Right upper quadrant	Palpable gallbladder (30% to 40% of cases)
—Radiation to right shoulder or scapula	
Nausea and vomiting	Minimal icterus to frank jaundice may be present
Recurrent attacks 1 to 6 hours after meals	
—Pathognomonic description of attacks: sharp pain that rises to peak of	Mild to marked hepatomegaly

intensity over 2 to 3
minutes and is
maintained for 20 to
30 minutes
—Attacks last for over
12 hours but usually
less than 48 hours
Fever (may be low
grade or high)
Abdominal distention
Anorexia and weight
loss

Differential Diagnosis:

Acute pancreatitis
Peptic ulcer with perforation
Nonulcer dyspepsia
Diverticulitis
Pyelonephritis
Right lower lobe pneumonia
Hepatic abscess
Hepatic neoplasm
Irritable bowel disease
Inflammatory bowel disease
Myocardial infarction
Intestinal obstruction
Hepatitis

Suggested Workup:

- Laboratory:
  - CBC: leukocytosis with left shift
  - LFTs:
    —Increased bilirubin (50% of patients)
    —Elevated AST (40%)
    —Elevated alkaline phosphatase
    (25%)
  - Elevated amylase (10%)

- Imaging studies:
  - Abdominal radiograph is of limited value; may show nonspecific changes:
    —Elevation of right hemidiaphragm
    —Calcified gallstones indicate cholelithiasis, but not infection
    —Gas in the gallbladder wall or lumen is diagnostic of emphysematous cholecystitis
  - Ultrasound is method of choice
    —Detects gallstones (95% sensitivity; 98% specificity)
    —Diagnoses inflammation of acute cholecystitis:
      –Thickened gallbladder wall
      –Gallbladder distention
      –Luminal sludge and dilatation
      –Pericholecystic fluid collection
  - CT scan is helpful to demonstrate abscess formation and to rule out neoplasms
  - Hepatobiliary scan with ^{99m}Tc-labeled iminodiacetate (IDA) derivative is a rapid and sensitive method for the diagnosis of acute cholecystitis
  - Oral cholecystography is contraindicated in acute cholecystitis

Definitive Diagnosis:

Acute cholecystitis   ICD-9-CM 575.0

Suggested Treatment:

- Empiric antimicrobial therapy is appropriate for
  - Severely ill patients
  - Elderly patients
  - Patients with emphysematous cholecystitis or other infectious complications

- Perforation
- Signs of peritonitis or peritoneal irritation
- Pericholecystic collection
- Cholangitis
- Gentamicin 1.7 mg/kg IV every 8 hours, or
    Tobramycin 1.7 mg/kg IV every 8
      hours, and
    Ampicillin 2 g IV every 6 hours, or
    Piperacillin 2 to 5 g IV every 6 hours
    (Penicillin allergy: Cefoperazone 1 to 2 g
      IV every 12 hours), and
    Clindamycin 600 to 900 mg IV every 6 to
      8 hours, or
    Metronidazole 500 mg IV every 6 to 8
      hours all for 7 to 10 days
- For mild infections:
    Cefoperazone 1 to 2 g IV every 12
      hours, or
    Ampicillin + sulbactam 1 to 2 g IV every
      6 hours, or
    Ticarcillin-clavulanate 3 g IV every 6
      hours, or
    Cefazolin 1 to 2 g IV every 8 hours, for 5
      to 7 days
- Surgery is immediately indicated for:
  - Gangrenous (emphysematous) cholecystitis
  - Perforation with peritonitis
  - Suspected pericholecystic abscess
  - Cholecystectomy with intraoperative cholangiography is the procedure of choice

Follow-Up:

- Follow closely in hospital and through surgery
- **Watch for:** signs and symptoms of
        - Perforation leading to peritonitis (10% to 15% of cases)
        - Pancreatitis

- Cholangitis
- Abscess formation
- Fistula formation (with intestine, colon, skin)
- Gangrene
- Empyema
- Hepatitis
- Gallstone ileus

ACUTE CHOLANGITIS

Presenting Symptoms:

SUBJECTIVE

Generally mild right upper quadrant or diffuse abdominal pain, acute onset

Charcot's triad:
—Fever
—Chills
—Jaundice

OBJECTIVE

Abdominal examination may be unrevealing or may show diffuse tenderness over liver

Prominent jaundice

Signs of shock may be present

Signs of CNS depression may be present

Differential Diagnosis:

Acute cholecystitis
Pyogenic liver abscess
Hepatitis
Acute pancreatitis
Perforated duodenal ulcer
Pelvic inflammatory disease
Peritonitis
Kidney stones
Hepatic abscess
Intestinal obstruction

Right lower lobe pneumonia
Pyelonephritis
Bacteremic shock of other cause

Suggested Workup:

- Laboratory:
    - CBC: marked leukocytosis with left shift
    - Increased bilirubin to levels greater than 4 mg/dL (90% of cases)
    - LFTs
      —Increased serum alkaline phosphatase
      —Increased serum AST
    - Blood cultures positive in 50% of patients
    - Biochemical evidence of disseminated intravascular coagulation (DIC) may be present
- Imaging studies:
    - Chest radiograph shows nonspecific findings that are rarely helpful
    - Oral cholecystography is of no value
    - Intravenous cholangiography is generally not helpful
    - Ultrasound is the method of choice to:
      —Evaluate gallbladder size
      —Detect the presence of gallstones
      —Monitor the degree of bile duct dilatation
    - ^{99m}Tc-labeled IDA derivative scanning can be used to diagnose obstruction of the common bile duct
- Invasive tests:
    - Percutaneous transhepatic cholangiography
    - ERCP
      —Both tests can be valuable in evaluating bile duct obstruction
      —Neither test can be performed safely in the acutely ill patient

Definitive Diagnosis:

Acute cholangitis   ICD-9-CM 576.1

Suggested Treatment:

- Antimicrobial therapy should be instituted immediately because cholangitis is frequently complicated by bacteremia and shock:
  - Ampicillin 1 g IV every 6 hours (Penicillin allergy: Ciprofloxacin 400 mg IV every 12 hours), and Tobramycin 1.7 mg/kg IV every 8 hours, and Metronidazole 500 mg IV every 8 hours for 7 to 10 days
- Surgery:
  - Decompression of common bile duct with intraoperative cholangiography is mandatory in all patients who do not respond immediately to antibiotics alone
  - Cholecystectomy should also be performed, followed by common duct exploration and T-tube drainage
  - Choledochoduodenostomy or cholecystoduodenostomy may be necessary in complicated cases

Follow-Up:

- Inpatient care with careful monitoring of hemodynamic parameters
- **Watch for:** signs and symptoms of
  - Bacteremia and shock
  - Hepatic abscess
  - Secondary sclerosing cholangitis
  - Perforation of gallbladder with peritonitis
  - Pancreatitis

Genitourinary, Gynecologic, and Sexually Transmitted Infections

7

INFECTIONS COVERED

URINARY TRACT INFECTIONS (UTIs) AND PYELONEPHRITIS

Presenting Symptoms:

SUBJECTIVE | OBJECTIVE

Lower Urinary Tract Infections

Urinary frequency and urgency

Dysuria; burning during urination

Hesitancy or slow stream

Suprapubic discomfort

Turbid, foul-smelling urine

Gross hematuria, especially at the end of the stream

Fever, chills uncommon

Lower abdominal pain on palpation

Elicit history of risk factors

—Previous UTIs

—Diabetes mellitus

—Incontinence of urine and/or stool

—Urinary tract instrumentation or indwelling catheter

—Underlying urinary tract abnormalities
  –Outlet obstruction
  –Tumor
  –Calculus
  –Stricture
  –Incomplete bladder emptying

—Immunocompromised host

—More frequent/ vigorous sexual activity

—Anal intercourse

—Use of barrier contraceptives

—Hospitalized patient

Upper Urinary Tract Infections/Pyelonephritis

Fever (usually over 38.5°C)
Chills
Flank pain
Lower UTI symptoms
Malaise
Myalgias
Nausea, vomiting
Anorexia
Symptoms of systemic toxicity/shock may be present
Lower abdominal/suprapubic tenderness on palpation
Unilateral/bilateral flank pain on percussion or palpation
Rebound/guarding on affected side
Elicit history of risk factors
—Underlying urinary tract abnormalities (as above)
—Diabetes mellitus
—Nephrolithiasis
—Immunocompromised host
—Elderly, institutionalized patient, especially with indwelling catheter
—Previous recent case of acute pyelonephritis

Perinephric Abscess

Fever of at least 2 weeks duration
Abdominal and flank pain
Lower UTI symptoms
Failed treatment for acute pyelonephritis
Abdominal pain
Unilateral flank tenderness on percussion or palpation
Palpable mass may be present in

> perinephric area or
> in retroperitoneum
> Elicit history of risk
> factors
> —Diabetes mellitus
> —Urinary tract calculi

Differential Diagnosis:

For lower UTIs
—Urethritis
—Epididymitis
—Vaginitis
—Sexually transmitted disease
—Tumors
  –Bladder
  –Ureter
  –Prostate
  –Urethra
—Lower urinary tract calculi
—Anatomic or physiologic abnormality, e.g.,
  ureterocele
—Prostatitis
—Drugs (especially cyclophosphamide,
  anticoagulants)
—Inflammatory bowel disease
For pyelonephritis
—Pelvic inflammatory disease (PID)
—Cholecystitis
—Lower lobe pneumonia
—Nephrolithiasis
—Perinephric abscess
—Renal infarction
—Renal vein thrombosis
—Renal artery dissection
—Obstructive uropathy
—Acute glomerulonephritis
—Acute hepatitis

—Acute pancreatitis
—Acute appendicitis
—Perforated abdominal viscus/peritonitis
For perinephric abscess
—Intrarenal abscess
—Pancreatic abscess or pseudocyst
—Retroperitoneal tumor
—Other, nonrenal retroperitoneal abscess

Suggested Workup:

- Uncomplicated UTI (sexually active woman with symptoms of urgency, dysuria, and frequency) may be treated (as indicated below) without urine culture
  - Urinalysis to document pyuria by microscopic examination (greater than 8 white blood cells (WBCs)/mm^3 of uncentrifuged urine) is sufficient to establish presumptive diagnosis of uncomplicated UTI
- More extensive evaluation required in patients at risk for complicated UTI:
  - Pregnancy
  - Nosocomially acquired infection
  - Patient with indwelling catheter or recent urologic instrumentation
  - Post-renal transplant
  - Documented renal calculi
  - Diabetes mellitus
  - Structural urologic anomalies
  - Vesicoureteral reflux
  - Neurogenic bladder
- Microbiologic examination of midstream urine specimen
  - Urinalysis: pyuria by microscopic examination

- Leukocyte esterase dipstick: up to 90% sensitivity and 95% specificity
- Nitrite dipstick: up to 85% sensitivity and 70% specificity
- Urine culture: greater than 10^5 bacteria/mL of urine confirms diagnosis of UTI, but lower counts may still indicate UTI in the presence of significant pyuria
- Ninety-five percent probability of UTI if two clean catch urine cultures demonstrate greater than 10^5 of the same bacterium/mL
- UTI still possible diagnosis with counts significantly less than 10^5/mL (e.g., 10^2 to 10^4/mL)—"Low colony-count UTI"
- Localization of site of infection (noninvasive): ACB test (antibody coating of bacteria) can be used to localize infection to the kidney (88% sensitivity; 76% specificity)
- Localization of site of infection (invasive): ureteral catheterization studies
- Blood cultures
- Imaging studies—indicated in patients suspected of:
  - Complicated episode of pyelonephritis
  - Underlying structural abnormality that may be surgically correctable
  - Intrarenal or perinephric abscess
  - Nonresponsive pyelonephritis
- Abdominal radiograph
  - Can detect urinary tract calculi, calcification, soft tissue masses, abnormal gas collections
  - Fifty percent of patients with perinephric abscess demonstrate characteristic changes
- Renal ultrasound
  - More sensitive than intravenous pyelogram (IVP) for detecting parenchymal changes associated with renal infection

- Detects renal swelling associated with pyelonephritis
- Detects perirenal abscesses greater than 2 to 3 cm
- Computed tomography (CT) of kidneys (with contrast)
  - Most sensitive technique for detecting intrarenal or perirenal suppuration
  - Provides better parenchymal delineation than IVP, but IVP is better for delineation of collecting system
- Radionuclide scans (gallium [^{67}Ga] or indium [^{111}In]-labeled WBCs)
  - May be useful in localizing inflammation or infection to kidneys
  - Where ultrasound or CT demonstrate a solid renal mass, these tests may suggest inflammatory nature of lesion
- Excretory urography
  - Generally supplanted today by ultrasound
  - May be useful in detecting unusual structural abnormalities or infectious processes
    —Renal scarring
    —Renal tuberculosis
    —Papillary necrosis
    —Granulomatous pyelonephritis
- Voiding cystourethrography: recommended (with ultrasound) in all boys after the first episode of UTI and in preschool girls after the second episode of UTI—will detect vesicoureteral reflux
- Intravenous pyelogram
  - Largely supplanted unless imaging of collecting system and detailed anatomic visualization of the upper tract are required

- • May be indicated where perinephric abscess is suspected
- Laboratory:
  - • Reagin test for *Chlamydia*

Definitive Diagnosis:

Acute cystitis   ICD-9-CM 595.1
Urinary tract infection   ICD-9-CM 599.0
Acute pyelonephritis   ICD-9-CM 590.10
Perinephric abscess   ICD-9-CM 590.2

Suggested Treatment:

- Asymptomatic bacteriuria:
  - • Generally, antimicrobial therapy is not needed, except for:
    —Preschool-age children
    —Pregnant women
    —Neutropenic patients
    —Patients undergoing urologic procedures (but NOT for patients with chronic indwelling catheters)
    —Postrenal transplant
    —Diabetes mellitus
    —Documented renal calculi
  - • Treatment can be delayed until two urine cultures have been obtained and the identity and antimicrobial susceptibility of the organisms determined; treatment is based on the results of those tests
- Acute UTI/cystitis—uncomplicated:
  - • Conventional therapy:
    Trimethoprim-sulfamethoxazole (TMP-SMX) DS 1 tablet orally twice a day for 7 to 10 days, or
    Ciprofloxacin 500 mg orally twice a day for 7 to 10 days

- Short-course therapy:
  - —TMP-SMX DS 1 tablet orally twice a day for 3 days, or
    - Norfloxacin 400 mg orally twice a day for 3 days, or
    - Ciprofloxacin 500 mg orally twice a day for 3 days
  - —**NOTE:** This is now the standard for most female patients and most pediatric patients with no suspicion of anatomic abnormality
  - —It is NOT recommended for male patients, pregnant patients, women with a history of previous UTIs, or any patient with more than 7 days of symptoms; 7 to 10 days of therapy is recommended for these patients
- One-day therapy:
  - —Amoxicillin 3 g orally for 1 dose, or
    - TMP-SMX DS orally for 1 dose, or
    - Tetracycline 2 g orally for 1 dose, or
    - Nitrofurantoin 200 mg orally for 1 dose, or
    - Ceftriaxone 0.5 g intramuscularly for 1 dose, or
    - Norfloxacin 800 mg orally for 1 dose
  - —**NOTE:** Reserved for women requiring treatment for postcoital cystitis and women presenting with frequency/ urgency/dysuria syndrome and no signs of upper tract disease; this regimen is associated with a failure rate of up to 65% and is generally inferior to the short-course therapy
- Acute UTI—complicated or recurrent:
  - Treat with agents above for 14 to 21 days

- If there is relapse after this treatment
  - —Evaluate men for bacterial prostatitis (see section on prostatitis)
  - —Renal ultrasound or IVP to rule out surgically correctable abnormality of the urinary tract
  - —If surgery is not indicated, consider antimicrobial therapy for 4 to 6 weeks
- If further relapse, consider therapy for up to 6 months
  - —No therapy may be needed in nonpregnant asymptomatic adults without obstructive uropathy
- Acute pyelonephritis:
  - Outpatient treatment: for patients with mild, uncomplicated disease, who can tolerate oral therapy, who are hemodynamically stable, and can report lack of improvement at an early stage
    - —TMP-SMX DS orally twice a day for 2 weeks, or
      - Ciprofloxacin 500 mg orally twice a day for 2 weeks, or
      - Cephalexin 200 to 500 mg orally every 6 hours for 2 weeks, or
      - Amoxicillin + clavulanate 500 mg orally every 8 hours for 2 weeks
  - Inpatient treatment: for majority of patients
    - —Uncomplicated
      - –TMP-SMX 2 to 20 mg/kg/day (based on TMP) intravenously (IV) given every 6 to 8 hours, or
        - Ceftriaxone 2 to 4 g IV every 24 hours, or
        - Cefotaxime 1 g IV every 6 hours, or
        - Cefoperazone 1 g IV every 12 hours, or
        - Ciprofloxacin 200 to 400 mg IV every 12 hours, or

       Gentamicin 1.5 mg/kg IV once, then 1 mg/kg IV every 8 hours, and

       Ampicillin 1 g IV every 4 hours, or (if *Pseudomonas* is suspected)

       Piperacillin 2 g IV every 6 hours given until fever is gone for 24 hours, then

    –TMP-SMX DS 1 tablet orally 2 times a day, or

       Amoxicillin 500 mg orally every 6 hours, or

       Ciprofloxacin 500 mg orally 2 times a day, or

       Cephalexin 500 mg orally 4 times a day for 14 days

   —Complicated, serious infections, with evidence of sepsis, or hospital-acquired

    –Ceftazidime 3 to 6 g/day IV given every 8 to 12 hours, or

       Ticarcillin-clavulanate 4 to 24 g/day (based on ticarcillin) IV given every 4 to 6 hours, or

       Aztreonam 1 to 2 g IV every 6 to 8 hours, or

       Imipenem 2 g/day IV given every 6 hours, and

       Gentamicin 1.5 mg/kg IV 1 time, then 1 mg/kg IV every 8 hours, or

       Ciprofloxacin 200 to 400 mg IV every 12 hours given until fever is gone for 48 hours, then

    –Oral therapy as above

- Surgical drainage for obstruction

- Prophylaxis for recurrent reinfections of the urinary tract:

  - Nitrofurantoin 50 mg orally each night at bedtime, or

       TMP-SMX $\frac{1}{2}$ tablet orally each night at bedtime, or

> Ciprofloxacin 250 mg orally each night at bedtime
- Monthly urine cultures as follow-up
- Bacteriuria of pregnancy:
  - Amoxicillin + clavulanate 0.5 g (based on amoxicillin) orally every 8 hours, or
    > Cephalexin 500 mg orally 4 times a day, or
    > Nitrofurantoin 50 to 100 mg orally every 6 hours for 3 to 7 days
- Perinephric abscess:
  - Antimicrobial therapy as for pyelonephritis
  - Surgical drainage should be considered where
    —Patient responds poorly to antimicrobial therapy alone
    —Pain and inflammation become severe
    —Renal function is threatened because of compression effect or external ureteral obstruction

Follow-Up:

- UTI can be managed as outpatient; most cases of pyelonephritis should be managed as inpatients
- UTI in men should be followed closely until patient is improved clinically; urinalysis should be repeated after treatment
- First or rare UTI in nonpregnant, young women or women who present with frequency/urgency/dysuria syndrome, and are cured after single-dose therapy requires no follow-up
- All other women should have post-treatment urine culture
- Patient with pyelonephritis should be retested at 2, 6, and 12 weeks after therapy with urine culture

- **Watch for:** signs and symptoms of
    - UTI → pyelonephritis
    - Pyelonephritis → urosepsis and shock
    - Renal abscess or perinephric abscess
    - Prostatitis
    - Recurrent infections
    - Chronic renal insufficiency
    - Renal scarring from recurrent infections

SYPHILIS

Presenting Symptoms:

SUBJECTIVE   OBJECTIVE

Primary Syphilis

Single painless papule in the genital area that erodes quickly into a nontender ulcer

May be slightly tender to the touch

Primary chancre appears an average of 21 days after sexual contact (3 to 90 day range)

Ulcer has a raised, hard border with a smooth, clean yellow base

There is little or no pain or bleeding when the ulcer is scraped

Ulcers are usually solitary, but may be multiple, especially in human immunodeficiency virus (HIV)-infected patient

| | Regional lymphadenopathy common |
| | Primary chancre heals with scarring in 3 to 6 weeks with no further symptoms in 75% of cases |

Secondary Syphilis

Symptoms begin 2 to 8 weeks after the appearance of the chancre in 25% of patients	Bilateral pink to red macular lesions beginning on trunk and proximal extremities, 3 to 10 mm in diameter, persisting from 3 to 4 days to 8 weeks, often evolving to papules and pustules (never vesicles)
Macular, maculopapular, papular, and/or pustular rash on trunk, extremities, palms and soles	
Patchy alopecia	Alopecia can involve head, eyebrows, and beard
Moist, pink, flat, warty growths in perianal area, vulva, scrotum, penis, thighs, and under breasts (condylomata lata)	Condylomata lata in intertriginous areas
Silvery gray erosive patches on all mucous surfaces	Mucous patches of mouth and throat, vulva, vagina, penis, cervix, and anal canal
Low-grade fever	Generalized painless lymphadenopathy
Malaise	
Pharyngitis, laryngitis	Meningismus (40% of patients)
Anorexia, weight loss	
Arthralgias	Cranial nerve (CN) II–VIII abnormalities
Headache	
Meningeal signs	Diplopia

Visual disturbances
Tinnitus
Vertigo
Nocturnal bone pain
Gastritis

Decreased vision
Anterior uveitis
(pathognomonically
worsened by
steroids)
Synovitis
Osteitis
Periosteitis
Mild
hepatosplenomegaly

Latent Syphilis

No clinical
manifestations of
syphilis

No clinical
manifestations of
syphilis
Positive serology for
syphilis
—Fluorescent
treponemal antibody
absorption (FTA-ABS)
—*Treponema pallidum*
hemagglutination
(TPHA) test
—Microhemagglutination-
T. pallidum (MHA-
TP) test
—*T. pallidum*
immobilization (TPI)
test
Patient may display
mucocutaneous
relapse during this
time (25% in first
year; 5% in second
year; less than 1%
after that)
Patients with late latent

syphilis (more than 4 years) are not infectious via sexual intercourse, but infection can still be transmitted in utero or via transfused blood

Late (Tertiary) Syphilis

Complaints of coronary artery disease, coronary insufficiency, and aortic regurgitation
—Chest pain
—Exertional dyspnea
—Signs of congestive heart failure
Complaints of neurosyphilis
—Hemiplegia; hemiparesis
—Seizures
—Personality changes
—Slurring of speech
—Pupils do not accommodate to light
—Tremors of face, tongue, hands, and legs
—Shooting or lightning pains in extremities
—Ataxia
—Loss of peripheral vision

Cardiovascular syphilis
—Signs of aortic regurgitation
—Signs of coronary artery stenosis
—Signs of nondissecting aortic aneurysms
Neurosyphilis (asymptomatic in up to 30% of patients)
—Hemiplegia; hemiparesis
—Focal or generalized seizures
—Aphasia
—Change in personality, sensorium, intellect, insight, and judgment
—Speech disturbances
—Argyll Robertson pupils
—"Gun barrel" vision (concentric constriction of visual fields)
—Tabes dorsalis

—Urinary/fecal incontinence
—Peripheral neuropathies
—Asymmetric deafness
Complaints of gummatous syphilis
—Superficial nodules to deep granulomatous lesions located anywhere on the body

—Romberg's sign
—Abnormalities of CN II through VIII (especially VII and VIII) leading to loss of facial expression and tremors of lips, tongue, and facial muscles
Granulomatous gummas

Congenital Syphilis (first 6 to 12 months)

Snuffles (rhinitis)
Diffuse desquamative rash
Saddle nose deformity
Anterior bowing of legs
Jaundice
Inflammation of umbilical cord (swollen and discolored red, white, and blue; "Barber's Pole" appearance)

Diffuse maculopapular desquamative rash with extensive epithelial sloughing, especially on palms, soles, around the mouth and anus
Vesicular rash and bullae may result
Generalized osteochondritis
—Saddle nose deformity
—Saber shins
Hepatosplenomegaly
Jaundice
Umbilical necrotizing funisitis

(after 6 to 12 months)

Photophobia
Eye pain

Frontal bossing
Short maxillas

Corneal inflammation
Deafness
Bilateral knee swelling
Widely spread, peg-
  shaped upper
  incisors

Saddle nose deformity
Protruding mandible
Interstitial keratitis
CN VIII deafness
Hutchinson's incisors
Mulberry molars
Clutton's joints
  (painless bilateral
  knee effusions with
  diffuse arthropathy)
Saber shins
Flaring scapulas
Circumcorneal
  inflammation
Corneal
  neovascularization

Differential Diagnosis:

Primary syphilis
—Chancroid
—Lymphogranuloma venereum
—Granuloma inguinale
—Herpes simplex genitalis
—Behçet's syndrome
—Traumatic suprainfected genital lesions
Secondary syphilis
—Pityriasis rosea
—Guttate psoriasis
—Drug eruption
—Hepatitis
—Glomerulonephritis due to immune complexes
  of another cause
—Anterior uveitis
—Arthritis
—Meningitis/encephalitis
—Epilepsy
Latent syphilis
—Previously treated syphilis

—False-positive serology for syphilis
  –Collagen vascular diseases (especially systemic lupus erythematosus or rheumatoid arthritis)
  –Thyroiditis
  –Hypergammaglobulinemia
  –Pregnancy
  –Multiple blood transfusions
  –Chronic liver disease
  –Drug addiction
  –Other spirochetal infection
    —Yaws
    —Pinta
    —Leptospirosis
    —Relapsing fever
    —Rat-bite fever
    —Lyme disease
  –Other infectious diseases
    —Leprosy
    —Tuberculosis
    —Pneumococcal pneumonia
    —*Mycoplasma* pneumonia
    —Subacute bacterial endocarditis
    —Scarlet fever
    —Rickettsial disease
    —Malaria
    —Trypanosomiasis
    —Measles
    —Chickenpox
    —Infectious mononucleosis
    —Early HIV infection

Suggested Workup:

- Laboratory:
  - Darkfield examination for *T. pallidum* of serous transudate from:
    —Primary chancre

- —Condyloma lata
- —Mucous patch
- —Dry skin lesion
- —Lymph node aspiration
- A lesion can be considered nonsyphilitic after three negative examinations
- Biopsy of lesion and testing with specific immunofluorescent or immunoperoxidase staining
- Serology:
  - Nonspecific nontreponemal reaginic tests (useful as an initial screen and to follow the efficacy of therapy)
    - —Venereal Disease Research Laboratories (VDRL) test (percent positive in primary, secondary, and late syphilis: 70%, 99%, 56%, respectively)
    - —Persistently positive VDRL after apparently adequate therapy may be biologically false reaction, persistent active infection, or reinfection, especially with a titer greater than $1:4$
    - —Rapid plasma reagin (RPR) test (80%, 99%, 56% positive in primary, secondary, and late syphilis, respectively)
      - –Should become nonreactive 1 year after successful therapy (2 years after therapy of secondary syphilis and 5 years after therapy for late syphilis)
    - —Automated reagin test (ART)
  - Specific treponemal tests (useful as a means to confirm the diagnosis of syphilis, but not for assessing the adequacy of therapy)
    - —FTA-ABS (fluorescent antibody absorbed test) (85%, 100%, 98% positive in primary, secondary, and late syphilis, respectively)
      - –Once positive, it remains so for life in 90% of patients

- –Difficult to quantitate
- –High sensitivity; poor specificity
- —TPHA (65%, 100%, 95% positive in primary, secondary, and late syphilis, respectively): less sensitive and more specific than FTS-ABS
- —MHA-TP (a microtiter adaptation of TPHA)
- —TPI (50%, 97%, 95% positive in primary, secondary, and late syphilis, respectively): expensive and time-consuming
- —Tests for neurosyphilis
  - –Cerebrospinal fluid (CSF)-VDRL
  - –Intrathecal *T. pallidum* antibody index) (ITPA)
  - –CSF-FTA unABS
  - –CSF-TPHA
- Polymerase chain reaction (PCR) test for syphilis (positive test is confirmatory)
  - Blood
  - CSF (confirmatory for neurosyphilis)

Definitive Diagnosis:

Syphilis	ICD-9-CM 097.9
Congenital syphilis	ICD-9-CM 090.9
Neurosyphilis	ICD-9-CM 094.9

Suggested Treatment:

- Early syphilis (primary or secondary or latent for less than 1 year):
  - HIV-negative (HIV−) patients or HIV-positive (HIV+) patients with CD4 count greater than 400:
    - Benzathine penicillin (PCN) G 2.4 million units (U) intramuscularly for 1 dose (Penicillin allergy: Doxycycline 200 mg orally twice a day for 15 days, or Erythromycin 500 mg orally 4 times a day for 15 days, or penicillin desensitization)

- HIV+ patients with CD4 count less than 400 and/or symptomatic:
  Benzathine PCN G 2.4 million U intramuscularly for 1 dose or
  2.4 million U intramuscularly weekly for 2 to 3 weeks, and
  Amoxicillin 3 g + probenecid 500 mg orally twice a day for 10 days
  (Penicillin allergy: Doxycycline 200 mg orally twice a day for 21 days, or
  Ceftriaxone 1 g intramuscularly daily for 14 days, or penicillin desensitization)
- Late syphilis or neurosyphilis:
  - Aqueous crystalline PCN G 2.0 to 4.0 million U IV every 4 hours for 10 days, or
    Procaine PCN G 2.4 million U/day intramuscularly + probenecid 500 mg orally 2 times a day for 10 to 14 days, or
    Amoxicillin 3 g + probenecid 500 mg orally twice a day for 15 days,
    (Penicillin allergy: Doxycycline 200 mg orally twice a day for 21 days, or
    Ceftriaxone 1 g/day intramuscularly/IV for 14 days, or
    Chloramphenicol 2 g IV or 500 mg orally every 6 hours for 30 days, or penicillin desensitization)
- Congenital syphilis:
  - Aqueous crystalline PCN G 50,000 U/kg/day IV given every 12 hours for 10 days, or
    Procaine PCN G 50,000 U/kg/day intramuscularly for 10 days
    (Penicillin allergy: penicillin desensitization)
  - Treatment is recommended for all infants born to syphilitic mothers

- Treatment of syphilis in pregnancy:
  - Same regimens as for nonpregnant patients
  - Only penicillin therapy reliably treats the infant
  - Penicillin-allergic patients should be desensitized

Follow-Up:

- Outpatient care is appropriate except where intravenous therapy or penicillin desensitization is contemplated
- All patients with early and congenital syphilis should have repeat quantitative nontreponemal serologic tests 3, 6, and 12 months after therapy
- All patients with secondary syphilis or syphilis for longer than 1 year should have repeat nontreponemal serologic testing 24 months after treatment
- All patients with neurosyphilis should have periodic CSF examinations and serology testing for at least 5 years
- All HIV+ patients with syphilis should have aggressive post-treatment serologic follow-up at 1, 2, 3, 6, 9, and 12 months
- Retreatment should be considered for any patient if:
  - Clinical signs and symptoms of syphilis persist or recur
  - There is a sustained level or increase in the titer of a nontreponemal serology test
  - Whenever a positive RPR test persists beyond 12 months in primary syphilis, 24 months in secondary or latent syphilis, and 5 years in late syphilis
  - There is a positive PCR test
- Trace and treat all sexual contacts of the patient

- Advise patient to avoid all sexual contact until treatment is completed
- **Watch for:** signs and symptoms of
    - Cardiovascular complications
        - —Coronary insufficiency
        - —Aortic regurgitation
        - —Aneurysms of ascending aorta
    - CNS complications
        - —Deafness
        - —Ataxia
        - —Paresis
        - —Seizure activity
        - —Loss of vision
        - —Change in sensorium
    - Membranous glomerulonephritis
    - Multiorgan system failure

GONORRHEA

Presenting Symptoms:

SUBJECTIVE	OBJECTIVE
In Men	
Purulent urethral discharge, scant to copious	Elicit history of sexual contact 2 to 5 days before onset of symptoms
Dysuria	symptoms
Testicular pain	Purulent urethral discharge
	Penile edema seen occasionally
	Epididymitis may be present
In Homosexual Men	
Purulent or bloody rectal discharge	Purulent or bloody rectal discharge

Tenesmus	Mucopurulent exudate
Rectal burning or discharge	and inflamed rectal mucosa on anoscopic exam

In Women

Vaginal discharge	Elicit history of sexual contact within 10 days of symptoms
Dysuria	
Vulvar pain and inflammation	Mucopurulent cervical exudate may be seen on pelvic examination
	Purulent discharge may be expressed from the urethra or Bartholin's gland ducts
	Cervical, fundal, or adnexal tenderness suggests PID (see section on pelvic diseases)

Pharyngeal Infections

Typically asymptomatic	Exudative pharyngitis with adenopathy rarely seen (less than 1%)

Ocular Autoinfection

Purulent exudate and pain in affected eye	Overtly purulent corneal exudate
	Corneal ulceration may be present

Disseminated Infection

Fever, chills	Signs of arthritis, tenosynovitis, or periarticular inflammation in
Migratory polyarthralgias	
Pain and swelling of	

hands and feet	knees, elbows, or
Painful skin lesions	distal joints, typically beginning as a migratory polyarthritis and evolving to a monoarticular septic arthritis with asymmetric involvement
	Discrete, hemorrhagic papules and pustules, occurring predominantly on the extremities

Differential Diagnosis:

Chlamydial infections
UTIs
Other bacterial vaginosis
Vaginal yeast infection
Trichomonas infection of vagina
Ecthyma gangrenosum
Sweet's syndrome
Meningococcemia
Infective arthritis
Reiter's syndrome

Suggested Workup:

- Laboratory:
  - Gram stain of exudate from infected mucosal surface
  - In men, urethral smear (collected with a swab inserted 2 to 3 cm into the urethra) has 95% sensitivity
  - In women, endocervical smear (collected by placing a swab in the external os, exercising care to avoid vaginal mucosa or secretions) has 80% to 90% sensitivity

- Culture of exudate on selective media for *Neisseria gonorrhoeae* (Thayer-Martin or Martin-Lewis)
- Culture of rectal specimens on selective media
  - Rectal specimen should be obtained by passing a swab 2 to 4 cm into the anal canal
  - Specimens heavily contaminated with feces should be discarded
- Culture of pharyngeal specimens: obtained by swabbing posterior pharynx and tonsillar pillars
- Blood culture: 50% sensitivity in disseminated disease
- Gram stain and culture of joint fluid: 50% sensitivity in patients with gonococcal arthritis

Definitive Diagnosis:

Acute gonorrhea   ICD-9-CM 098.0

Suggested Treatment:

- Uncomplicated anogenital gonorrhea in adults:
  - Ceftriaxone 250 mg intramuscularly for 1 dose, or
    Ceftizoxime 500 mg intramuscularly for 1 dose, or
    Cefixime 400 mg orally for 1 dose, or
    Ciprofloxacin 500 mg orally for 1 dose, or
    Ofloxacin 400 mg orally for 1 dose
  FOLLOWED BY
  - Azithromycin 1 g orally for 1 dose, or
    Doxycycline 100 mg orally 2 times a day for 7 days, or
    Erythromycin 500 mg orally 4 times a day for 7 days
- Uncomplicated anogenital gonorrhea in pregnant women:
  - Ceftriaxone 250 mg intramuscularly once

FOLLOWED BY
- Erythromycin 500 mg orally 4 times a day
  for 7 to 10 days
- Ascending genital infection in women (PID;
  see also pelvic diseases section):
  - Hospitalized patients:
    —Cefoxitin 2.0 g IV every 6 hours, or
      Cefotetan 2.0 g IV every 8 hours, and
      Doxycycline 100 mg IV/orally every
        12 hours for 48 hours past the time
        the patient substantially improves,
        FOLLOWED BY Doxycycline
        alone for a total of 14 days of
        therapy; or
    —Clindamycin 900 mg IV every 8
      hours, and
        Gentamicin 2.0 mg/kg IV 1 time, then
        1.5 mg/kg IV every 8 hours for 48
        hours past the time the patient
        substantially improves,
        FOLLOWED BY
      Doxycycline 100 mg orally twice a
      day, or
      Clindamycin 450 mg orally 4 times a
        day for a total of 14 days of therapy
  - Outpatients:
    —Cefoxitin 2.0 g intramuscularly +
      probenecid 1.0 g orally 1 time, or
        Ceftriaxone 250 mg intramuscularly 1
          time, or
        Ceftizoxime 2.0 g intramuscularly 1
          time, or
        Cefotaxime 2.0 g intramuscularly 1
          time, FOLLOWED BY
        Doxycycline 100 mg orally 2 times a
          day for 14 days; or

—Ofloxacin 400 mg orally twice a day for 14 days, and

Clindamycin 450 mg orally 4 times a day, or

Metronidazole 500 mg orally twice a day for 14 days

- Disseminated gonococcal infection:
  - Ceftriaxone 1.0 g intramuscularly/IV every day until there is significant clinical improvement (typically no less than 7 days), FOLLOWED BY
  - Cefixime 400 mg orally twice a day, or
  - Ciprofloxacin 500 to 750 mg orally twice a day, or
  - Cefaclor 500 mg orally every 8 hours, or
  - Cefuroxime 250 mg orally twice a day for a total of 10 to 14 days of therapy
- Gonorrhea in children: Ceftriaxone 25 to 50 mg/kg intramuscularly (up to 125 mg) 1 time—continue treatment for 7 to 10 days if disseminated disease or gonococcal conjunctivitis are present

Follow-Up:

- Most patients can be managed as outpatients
- In-hospital care appropriate for patients with disseminated disease, PID, gonococcal meningitis or endocarditis, or infants with pneumonia or conjunctivitis
- Repeat cultures from mucosal sites 1 to 2 weeks after completing therapy
- Encourage testing for syphilis and HIV infection
- Patients should refrain from sexual activity until after follow-up examination and testing and treatment of sexual partner(s)
- Discuss "safe sex" practices with patient; encourage condom use

- **Watch for:** signs and symptoms of
  - Gonococcal meningitis
  - Gonococcal endocarditis with destruction of cardiac valves, especially aortic
  - Gonococcal conjunctivitis with eventual corneal scarring
  - Gonococcal arthritis with destruction of joint articular surfaces
  - Disseminated disease
  - Urethral stricture in men
  - Tubal scarring and infertility in women
  - Syphilis or HIV infection
  - Hepatitis B infection
  - Other sexually transmitted diseases (STDs)

SEXUALLY TRANSMITTED NONGONOCOCCAL URETHRITIS

Presenting Symptoms:

SUBJECTIVE	OBJECTIVE
Many patients may be asymptomatic carriers	Scanty urethral discharge on "milking" of the urethra
Dysuria	
Scanty urethral discharge	May be epididymal tenderness
Suprapubic discomfort	May be signs of bartholinitis
Urethral itching or tenderness of urethral meatus	Elicit history of risk factors
Dyspareunia	—Sexual promiscuity

Symptoms of proctitis —Lower
socioeconomic group
—History of STDs

Differential Diagnosis:

Gonococcal urethritis
Postgonococcal urethritis
Epididymitis
Cervicitis
PID
Reiter's syndrome
Lymphogranuloma venereum
Proctitis
Syphilis
UTI
Intraurethral growth (e.g., polyps, warts)
Atrophic vaginitis
Vaginal hypersensitivity reaction
Chronic amphetamine use (women)
Stevens-Johnson syndrome

Suggested Workup:

- Microbiology:
  - Gram stain and culture of urethral
    discharge
    —Polymorphonuclear leukocytes (PMNs)
      with intracellular diplococci → *N.
      gonorrhoeae*
    —Sheets of PMNs without bacteria →
      Chlamydia trachomatis
  - Urinalysis and urine culture
- Cytology: Cytology brush scraping of urethra,
  transported in sucrose-phosphate antibiotic-
  supplemented media—diagnostic for
  Chlamydia
- Laboratory:
  - VDRL
  - HIV testing

- Reagin test for *Chlamydia*
  - PCR for *Chlamydia* if confirmatory testing is required
- Invasive testing reserved for patients with persistent symptoms despite adequate antimicrobial therapy:
  - Urethrogram
  - Urethrocystoscopy to rule out intraurethral growths or foreign bodies

Definitive Diagnosis:

Nongonococcal urethritis   ICD-9-CM 099.40

Suggested Treatment:

- Primary uncomplicated infection with *C. trachomatis:*
  - Doxycycline 100 mg orally twice a day for 7 days, or
  - Azithromycin 1 g orally 1 time, or
  - Erythromycin 250 mg orally 4 times a day for 14 days or 500 mg orally 3 times a day for 7 days, or
  - Ofloxacin 300 mg orally twice a day for 7 days
- *Chlamydia* in pregnancy:
  - Amoxicillin 500 mg orally 3 times a day for 10 days, or
  - Erythromycin 250 mg orally 4 times a day for 14 days or 500 mg orally 3 times a day for 7 days

Follow-Up:

- Outpatient care is appropriate
- Repeat cultures (for patients with positive cultures in the first place) several days after completing treatment
- Identify and treat all sexual partners
- Counsel regarding condom use

- **Watch for:** signs and symptoms of
  - Chronic pelvic pain
  - Urethral stricture formation
  - PID
  - Problems with future pregnancies
    - Infertility
    - Ectopic pregnancy

CHANCROID

Presenting Symptoms:

<u>SUBJECTIVE</u>

Tender papule in genital area that later forms a pustule and then erodes into an ulcer within 24 hours after appearance

Painful "swollen glands" in inguinal region

Ulcers may be single or multiple

<u>OBJECTIVE</u>

Painful, nonindurated, ragged ulcers with erythematous base

Ulcers bleed easily on manipulation

Men usually have single ulcers located on the shaft of the penis, the glans, or the meatus

Women typically have multiple lesions located on the fourchette, labia, vestibule, clitoris, cervix and anus

Ulcers vary in size from 1 mm to 5 cm in diameter

Tender unilateral inguinal lymphadenopathy is common

> If untreated, ulcers may become confluent and suppurative with periadenitis (bubo formation); the abscesses may rupture to form draining sinuses
>
> Elicit history of sexual intercourse with suspect carrier an average of 5 to 7 days before appearance of symptoms

Differential Diagnosis:

Syphilis
Herpes simplex ulcerative disease
Lymphogranuloma venereum
Granuloma inguinale
Malignancy

Suggested Workup:

- Microbiology:
    - Collect ulcer exudate for Gram stain and culture
    - Aspirate bubo for Gram stain and culture—*Haemophilus ducreyi*
    - Collect ulcer exudate and/or aspirate bubo for darkfield examination for *T. pallidum* to exclude syphilis
- Laboratory:
    - VDRL to exclude syphilis
    - Immunofluorescence test for *H. ducreyi*

Definitive Diagnosis:

Chancroid   ICD-9 CM 099.0

Suggested Treatment:

Erythromycin 500 mg orally 4 times a day for 7
days, or
Azithromycin 1 g orally for 1 dose, or
Ceftriaxone 250 mg intramuscularly 1 time (high
failure rate in men with concomitant HIV
infection), or
Ciprofloxacin 750 mg orally for 1 dose, or 500 mg
orally twice a day for 3 days

Follow-Up:

- Outpatient treatment is satisfactory; follow
  until all clinical signs of infection are resolved
- If baseline VDRL is negative, repeat 3 months
  later
- Needle aspiration of suppurated or fluctuant
  nodes should be performed to prevent
  rupture, sinus formation, and scarring
- Identify all sexual partners of patient and treat
  with antibiotic regimen
- Educate patient and sexual partners regarding
  condom use and not to engage in sexual
  intercourse until infection is resolved
- **Watch for:** signs and symptoms of
    - Phimosis
    - Balanoposthitis
    - Rupture of buboes
    - Chronic abscess formation
    - Draining sinus formation
    - Genital scarring
    - HIV infection
    - Relapse (5% even with adequate
      treatment)

VULVOVAGINITIS

Presenting Symptoms:

SUBJECTIVE	OBJECTIVE
Bacterial Vulvovaginitis	
Unpleasant vaginal odor	Mild vaginal inflammation
—Musty or fishy	Labia and vulva generally not erythematous
—Exacerbated by sexual intercourse	
Vaginal discharge, usually thin, gray, and modest	Vaginal walls usually appear uninflammed, but may be covered with thin, gray discharge that appears floccular and contains bubbles; discharge usually not copious enough to pool in the vagina or posterior fornix
Mild vulvovaginal irritation	
Dysuria and dyspareunia are rare	
	Normal endocervix
	Bimanual examination generally normal
Fungal Vulvovaginitis	
Intense vulvar itching	Labia pale or erythematous, often with excoriations
Thick, curdy vaginal discharge	
Erythema of vulva and perineum	Posterior portion of introitus typically exhibits shallow, linear ulcerations
Dyspareunia common	
Vulvar rather than urethral dysuria	Tiny satellite papules or pustules are seen often

Curdy, thick vaginal discharge

Trichomoniasis

Yellow-green frothy vaginal discharge	Copious, loose discharge
Vulvovaginal irritation	Cases divided:
Dysuria common	—50% with normal-appearing vulva
Fishy vaginal odor	
Dyspareunia common	—50% with vulvovaginal inflammation/erythema
Suprapubic discomfort	
Symptoms often begin or are exacerbated during menstruation	Vaginal hyperemia is typical
	"Strawberry cervix" (due to punctate hemorrhages) seen in 2% to 5% of cases, but visualized in up to 50% by colposcopy

Differential Diagnosis:

Cervicitis
Vulvovaginitis of another etiology
Gonorrhea
Contact dermatitis/vaginitis
Chlamydial infection

Suggested Workup:

- Microbiology
  - Vaginal secretions are collected for:
    —Wet mount
      –Clue cells (vaginal epithelial cells studded with coccobacilli) → bacterial infection

> –Presence of motile *Trichomonas vaginalis* with no clue cells (i.e., normal epithelial cells) → trichomoniasis
> —pH determination
> > –pH greater than 4.5 in trichomoniasis
> > –pH less than 4.5 in candidal vulvovaginitis
> > –pH greater than 4.5 in bacterial vulvovaginitis
> —10% potassium hydroxide (KOH) smear
> > –Yeast, spores, and/or pseudohyphae present → candidal infection
> > –Positive Whiff test: (transient amine or fishy odor) → bacterial vulvovaginitis;
> > –Negative results: → trichomoniasis
> —Gram stain
> > –Clumps of coccobacilli with no large rods (normal *Lactobacillus* flora of vagina) → bacterial
> > –Negative results → trichomoniasis or fungal infection
> —Culture
> > –For *Trichomonas* on Diamond's medium has an 85% to 90% sensitivity
> > –For *Candida* on Sabouraud's or Nickerson's media is usually not necessary if KOH smear is positive
> > –For *Gardnerella vaginalis* has a 92% to 98% sensitivity for bacterial vulvovaginitis

- Serology (generally not recommended for diagnostic workup of individual patients)
  - Trichomoniasis—enzyme-linked immunosorbent assay (ELISA) and fluorescent antibody tests are available and have 85% to 90% sensitivity
  - Candidal infection—latex agglutination test has only 60% sensitivity

- Pap smear: can be used to distinguish between candidal vulvovaginitis and trichomoniasis
- HIV testing recommended in severe cases of candidal infection

Definitive Diagnosis:

Bacterial vulvovaginitis/ vaginosis	ICD-9-CM 616.10
Candidal vulvovaginitis	ICD-9-CM 112.1
Trichomonal vulvovaginitis	ICD-9-CM 131.01

Suggested Treatment:

- Bacterial vulvovaginitis:
    - Metronidazole 250 mg orally 3 times a day or 500 mg orally twice a day for 7 days, or
    - Metronidazole 2 g orally for 1 dose, or
    - Clindamycin 300 mg orally twice a day for 7 days, or
    - Cephalexin 250 mg orally 4 times a day for 7 days (primarily anecdotal data), or
    - Cefadroxil 500 mg orally 2 times a day for 7 days, or
    - Clindamycin 2% vaginal cream 5 g vaginally each night at bedtime for 7 days, or
    - Metronidazole 0.75% vaginal gel 5 g vaginally twice a day for 5 days
- Candidal vulvovaginitis:
    - Single dose:
        Miconazole 1200 mg vaginal suppository, or
        Clotrimazole 500 mg vaginal
            suppository, or 10% cream 5 g
            vaginally, or 6.5% cream 4.6 g
            vaginally
    - Three-day course:
        Miconazole 200 mg vaginal suppository
            each night at bedtime, or
        Clotrimazole 200 mg vaginal suppository
            each night at bedtime, or

Butoconazole 2% cream 5 g vaginally
each night at bedtime, or
Tioconazole 2% cream 5 g vaginally each
night at bedtime, or
Econazole 150 mg vaginal suppository
each night at bedtime, or
Terconazole 0.8% cream 5 g vaginally or
80 mg vaginal suppository each night
at bedtime
- Seven-day course:
    Miconazole 2% cream 5 g vaginally or
        100 mg vaginal suppository each night
        at bedtime, or
    Clotrimazole 100 mg vaginal suppository
        or 1% cream 5 g vaginally each night
        at bedtime, or
    Terconazole 0.4% cream vaginally each
        night at bedtime
- Fourteen-day course:
    Nystatin 100,000 U vaginal suppository
        each night at bedtime
- Oral medication is not approved by the
    Food and Drug Administration (FDA) for
    this use, but may be tried in resistant or
    recurrent, hard to treat cases:
    Ketoconazole 200 mg orally twice a day
        for 3 to 5 days or 200 mg orally once
        a day for 3 days or 150 mg orally for
        1 dose, or
    Fluconazole 200 mg orally twice a day
        for 1 day or 150 mg orally for 1
        dose, or
    Itraconazole 200 mg orally twice a day
        for 1 day or 200 mg orally once a day
        for 3 days
- Trichomoniasis: Metronidazole 2 g orally
    1 time, or 250 mg orally 3 times a day or
    500 mg orally 2 times a day for 7 days

Follow-Up:

- Outpatient care is appropriate
- Monitor patient symptoms after therapy is completed
- Repeat pelvic exam if symptoms persist after treatment
- Examine and treat all sex partners
- Workup immunodeficiency (e.g., HIV infection) in patients with recurrent or severe cases of candidal vulvovaginitis
- **Watch for:** signs and symptoms of
    - Recurrent infection
    - Incompletely treated infection
    - Ascending infection (rare)
    - PID
    - Pelvic abscess
    - Secondary bacterial infections of vulva or vagina
    - Development of metronidazole resistance by *Trichomonas*—can try:
      —Metronidazole 2 g orally daily plus 500 mg tablet broken and inserted vaginally for 3 to 14 days
      —Timidazole (not available in the United States) 2 g orally daily for 2 days
      —Metronidazole 2 g IV given every 6 to 8 hours

CERVICITIS

Presenting Symptoms:

SUBJECTIVE	OBJECTIVE
Frequently asymptomatic	Mucopurulent discharge from the cervix
May be a yellow, foul vaginal discharge	Cervical tenderness on palpation

Evidence of erosion or
erythema around the
cervical os
Easily induced
endocervical mucosal
bleeding
Cervical ulcers (herpes
cervicitis only)
Elicit history of risk
factors
—Multiple sex
partners
—Previous STDs
—Postpartum period

Differential Diagnosis:

Vaginitis ascending into the cervix
Cervical ectropion
Cervical malignancy

Suggested Workup:

- Microbiology:
  - Endocervical swab for Gram stain and
    culture
  - Presence of greater than 10 WBCs high
    power field (hpf) suggests cervicitis
  - Gram stain and culture should identify
    C. trachomatis or *N. gonorrhoeae*
  - Endocervical swab for wet mount—can
    detect *T. vaginalis*
  - Endocervical swab for culture for herpes
    simplex (may be present even without
    cervical ulceration)
- Laboratory:
  - VDRL to rule out concurrent syphilis
  - HIV testing
- Colposcopy: generally reserved for chronic
  cases that fail to respond to antimicrobial
  therapy, or in patients with suspicious areas

Definitive Diagnosis:

Acute cervicitis   ICD-9-CM 616.0
Gonococcal cervicitis   ICD-9-CM 098.15
Chlamydial cervicitis   ICD-9-CM 099.53
Trichomonal cervicitis   ICD-9-CM 131.09

Suggested Treatment:

- Empiric therapy for infectious cervicitis without specific culture results, or for gonococcal cervicitis:
    - Ceftriaxone 250 mg intramuscularly once, FOLLOWED BY
    - Doxycycline 100 mg orally twice a day for 7 days, or
    - Azithromycin 1 g orally for 1 dose, or
    - Erythromycin 500 mg orally 4 times a day for 7 days, or
    - Ofloxacin 400 mg orally twice a day for 7 days
- Chlamydial cervicitis: as above, but without Ceftriaxone
- Trichomonal cervicitis: Metronidazole 2 g orally for 1 dose
- Herpes cervicitis: Acyclovir 200 mg orally 5 times a day for 7 to 10 days

Follow-Up:

- Outpatient treatment is appropriate
- May repeat Gram stain and cultures after treatment, especially in high-risk patients (generally not required for most patients)
- Evaluate and treat all recent sex partners
- Advise abstinence until treatment is complete
- Advise condom use
- Reinforce need for annual Pap tests
- **Watch for:** signs and symptoms of
    - PID
    - Chronic cervicitis

- Development of cervical dysplasia
- Other STDs
  - —Syphilis
  - —HIV infection
  - —Human papillomavirus (HPV) infection

CONDYLOMA ACUMINATA

Presenting Symptoms:

<u>SUBJECTIVE</u>
Fleshy, gray-colored finger-like projections on the skin in the genital area
Pruritus
Irritation
Burning
Tenderness

<u>OBJECTIVE</u>
Flesh- to gray-colored, hyperkeratotic, exophytic papules
Sessile or pedunculate on a short, broad stalk
May be smooth or jagged, cauliflower-like lesions
Men typically have smooth, papular lesions on the penile shaft or urethral meatus; scrotal lesions are rarely seen, and perianal involvement varies according to sexual practice (high in homosexual men and low among heterosexuals)
Women typically have flatter, irregularly-

> shaped lesions distributed over the posterior introitus, labia, clitoris, periurethral area, perineum, vagina, cervix, and anus
>
> Elicit history of unprotected homosexual or heterosexual activity

Differential Diagnosis:

Condyloma lata (syphilis)
Lichen planus
Seborrheic keratosis
Molluscum contagiosum
Keratomas
Scabies
Verrucous carcinoma (women only)
Cervical intraepithelial neoplasia

Suggested Workup:

- Laboratory: VDRL to rule out syphilis
- Colposcopy:
  - Soak examined tissues with 5% acetic acid
    —Vulva, vagina, or cervix is "painted" with solution
    —Penis is wrapped with gauze soaked in solution
  - Warts will appear as tiny white papules
  - Epithelial hyperplasia without warts will appear as a shiny white area with no papules
  - Examination under a 10× power lens may be as useful as a colposcope, especially in male patients or female patients with

external lesions; colposcopy is
recommended for examination of the
vagina and cervix
- Anoscopy: examination as for colposcopy
- Pap smear
- Biopsy usually not necessary, but may be
indicated for persistent, treatment-resistant
warts—special techniques available for
identifying human Papilloma virus (HPV) in
biopsy material

Definitive Diagnosis:

Condyloma acuminatum   ICD-9-CM 078.1

Suggested Treatment:

- Inflammatory, immunostimulatory therapy
(best for early external lesions):
  - Podophyllin 20% to 25% in benzoin applied
topically for 2 to 3 minutes, then repeated
with a second coat; treated areas should be
washed 3 to 4 hours later with soap and
water; treatment can be repeated every 10
days for up to 4 cycles, or
  - Podofilox purified podophyllin, applied
twice a day for 3 days, then rest for 4 days,
then repeat cycle as needed (purified
material causes less severe local
inflammation than podophyllin), or
  - 5-Fluorouracil 2% to 5% solution or cream
applied topically daily until erythema or
desquamation develops, then not again
until healing ensues (severe local responses
can result in poorly healed vaginal lesions
with strictures and scarring)
- Ablative therapy (can be used for external
lesions of any age and, to a limited extent, for
internal lesions):
  - Trichloroacetic acid applied topically to
lesions and in a 1 to 2 mm margin around

the base of each lesion; there is no need to wash off the acid after application
—Healing occurs after 10 to 14 days
—May be repeated 3 to 4 weeks later
- Cryotherapy with liquid nitrogen applied topically to lesions in 5- to 10-second bursts; may require treatment for 2 to 3 days
- Carbon dioxide laser surgery
- Antiviral therapy:
  - Interferon-α_{2a} or -α_{2b} or -α_{n3} 0.25 to 1.0 million U injected intralesionally with a 30G needle 2 to 3 times a week for 3 to 4 weeks; cycle may be repeated for resistant lesions after a 1-month rest period, or
  - Interferon-α_{2a} or -α_{2b} or -α_{n3} 2 to 3 million U intramuscularly or subcutaneously every other day for 4 to 6 weeks, or (for resistant disease) 2 to 3 million U intramuscularly/ subcutaneously every day for 2 weeks, then 3 times a week or every other day for 2 to 4 weeks (therapy should be continued for at least 1 week after lesions have resolved)
- Combination therapy (for severe, extensive, or diffuse disease): Podophyllin or ablative therapy, followed by intermittent use of 5-Fluorouracil or interferon
- Surgical excision is reserved for very large warts that are resistant to more conservative treatment

Follow-Up:

- Follow as outpatient every 2 weeks until lesions are healed
- Biopsy persistent warts that are resistant to treatment
- Annual Pap smear test for all infected women for an indefinite period

- Monitor patient's sex partners
- Infected men should be instructed to wear condoms until all lesions are healed
- Infected women should abstain from sexual intercourse until all lesions are healed
- May consider circumcision in infected men to prevent recurrence
- **Watch for:** signs and symptoms of
  - Cervical dysplasia
  - Cervical, penile, or rectal carcinoma
  - Uretrhral obstruction (more common in men)
  - Vaginal strictures
  - Scarring of genital area

PELVIC INFECTIONS

Presenting Symptoms:

SUBJECTIVE	OBJECTIVE
Pelvic Inflammatory Disease	
May be asymptomatic	Direct lower quadrant
Abdominal pain	abdominal
Fever and malaise	tenderness
Vaginal discharge	Cervical motion
Dysuria	tenderness
Proctitis	Adnexal tenderness
Nausea, vomiting	Mucopurulent
	cervicitis
	Fever
	Unilateral or bilateral
	adnexal mass(es)
	(less common)
Pelvic Cellulitis	
Lower abdominal and	History of
pelvic pain occurring	hysterectomy 2 to 3
on second or third	days prior to onset

postoperative day
after hysterectomy
Fever

of symptoms
Direct tenderness over
parametrial area by
abdominal and
bimanual
examination

Pelvic Abscess

Lower abdominal pain
occurring weeks
after pelvic surgery
Fever with typical
spike in late
afternoon

Palpable mass high in
the pelvis

Intrapartum Chorioamnionitis

Fever
Uterine tenderness

Elicit risk factors
—Prolonged duration
of labor
—Premature rupture
of membranes for
prolonged time
—Preexisting bacterial
vaginosis
—Multiple vaginal
examinations
Fever
Tachycardia
Fetal heart rate
abnormalities

Postpartum Endometritis (Puerperal Fever)

Fever on the first or
second day
postpartum with
chills
Lower abdominal pain
Foul-smelling lochia

Elicit risk factors
—Indigent patients
—Prolonged
membrane rupture
—Midforceps delivery
—Maternal soft tissue
trauma

—Maternal anemia
—Diabetes
—Drug addiction
—History of STDs
—UTI
—Malnutrition
Fever 1 to 2 days
  postpartum
Uterine tenderness on
  abdominal or
  bimanual
  examination
Peritoneal signs may
  be present

Postabortion Infection

Fever and chills within
  4 days of procedure
Abdominal pain
Vaginal bleeding with
  passage of placental
  tissue

Elicit risk factors
—Long duration of
  pregnancy
—Technical difficulties
  with procedure
—Preexisting STD
Fever within 4 days of
  procedure
Tachycardia, tachypnea
Abdominal tenderness
  on examination
Sanguinopurulent
  discharge and
  uterine tenderness
  on pelvic
  examination
Hypotension and frank
  shock may be
  present
There may be evidence
  of disseminated

intravascular
coagulation (DIC)
—Jaundice
—Gross hematuria

Differential Diagnosis:

Appendicitis
Ectopic pregnancy
Torsion of the ovary
Ruptured ovarian cyst
Endometriosis
Inflammatory bowel disease
Irritable bowel syndrome
Septic pelvic thrombophlebitis
Osteomyelitis pubis
Ischemic bowel
Ovarian vein thrombophlebitis
Noninfectious surgical complications
Noninfectious fever (e.g., drug fever, breast
   engorgement in the puerperal period)

Suggested Workup:

- PID:
    - Endocervical swab for Gram stain
      and culture—may be able to detect
      N. gonorrhoeae and *C. trachomatis*
    - Endometrial transvaginal ultrasound—may
      show thickened, fluid-filled tubes
    - Endometrial biopsy—may show plasma
      cell endometritis (67% specificity for PID)
    - Laporoscopy and culdocentesis are
      generally reserved for patients with
      atypical clinical presentations or for those
      who have failed empiric therapy
    - Nonspecific laboratory findings:
      —Complete blood count (CBC) → WBC
        greater than $10{,}500/\text{mm}^3$

- —Erythrocyte sedimentation rate (ESR) greater than 15 mm/hour
- Pelvic cellulitis:
  - Swab of vaginal cuff for Gram stain and culture (care must be taken to avoid contamination with vaginal flora)
- Pelvic abscess:
  - Imaging studies
  - Ultrasound and/or CT scan of abdomen and pelvis
    - —Confirm the presence of a mass
    - —Determine if mass is loculated
    - —Establish anatomy (i.e., is mass related to an intraperitoneal structure?)
    - —Determine if mass is drainable percutaneously
- Intrapartum chorioamnionitis:
  - Obtain amniotic fluid for
    - —Gram stain and culture
    - —Leukocyte esterase activity $(1+/2+ \rightarrow$ infection likely)
    - —Glucose concentration (less than 16 mg/dL $\rightarrow$ infection likely)
- Postpartum endometritis:
  - Transvaginal uterine cultures
  - Blood cultures
  - Rapid antigen detection test for *Chlamydia*
  - Abdominal/pelvic ultrasound to look for abscess
- Postabortion infection:
  - Collect cervical swab for Gram stain and culture
  - Blood cultures
  - CBC
  - Urinalysis
  - Chest radiograph
  - Abdominal and pelvic radiographs

- Pelvic ultrasound to confirm presence of retained products of conception

Definitive Diagnosis:

Pelvic inflammatory disease — ICD-9-CM 614.9
Pelvic cellulitis — ICD-9-CM 614.4
Pelvic abscess — ICD-9-CM 614.3
Intrapartum chorioamnionitis — ICD-9-CM 658.4
Postpartum endometritis — ICD-9-CM 670
Postabortion infection — ICD-9-CM 635.0
Postabortion infection with shock — ICD-9-CM 635.5

Suggested Treatment:

- PID:
  - Inpatient:[1]
    —Cefoxitin 2 g IV every 6 hours or Cefotetan 2 g IV every 12 hours, and Doxycycline 100 mg orally/IV every 12 hours for at least 48 hours after patient clinically improves, then Doxycycline 100 mg orally twice a day for a total of 10 to 14 days, or
    —Clindamycin 900 mg IV every 8 hours, and Gentamicin 2 mg/kg intravenous loading dose, then 1.5 mg/kg IV

[1] Centers for Disease Control and Prevention (CDC) recommends hospitalization for patients with acute PID in the following situations: diagnosis is uncertain; surgical emergencies cannot be excluded (appendicitis, ectopic pregnancy); pelvic abscess or tubo-ovarian abscess are suspected; patient is pregnant; patient is an adolescent; patient is unable to tolerate an outpatient regimen; patient has failed to respond to outpatient therapy; clinical follow-up within 72 hours of starting antibiotic treatment cannot be arranged.

      every 8 hours for at least 48 hours
after patient clinically improves, then
Doxycycline 100 mg orally twice a
day, or
Clindamycin 450 mg orally 4 times a
day for a total of 14 days of therapy

- Outpatient:
—Cefoxitin 2 g intramuscularly plus
concurrent probenecid 1 g orally, or
Ceftriaxone 250 mg intramuscularly, or
Ceftizoxime 2 g intramuscularly, or
Cefotaxime 2 g intramuscularly, and
Doxycycline 100 mg orally twice a day
for 14 days, or
—Ofloxacin 400 mg orally twice a day for
14 days, and
Clindamycin 450 mg orally 4 times a
day for 14 days, or
Metronidazole 500 mg orally 2 times a
day for 14 days
- Pelvic cellulitis: Clindamycin 900 mg IV every
8 hours, and Gentamicin 2 mg/kg intravenous
loading dose, then 1.5 mg/kg IV every 8
hours until patient has been afebrile for 24 to
36 hours, then careful outpatient monitoring
without additional oral therapy
- Pelvic abscess:
  - Clindamycin 900 mg IV every 8
hours, or
Metronidazole 1 g IV every 12 hours, and
Gentamicin 2.0 mg/kg intravenous
loading dose, then 1.5 mg/kg IV
every 8 hours until patient has
been afebrile and CBC has normalized
for 48 to 72 hours, then
Metronidazole 500 mg orally twice a day
for 7 days

- Surgical drainage is indicated when antibiotics alone are not successful in treatment—accessibility of abscess by percutaneous drainage under CT guidance or by colpotomy should help guide decision regarding surgical options
- Intrapartum chorioamnionitis:
  - Ampicillin 500 mg IV every 4 hours (Penicillin allergy: Erythromycin 500 mg IV every 4 to 6 hours), and Gentamicin 2.0 mg/kg intravenous loading dose, then 1.5 mg/kg IV every 8 hours
  - If cesarean delivery is contemplated, add to the above: Clindamycin 900 mg IV every 8 hours until patient has been afebrile for 72 hours
- Postpartum endometritis:
  - Clindamycin 900 mg IV every 8 hours, and Gentamicin 2.0 mg/kg intravenous loading dose, then 1.5 mg/kg IV every 8 hours until patient is afebrile, pain free, and CBC has normalized for 24 hours, or
  - Ampicillin 1 to 2 g IV every 6 hours (Penicillin allergy: Erythromycin 500 mg IV every 4 to 6 hours), and Metronidazole 7.5 mg/kg IV every 6 hours, and Gentamicin 2.0 mg/kg intravenous loading dose, then 1.5 mg/kg IV every 8 hours until patient has been afebrile for 24 to 48 hours
  - Oral therapy after discharge is unnecessary UNLESS the patient has had a positive culture for *Chlamydia*, then add: Doxycycline 100 mg orally 2 times a day for 10 days

- Mild to moderate infection may be treated with
  —Cefotetan 1 g IV every 12 hours, or
    Cefoxitin 1 g IV every 4 to 6 hours, or
    Ticarcillin + clavulanic acid 3 g ticarcillin IV every 6 hours
- Postabortion infection:
  - Mild postabortion endometritis: Doxycycline 100 mg orally twice a day for 10 to 14 days
  - Serious infection/septic shock
    Ampicillin 2 g IV every 6 hours, and
    Clindamycin 900 mg IV every 8 hours, and
    Gentamicin 2.0 mg/kg intravenous loading dose, then 1.5 mg/kg IV every 8 hours, or
    Aztreonam 2 g IV every 8 hours
  - Curettage to remove infected tissue is essential in all but the mildest of postabortal infections

Follow-Up:

- Patient monitoring must be individualized according to severity of infection, and generally depends on:
  - Need for intravenous antibiotics
  - Need for surgical intervention
  - Pregnancy
  - Presence of bacteremia
  - Evidence of sepsis/septic shock
- In all cases, close observation of clinical status is necessary, particularly with respect to:
  - Patterns of pulse and fever
  - Pain
  - Findings of general systemic toxicity
  - Level of peritoneal signs
  - WBC count

- Appropriate patient counseling
  - Use of contraceptives to avoid pregnancy
  - Use of condoms to avoid STDs
  - Appropriate prenatal care
- Consider prophylactic antibiotics for future pregnancies in patients with intrapartum chorioamnionitis and postpartum endometritis
- **Watch for:** signs and symptoms of
    - Abscess formation
      —Tubo-ovarian
      —Adnexal
    - Peritonitis
    - Shock
    - Recurrent infections
    - Chronic pelvic pain and/or dyspareunia caused by adhesions, chronic salpingitis, or recurrent infections
    - Infertility or ectopic pregnancies in the future

PROSTATITIS

Presenting Symptoms:

SUBJECTIVE	OBJECTIVE
Acute Bacterial Prostatitis	
Urinary frequency	Lower abdominal or
Dysuria	suprapubic
Fever, chills	tenderness
Low back pain	Exquisitely tender,
Symptoms of systemic	tense prostate on
toxicity are common	rectal examination
Scrotal or inguinal pain	Bladder outlet
Ejaculatory pain or	obstruction may be
discomfort	evident
	Systemic symptoms

include fever, pain,
rigors and signs of
bacteremia

Chronic Bacterial Prostatitis

Generally asymptomatic

Dysuria or irritative
  voiding may be
  present

Ejaculatory pain or
  discomfort

Perineal or low
  back pain

Normal abdominal and
  prostate examination

No systemic symptoms

Differential Diagnosis:

Cystitis
Urethritis
Pyelonephritis
Prostate cancer
Bladder cancer
Acute urinary retention
Obstructive nephrolithiasis
Nonbacterial prostatitis
—Neuromuscular dysfunction
—Bladder neck dysfunction
—Allergy to environmental agents
Prostatodynia

Suggested Workup:

- Fractional urine examination:
  - Voided bladder $(VB)_1$ = initial 5 to 10 mL
    of urinary stream
  - VB_2 = midstream specimen after 200 mL of
    urine are discarded
  - EPS = expressed prostate secretion
    (secretions expressed from prostate by
    digital massage after VB_2)
  - VB_3 = first 5 to 10 mL of urinary stream
    immediately after prostatic massage

- Urinalysis, culture, and antibiotic sensitivity on all four specimens
  - Unequivocal diagnosis of acute bacterial prostatitis requires that the bacterial colony count in VB_3 exceed that in VB_1 by at least 10-fold
  - Strong evidence for acute bacterial prostatitis is greater than 10 to 15 WBC/high power field or positive bacterial culture in EPS or VB_3, but not in VB_1 or VB_2
- EPS culture: useful in diagnosing chronic bacterial prostatitis
- Imaging studies: prostatic ultrasound or CT—if prostatic malignancy, calculus, or abscess is suspected
- Invasive procedures:
  - Needle biopsy of prostate
    —Culture and sensitivity testing
    —Cytology for malignancy
  - Cystoscopy—evaluate for bladder cancer
- Urodynamic testing for prostatodynia

Definitive Diagnosis:

Acute bacterial prostatitis   ICD-9-CM 601.0
Chronic bacterial prostatitis   ICD-9-CM 601.1

Suggested Treatment:

- Acute bacterial prostatitis:
  - Outpatient: TMP-SMX DS 1 tablet orally twice a day for 30 days
  - Inpatient (bacteremic or toxic patient)
    Ampicillin 50 mg/kg IV every 6 hours (Penicillin allergy: Erythromycin 1 g IV every 6 hours), and
    Gentamicin 1.7 mg/kg IV every 8 hours for 7 to 10 days, then to oral therapy above for balance of 30 days

- Chronic bacterial prostatitis:
  - Ciprofloxacin 500 mg orally twice a day for 3 to 4 months, or
  - Norfloxacin 400 mg orally twice a day for 3 to 4 months
- Supportive care:
  - Hydration
  - Analgesics
  - Bed rest
  - Suprapubic cystostomy for urinary retention (transurethral catheter is to be avoided)

Follow-Up:

- Outpatient care if patient is nontoxic
- Inpatient care is appropriate if patient is uroseptic, immunocompromised, or has abscess
- Urinalysis and culture 30 days after treatment (may require multiples of 30 days for infection to clear in patient with chronic bacterial infection)
- Consider chronic suppression therapy in patient with chronic prostatitis and recurrent acute exacerbations
- **Watch for:** signs and symptoms of
  - Prostatic abscess
  - Sepsis
  - Urinary retention
  - Prostatic infarction
  - Chronic disease
  - Granulomatous prostatitis

EPIDIDYMITIS

Presenting Symptoms:

SUBJECTIVE	OBJECTIVE
Painful swelling of the scrotum, usually	Elicit history of risk factor:

abrupt in onset over several hours
Dysuria or irritative lower urinary tract symptoms
Urethral discharge
Fever

—Past history of genitourinary tract disease or prostatitis
—History of urethral stricture
—Recent sexual exposure
—Recent history of genitourinary tract manipulation
Generally unilateral, tender swelling and erythema of the posterior aspect of the scrotum
May involve ipsilateral testis so that testis becomes indistinguishable from epididymis
Induration and thickening of scrotal wall
Hydrocele usually present
Urethral discharge present on inspection or with urethral stripping

Differential Diagnosis:

Torsion of the testis
Orchitis
Testicular tumor
Testicular trauma
Epididymal cyst
Spermatocele

Hydrocele
Varicocele
Sexually transmitted urethritis

Suggested Workup:

- Urinalysis: pyuria
- Microbiology: Gram stain and culture urethral discharge
    - *Pseudomonas* most typical for nonspecific epididymitis
    - *C. trachomatis* and *N. gonorrhoeae* most common for sexually transmitted epididymitis
- Ultrasound of scrotum (especially color-flow Doppler): can be used to rule out abscess, tumors, hematoma caused by trauma

Definitive Diagnosis:

Nonvenereal epididymitis   ICD-9-CM 604.90
Chlamydial epididymitis   ICD-9-CM 099.54
Gonococcal epididymitis   ICD-9-CM 098.0

Suggested Treatment:

- Sexually transmitted epididymitis:
    - Doxycycline 100 mg orally twice a day for 10 days, or
    - Tetracycline 500 mg orally 4 times a day for 10 days
- Nonspecific bacterial epididymitis:
    - TMP-SMX DS 1 tablet orally twice a day for 10 to 14 days, or
    - Ciprofloxacin 500 mg orally twice a day for 10 to 14 days, or
    - Norfloxacin 400 mg orally twice a day for 10 to 14 days

- Septic or toxic patient:
    - Ceftriaxone 1 to 2 g IV/intramuscularly every 24 hours, and
    - Gentamicin 1 mg/kg IV every 8 hours
- Supportive measures:
    - Bed rest
    - Scrotal elevation
    - Local ice packs

Follow-Up:

- Usually outpatient care is appropriate, unless patient is septic or surgery is scheduled
- Office visits until all signs of infection have cleared
- Consider surgical measures in specific circumstances
    - Aspiration of hydrocele for diagnosis and to relieve discomfort
    - Vasostomy to drain infected material
    - Scrotal exploration if torsion of testis is suspected
    - Where response to antibiotics is poor, consider
      —Drainage of abscesses
      —Epididymectomy or epididymo-orchiectomy in severe cases threatening sepsis
- **Watch for:** signs and symptoms of
    - Testicular infarction
    - Scrotal abscess
    - Pyocele
    - Chronic draining scrotal sinus
    - Chronic epididymitis
    - Fournier's gangrene
    - Recurrent epididymitis
    - Infertility

BALANITIS

Presenting Symptoms:

SUBJECTIVE

Penile itching and burning

Dysuria

Inflammation of glans penis

OBJECTIVE

Drainage from glans penis

Erythema

Prepuce swelling

Ulceration and thrush-like plaques on glans penis

Plaques may be spread to thighs, gluteal folds, buttocks, and scrotum

Plaques may be surrounded by small, discrete papules (satellite lesions)

Note uncircumcised male as risk factor

Note diabetic as risk factor

Elicit history of sexual intercourse with partner having vaginal candidiasis as risk factor

Differential Diagnosis:

Leukoplakia

Lichen planus

Psoriasis

Reiter's syndrome

Lichen sclerosus et atrophicus

Erythroplasia of Queyrat

Malignancy

Suggested Workup:

- Laboratory:
  - VDRL
  - Serum glucose
- Microbiology:
  - Gram stain and culture of drainage
  - Wet mount for fungi
- Biopsy: reserved for persistent disease that does not respond to treatment

Definitive Diagnosis:

Balanitis   ICD-9-CM 607.1

Suggested Treatment:

- Fungal infection:
  - Clotrimazole 1% topically 2 times a day to affected area, or
  - Nystatin topically 2 to 4 times a day to affected area until healed
- Bacterial infection:
  - Bacitracin ointment topically 4 times a day to affected area, or ™Neosporin ointment topically 4 times a day to affected area until healed
  - If resistant to topical therapy,
    Ciprofloxacin 250 to 500 mg orally twice a day for 10 days, or
    TMP-SMX DS 1 tablet orally twice a day for 7 to 10 days

Follow-Up:

- Outpatient follow-up every 1 to 2 weeks until there is good clinical response
- Consider biopsy if condition persists despite treatment to rule out malignancy

- Consider circumcision to prevent recurrence
- **Watch for:** signs and symptoms of
    - Meatal stenosis
    - Premalignant changes from chronic irritation
    - UTI

Joints and Osteomyelitis — 8

INFECTIOUS ARTHRITIS

Presenting Symptoms:

SUBJECTIVE

Joint pain, acute onset

Diminished joint motion

Joint swelling

Mild fever; occasional chills

Malaise

Rash may be present

OBJECTIVE

Predominantly monoarticular joint swelling, erythema, and effusion, with loss of motion

Most commonly affected joints— knee > hip > ankle or elbow > wrist or shoulder > interphalangeal or metacarpal joints

Tenosynovitis usually present

Polyarticular involvement may be seen in viral or *Mycoplasma* arthritis

Cutaneous lesions may be pustular (gonococcal arthritis) or petechial (meningococcal arthritis)

Definitive Diagnosis:

Gout

Pseudogout

Reiter's syndrome

Psoriatic arthritis

Ankylosing spondylitis

Juvenile rheumatoid arthritis

Type IIa hyperlipoproteinemia

Rheumatoid arthritis
Rheumatic fever
Acquired immunodeficiency disease (AIDS)
Cellulitis
Neuropathic arthropathy
Lyme arthritis
Sarcoidosis
Trauma/foreign body
Sickle cell crisis

Suggested Workup:

- Laboratory:
    - Markedly elevated erythrocyte sedimentation rate (ESR)
    - Complete blood count (CBC) → anemia
        —White blood cell (WBC) normal in adults; elevated in children
    - Rheumatoid factor: positive in viral arthritis and with concurrent bacterial endocarditis
    - Antitechoid acid antibody-positive in staphylococcal arthritis (rarely used)
    - Blood cultures: positive in more than 50% of patients with nongonococcal arthritis
    - Urine culture
- Examination of synovial fluid (analysis should proceed promptly after arthrocentesis is performed; no delay should be allowed):
    - Laboratory analysis: (Table 8.1)
    - Joint fluid smears: Gram stain shows organism in 40% to 90% of the cases
    - Joint fluid culture (aerobic and anaerobic):
        —Positive in 90% of cases of bacterial arthritis
        —Positive in 80% of cases of mycobacterial arthritis

Table 8.1.

Laboratory Analysis of Synovial Fluid

Condition	Appearance	WBCs/mm^3	Glucose Ratio (synovium:blood)
Normal joint	Clear and colorless	<1,000 (Monos)	0.8–1.0
Bacterial arthritis	Turbid or purulent	>50,000 (>90% PMNs)	<0.5
Fungal arthritis	Serosanguinous	10–20,000 (70% PMNs)	<0.5
Mycobacterial arthritis	Cloudy	10–20,000 (50% PMNs)	0.5–1.0
Inflammatory arthritis	Serosanguinous	<10,000 (Monos)	0.8–1.0

WBCs = white blood cells; Monos = mononuclear leukocytes; PMNs = polymorphonuclear leukocytes

- —Fungal culture
- —Thayer Martin culture for *Neisseria*
- Polymerase chain reaction (PCR) for specific bacteria
- Imaging studies:
  - Radiograph of affected joint(s)
    - —Generally of little value less than 10 days into infection
    - —May show distention of joint capsule, periarticular soft tissue swelling, and a joint effusion with joint space widening
    - —May be useful to rule out contiguous osteomyelitis
  - Radionuclide scans (Technetium [Tc], gallium [Ga], or indium [In]): will identify areas of inflammation, but cannot definitively distinguish infectious arthritis from other forms of noninfectious arthropathies
  - Computed tomography (CT) scan:
    - —Can identify sequestration, effusion, and joint destruction
    - —Will detect abscess if present
    - —Cannot distinguish between infectious and noninfectious joint effusions
  - Magnetic resonance imaging (MRI)
    - —Can identify joint effusion, but cannot distinguish between infectious and noninfectious causes
    - —Will detect cartilage damage and soft tissue involvement
    - —Will detect contiguous osteomyelitis

Definitive Diagnosis:

Infectious arthritis   ICD-9-CM 711.9

Suggested Treatment:

- The choice of antimicrobial therapy is initially empiric, guided by the patient's age and the results of the Gram stain of the synovial fluid; the eventual choice of drug should be guided by the synovial fluid culture and sensitivity results

- Treatment for infectious arthritis is usually 2 weeks for *Streptococcus,* Gram-negative cocci, or *Haemophilus,* and 3 weeks for *Staphylococcus* or Gram-negative bacilli; if there is an underlying structural joint disease or the infection is difficult to eradicate (e.g., infections with *Staphylococcus aureus* or Gram-negative bacilli), intravenous therapy is given either for 4 weeks or for 2 weeks followed by an additional 4 to 6 weeks of an oral quinolone (e.g., Ciprofloxacin 500 mg orally 2 times a day) or Dicloxacillin 1 to 2 gram/day orally given every 6 hours
- Children under 5 years of age:
  - Gram-positive cocci:
    Penicillin (PCN) G 100,000 units (U)/ kg/day intravenously (IV) given every 4 to 6 hours, or
    Nafcillin 150 mg/kg/day IV given every 6 hours
    Penicillin allergy: Cefotaxime 100 mg/ kg/day IV given every 6 hours, or Ceftriaxone 100 mg/kg/day IV given every 12 hours
  - Gram-negative bacilli:
    Cefuroxime 100 mg/kg/day IV given every 8 hours, or
    Cefotaxime 200 mg/kg/day IV given every 6 hours, or
    Ceftriaxone 100 mg/kg/day IV given every 12 hours
- Children over 5 years of age and adults:
  - Gram-positive cocci:
    PCN G 250,000 U/kg/day IV given every 6 hours (5 to 13 years old);

> 1.2 million U/day IV given every 4 to 6
> hours (over 13 years old), or
> Nafcillin 150 mg/kg/day IV given every
> 6 hours (5 to 13 years old); 1 to 2 g IV
> every 4 hours (over 13 years old), or
> Penicillin allergy: Cefotaxime or
> Ceftriaxone as above (5 to 13 years
> old);
> Cefotaxime 1 g IV every 8 hours, or
> Ceftriaxone 2 g IV every 24 hours
> (over 13 years old)

- Gram-negative bacilli: Cefotaxime or
  Ceftriaxone as above
- Sexually active young adults:
  - Ceftriaxone 2 g IV/intramuscularly every
    24 hours for 10 to 14 days
  - If there is significant clinical improvement
    after 3 to 5 days of intravenous therapy,
    patient may be switched to oral therapy:
    Doxycycline 100 mg orally 2 times a day
    for 10 days
- Elderly patients:
  - Ampicillin + sulbactam 1.5 to 3.0 g
    (ampicillin) IV every 6 hours, or
    Ticarcillin + clavulanate 3 g (ticarcillin)
    IV every 6 hours, or
    Imipenem 0.5 to 1.0 g IV every 6 hours
    (may need to lower dose based on
    patient's renal function)
- Viral arthritis:
  - Generally self-limited, requiring no
    antimicrobial therapy
  - Oral anti-inflammatory drugs may be used
    for relief of pain and inflammation
  - If no resolution in 2 to 3 weeks, reassess
- Mycobacterial arthritis:
  - May be seen in patients with AIDS or other
    forms of immunosuppression

- Empiric therapy should be started pending results of culture and sensitivity testing:
  —Isoniazid 300 mg orally once daily, and Rifampin 600 mg orally once daily, and Pyrazinamide 25 to 35 mg/kg/day orally given once or twice a day, and Ethambutol 15 mg/kg/day orally
- Therapy can be reduced to the two drugs to which the infectious agent is susceptible; treatment should be continued for 18 to 24 months
- Surgery: surgical drainage and continuous flushing of infected joint should be considered when *S. aureus* or gram-negative bacilli is found or suspected as etiologic agent(s)

Follow-Up:

- Hospitalization is usually required, at least initially for parenteral therapy
- Repeat arthrocentesis as joint effusion reaccumulates
- Persistence of effusion beyond 7 days of antimicrobial therapy is evidence that surgical drainage is required, especially if weight-bearing joints are involved, or infection is caused by *S. aureus* or Gram-negative bacilli
- Joint immobilization is not necessary, although weight bearing should be avoided until signs of inflammation and pain have resolved
- Passive motion exercises should be instituted early, followed by active exercises as the inflammation diminishes
- Re-evaluate clinically and by radiograph 1 and 4 weeks after antibiotics are completed
- **Watch for:** signs and symptoms of
  - Osteomyelitis
  - Septic necrosis
  - Ankylosis
  - Postinfectious synovitis

- Mechanical dysfunction of joint
  - Limited range of motion
  - Joint dislocation or fusion
  - Shortening of limb (especially in children)
- Sepsis (especially in elderly population)

OSTEOMYELITIS

Presenting Symptoms:

<u>SUBJECTIVE</u>

<u>OBJECTIVE</u>

Hematogenous Osteomyelitis

SUBJECTIVE	OBJECTIVE
Mainly infants and children present with these symptoms	Tibia and femur of infants and children are most often involved
Abrupt onset of high fever	Local cellulitis often present
Irritability	
Malaise	Local edema
Restriction of movement of the involved extremity	Elicit history of preceding minor trauma with hematoma formation

Vertebral Osteomyelitis

SUBJECTIVE	OBJECTIVE
Adult with history of acute systemic infection prior to onset of vertebral symptoms	Lumbar (45%), thoracic (35%), or cervical spine (20%) involvement most common
—Genitourinary tract	Localized pain and tenderness of the involved bone segments
—Skin and soft tissue	
—Respiratory tract	
—Infected intravenous sites	
—Endocarditis	Motor and sensory neurologic defects in
—Dental infections	up to 15% of cases

Pain of the involved bone segments that progresses over several weeks to months

Fever in 50% of cases

Prior systemic infection with insidious onset of progressive vertebral bone pain should arouse suspicion

Contiguous Focus Osteomyelitis

Adult with history within 1 month previously of

—Trauma

—Surgery

—Internal fixation of a fracture

—Prosthetic device implantation

—Soft tissue infection (e.g., decubitus ulcer)

—Septic arthritis

—Septic bursitis

Low-grade fever

Pain of the involved bone

Drainage from affected site

Loss of bone stability

Evidence of bone necrosis

Evidence of soft tissue damage

Contiguous Focus Osteomyelitis with Generalized Vascular Insufficiency

Adult with history of diabetes mellitus is common

History of minor trauma to the feet, often with infectious sequelae

—Ingrown toenail

Small bones of the feet are most commonly involved

Decreased dorsalis pedis and posterior tibialis pulses

Poor capillary refill in toes

—Foot ulcer   Decreased sensation in
—Cellulitis   feet
—Deep space infection
Fever usually absent
Systemic toxicity rare

Chronic Osteomyelitis

Chronic bone pain and drainage   Nonhealing ulcer or draining sinus
Low-grade fever   Swelling and erythema may be present
Localized skin abscess may be present

Definitive Diagnosis:

Aseptic bone infarction
Neuropathic joint disease
Fractures
Gout
Infectious arthritis
Trauma
Bone cancer
Amyloidosis

Suggested Workup:

- Laboratory:
  - CBC → elevated WBCs (usually less than 15,000/mm^3)
  - ESR elevated
- Microbiology:
  - Blood cultures
  - Culture and antibiotic sensitivity of
    - —Material collected during debridement surgery
    - —Deep bone biopsy
    - —Needle aspiration of bone lesion
  - Draining sinus tract material may give misleading culture and sensitivity results, as this reflects soft tissue infection

- Imaging studies:
  - Radiographs
    - —Detect lesions 2 to 3 weeks after the start of infection
    - —Poor at differentiating infection from infarction or tumor
    - —Radiographic improvement lags behind clinical recovery
  - Radionuclide studies
    - —^{99m}Tc scan
      - –May be positive within 48 hours following initiation of bone infection
      - –May give false-negative results in osteomyelitis where there is impaired blood supply to the infected area
      - –Poor at differentiating infection from infarction or tumor
      - –Good at differentiating between bone and soft tissue inflammation
    - —^{67}Ga scan
      - –Poor at differentiating between bone and soft tissue inflammation
      - –Good in diagnosis of only advanced cases of osteomyelitis
    - —^{111}In scan
      - –Only 40% sensitivity
      - –False-positive results in bone infarction
  - CT scan
    - —Good in early detection and for diagnosis of hematogenous osteomyelitis (can see intramedullary gas)
    - —Can identify areas of necrotic bone and soft tissue involvement
    - —May help in plotting surgical approach for debridement
  - MRI scan
    - —Most sensitive technique, especially for differentiating bone and soft tissue

infections, and between infection, infarction, and tumor

Definitive Diagnosis:

Acute osteomyelitis   ICD-9-CM 730.0
Chronic osteomyelitis   ICD-9-CM 730.1

Suggested Treatment:

- Effective treatment depends on appropriate culture and sensitivity testing of isolated infecting organism(s); it is usually practical to delay antimicrobial therapy until antibiotic sensitivity results are available
- In acutely ill or toxic patients, empiric antibiotic therapy may be selected on the basis of the most likely infecting organisms:
  - Hematogenous osteomyelitis in infants: *S. aureus, Streptococcus agalactiae,* or *Escherichia coli;* in children over 1 year of age: *S. aureus, Streptococcus pyogenes,* and *Haemophilus influenzae*
  - Vertebral osteomyelitis: *S. aureus, Pseudomonas aeruginosa*
  - Contiguous focus osteomyelitis: *S. aureus,* Gram-negative bacilli, anaerobes
  - Contiguous focus osteomyelitis with generalized vascular insufficiency: *Staphylococcus* spp., *Streptococcus* spp., *Enterococcus,* Gram-negative bacilli, anaerobes
- Antimicrobial therapy based on isolated pathogens (parenteral therapy is generally continued for 4 to 6 weeks through indwelling catheter):
  - Gram-positive cocci (*Staphylococcus* and *Streptococcus*):
    —Nafcillin 2 g IV every 6 hours, or
      Oxacillin 2 g IV every 6 hours, or
      Ampicillin 2 g IV every 6 hours

    —Penicillin allergy: Cefazolin 2 g IV every
    8 hours, or
        Vancomycin 1 g IV every 12 hours
        (also indicated for Methicillin-
        resistant *S. aureus* [MRSA])
    —If isolated organism(s) is shown to be
    susceptible, may use oral therapy
    instead:
        Ciprofloxacin 750 mg orally every 12
        hours for 6 to 8 weeks, or
        Ofloxacin 400 mg orally every 12
        hours for 6 to 8 weeks

- Gram-negative bacilli (*P. aeruginosa*):
  - —Piperacillin 3 g IV every 6 hours, or
    Mezlocillin 3 g IV every 6 hours, or
  - —Penicillin allergy: Ceftazidime 2 g IV
    every 12 hours, or
    Ceftriaxone 2 g IV every 24 hours, or
  - —Highly resistant strains:
    Amikacin 15 mg/kg/day IV given
    every 8 to 12 hours, or
    Tobramycin 5 mg/kg/day IV given
    every 8 hours
  - —If isolated organism(s) is shown to be
    susceptible, may use oral therapy
    instead: Ciprofloxacin or Ofloxacin as
    above
- Gram-negative bacilli (*Enterobacteriaceae*):
  - —Ticarcillin + clavulanate 3.0 g (ticarcillin)
    IV every 6 hours
  - —Penicillin allergy: Ceftriaxone 2 g IV
    every 24 hours, or
    Ceftazidime 2 g IV every 12 hours, or
    Cefoperazone 2 g IV every 12 hours
  - —If isolated organism(s) is shown to be
    susceptible, may use oral therapy
    instead: Ciprofloxacin or Ofloxacin as
    above

- Anaerobes:
  - —Imipenem + cilastatin 1.0 g IV every 6 hours, or

      Clindamycin 900 mg IV every 8 hours, or

      Metronidazole 500 mg IV every 8 hours
- Surgical therapy as an adjunct to antimicrobial therapy depends on the Cierny and Mader Classification of the infection:
  - Stage I—Medullary osteomyelitis:
    - —Necrosis limited to medullary contents and endosteal surfaces
    - —Usually as a result of hematogenous spread
    - —Pediatric cases usually treated with antibiotics alone
    - —Adult cases may be treated with unroofing and intramedullary reaming
  - Stage II—Superficial osteomyelitis:
    - —Necrosis limited to exposed surfaces
    - —Usually caused by contiguous focus infection
    - —Treated with superficial debridement and coverage with microvascular flap
  - Stage III—Localized osteomyelitis:
    - —Full thickness cortical lesion
    - —Well-marginated and stable lesion before and after debridement
    - —Usually from trauma or evolving Stage I or II
    - —Treated with debridement, dead space management, temporary stabilization, and possible bone graft
  - Stage IV—Diffuse osteomyelitis
    - —Circumferential and/or permeative lesion
    - —Usually from trauma or evolving Stage I, II, or III

- —Treated with segmental resection, stabilization by orthopedic rod internal fixation, debridement, dead space management, and possible ablation
- Optimal treatment protocols and prognosis are based on this classification system, as well as on systemic or local host factors that affect immune competence, metabolism, and local vascularity:
  - Class A
    - —Normal host
    - —Best outcome and prognosis
  - Class B
    - —Local (B_l) or systemic (B_s) compromise
      - –Malnutrition
      - –Renal or liver failure
      - –Diabetes mellitus
      - –Chronic hypoxia
      - –Malignancy
      - –Age extreme
      - –Immunodeficiency
      - –Tobacco use
    - —Must treat underlying medical condition as well as infection
  - Class C
    - —Treatment of bone infection may be worse than infection itself
    - —Consider amputation, especially in patients with severe vascular insufficiency and/or gangrenous infection

Follow-Up:

- Majority of patients should be followed in hospital for initial treatment with parenteral antibiotics and possible surgical therapy
- Bedrest with immobilization of involved bone and joint

- Monitor clinical response and ESR; results on imaging studies may lag behind clinical status
- Consider hyperbaric oxygen therapy, especially for chronic refractory infections (not well-supported in the literature)
- **Watch for:** signs and symptoms of
  - Abscess formation
  - Bacteremia and sepsis
  - Fracture
  - Postoperative infections
  - Chronic osteomyelitis
  - Vascular compromise of limb

BONE AND JOINT PROSTHETIC INFECTIONS

Presenting Symptoms:

SUBJECTIVE	OBJECTIVE
History of joint replacement (usually hip or knee)	Clinical presentations vary
Joint pain	Most: long indolent course with progressive joint pain, but no fever or inflammation (hematogenous metastasis, often months or years after implantation)
Fever (less than 50%)	
Swelling in joint (less than 50%)	
Drainage from wound site (less than 50%)	
	Some: acute, fulminant illness with fever, local swelling, erythema, and pain, and systemic toxicity or shock (usually complication of implantation surgery)

> Purulent drainage from
> overlying cutaneous
> sinuses may be seen
> Elicit risk factors
> —Diabetes mellitus
> —Steroid treatment
> —Wound hematomas
> —Ischemic wounds

Differential Diagnosis:

Hemarthrosis
Mechanical loosening of prosthesis
Dislocation of prosthesis
Aseptic arthritis

Suggested Workup:

- History and physical:
  - Constant joint pain: suggests infection
  - Pain only with motion and weight bearing: suggests mechanical loosening
- Radiographs of affected areas can reveal abnormalities suggestive of septic prostheses
  - Abnormal bone lucencies
  - Positional changes in prosthesis
  - Cement fractures
  - Periosteal reaction
  - Abnormal stress views
- Joint arthrography:
  - Abnormal communications between the joint space
  - Defects in bone-cement interface
- Radionuclide scanning (Ga, In, Tc): nonspecific and not helpful in distinguishing infection from mechanical loosening
- Arthrocentesis:
  - Gram stain and culture (85% to 98% sensitivity)

—Inability to obtain intra-articular fluid can be circumvented by irrigating the joint with sterile saline without antiseptic preservatives; irrigation fluid can then be cultured
- WBC count of joint fluid ($\uparrow$ in infection)
- Glucose concentration ($\downarrow$ in infection)
- Protein concentration ($\uparrow$ in infection)
- Arthrotomy: culture of periprosthetic tissue for pathogens
- Laboratory:
  - Blood cultures
  - Workup any suspected primary infection if hematogenous spread from a distant site is suggested by the clinical presentation

Definitive Diagnosis:

Infection/inflammation of ICD-9-CM 996.66 internal joint prosthesis

Suggested Treatment:

- Standard protocol (90% to 97% success rate):
  - Surgical removal of prosthesis and cement, with thorough debridement of wound site
  - Antimicrobial therapy for 6 weeks, chosen on the basis of culture and susceptibility studies performed on material collected at surgery; empiric treatment may be started while waiting for these results:
    —Vancomycin 1 g IV every 12 hours, and Gentamicin 1.5 mg/kg IV every 8 hours, or Ceftazidime 1 to 2 g IV every 8 hours, or Ceftriaxone 2 to 4 g IV every 24 hours, or Imipenem 1 g IV every 6 hours

- Reimplantation of new prosthesis at the conclusion of antimicrobial therapy
- Alternative protocol (70% to 80% success rate):
  - Surgical removal of prosthesis and cement, with immediate reimplantation of a new prosthesis
    —Methylmethacrylate cement impregnated with gentamicin or tobramycin is used for the reimplantation procedure
  - Systemic antibiotics have typically not been administered in this protocol, but the 6-week regimen described above should be seriously considered
- Suppressive antibiotic therapy where removal of implanted prosthesis is not available
  - Contraindicated due to the medical or surgical condition of the patient
  - Patient refusal
  - Lifelong suppressive antibiotic therapy may be used in such situations to preserve the usefulness of the joint replacement
  - Oral regimens used with some success (63% success rate in patients with relatively avirulent infection and a prosthesis that has not loosened):
    —Ciprofloxacin 250 mg orally 2 times a day, and
       Metronidazole 250 mg orally every 12 hours, or
       Clindamycin 150 mg orally every 6 hours, or
    —Cefixime 200 mg orally every 12 hours, and
       Clindamycin 150 mg orally every 6 hours
- Antibiotic prophylaxis for patients with prosthetic joints in anticipation of bacteremic events:

- Prophylactic antibiotics in advance of various surgical procedures is controversial; there are no data available with which to determine the cost effectiveness of such an approach, and a clinical decision must be made in each patient individually based on perceived risk factors
- Suggested regimens include:
  —Dental, oral, or upper respiratory tract procedures
    –Amoxicillin 3.0 g orally 1 hour before and 1.5 g orally 6 hours after procedure
    –Penicillin allergy: Erythromycin 1.0 g orally 1 hour before and 500 mg orally 6 hours after procedure, or
      Clindamycin 300 mg orally 1 hour before and 150 mg orally 6 hours after procedure
  —Genitourinary procedures
    –Patient able to take oral medication: as above
    –Patient unable to take oral medication: Ampicillin 2.0 g IV, and
      Gentamicin 1.5 mg/kg IV 30 minutes before and 8 hours after procedure
    –Penicillin allergy: Vancomycin 1.0 g IV, and
      Gentamicin 1.5 mg/kg IV 30 minutes before and 8 hours after procedure
  —Gastrointestinal procedures: as for dental procedures above

Follow-Up:

- Careful surgical monitoring after debridement and reimplantation is necessary
- For patients on chronic suppressive antibiotic therapy, periodic radiologic monitoring for

progressive bone resorption at the bone-cement interface is required
- **Watch for:** signs and symptoms of
    - Osteomyelitis
    - Extension of a localized septic process into adjacent tissue compartments
    - Systemic infection
    - Side effects of chronic antibiotic administration

Parasites, Rickettsiae, and Spirochetes

9

AMEBIASIS

Presenting Symptoms:

SUBJECTIVE

OBJECTIVE

Intestinal Disease

In noninvasive infection, patients may be asymptomatic or complain of mild diarrhea and colicky lower abdominal discomfort

In invasive infection, patients will complain of

—Gradual onset of severe abdominal pain over 1 to 3 weeks

—Diarrhea

—Dysentery

—Rectal pain

—Weight loss

—Bloody stools

—Fever (30%)

Abdominal distention and pain on palpation

Liver enlarged and tender to percussion

Heme-positive stools

Rectal bleeding

Perianal lesions

Systemic toxicity may be present in severe cases

Extraintestinal Disease

Fever

Right upper quadrant abdominal pain

Diarrhea

Weight loss

Nausea and vomiting

Most frequently manifested as an amebic liver abscess

History of symptomatic intestinal amebic infection frequently not present

Right upper quadrant
abdominal point
tenderness over the
liver
Hepatomegaly (50%)
Dullness to percussion
and rales at the right
lung base are
common
Pleural effusion and
atelectasis suggest
pleuropulmonary
amebiasis as a
complication (not an
extension) of liver
abscess
Pericardial friction rub
(in patients with
amebic pericarditis
caused by extension
from liver)
Peritoneal signs (in
patients with amebic
pericarditis caused
by extension from
liver)

Differential Diagnosis:

Campylobacter colitis
Shigellosis
Salmonellosis
Yersinia colitis
Pseudomembranous colitis
Ulcerative colitis
Crohn's disease
Ischemic colitis
Pyogenic liver abscess

Viral hepatitis
Giardiasis
Viral gastroenteritis
Enterotoxigenic *Escherichia coli* infection
Cryptosporidiosis
Isosporiasis
Malabsorption syndrome
Functional bowel disease
Hepatoma

Suggested Workup:

- Microbiology:
  - Examination of stool for ova and parasites
    —Finding of either trophozoite or cyst form
      of *Entamoeba histolytica* confirms
      diagnosis
    —Prior to collecting stool, avoid giving
      patient substances that interfere with
      stool examination
      –Barium
      –Bismuth
      –Antibiotics (tetracycline, erythromycin)
      –Antacids
      –Laxatives
      –Enemas
    —At least three separate stools should be
      examined before intestinal amebiasis can
      be ruled out
  - Stool examination for amebic antigens
    (shortly to be widely commercially
    available)
  - Stool culture to rule out bacterial pathogens
    (especially *Campylobacter*)
- Serology:
  - Anti-amebic antibody by indirect
    hemagglutination
    —Sensitivity—85% to 95%

  —May remain positive in highly endemic areas
- Anti-amebic galactose adhesin antibody (enzyme-linked immunosorbent assay [ELISA] test)
  —Specificity—99%
- Imaging studies:
  - Abdominal ultrasound
    —Rapid and low cost for detecting liver abscess
    —Sensitivity for abscess nearly as good as computed tomography (CT) or liver scan
  - Abdominal CT scan
    —Sensitive in detecting liver abscess
    —Not specific in diagnosing amebic liver abscess
    —Can differentiate abscess from liver tumor
  - Magnetic resonance imaging (MRI) scan—sensitivity and specificity similar to CT scan
  - Gallium (^{67}Ga) scan—can differentiate amebic from pyogenic liver abscess
  - Technetium-99m (^{99m}Tc) liver scan—largely replaced by CT scan
- Invasive testing:
  - Proctoscopy, flexible sigmoidoscopy, or colonoscopy with biopsy or scrapings to diagnose intestinal amebiasis
    —Appropriate for patients with:
      –Negative stool but positive antibody test
      –Acute presentations with high index of suspicion, but negative stool and/or antibody tests

- CT- or ultrasound-guided skinny-needle
  aspiration of hepatic abscess
  —Material should be examined for amebae
    and sent for bacterial culture
  —Risk/benefit ratio should be considered
    –Peritoneal spillage $\rightarrow$ amebic peritonitis
    –Most cases can be diagnosed and
      treated without aspiration

Definitive Diagnosis:

Acute amebic dysentery   ICD-9-CM 006.0
Amebic nondysenteric colitis   ICD-9-CM 006.2
Amebic liver abscess   ICD-9-CM 006.3
Unspecified amebiasis   ICD-9-CM 006.9

Suggested Treatment:

- Asymptomatic cyst passers:
  - Diloxanide furoate 500 mg orally 3 times a
    day for 10 days
      (Pediatric: 20 mg/kg/day orally given 3
        times a day for 10 days), or
  - Paromomycin 25 to 30 mg/kg/day orally
    for 5 to 10 days
      (Pediatric: same dosage as for adults), or
  - Tetracycline 250 mg orally 4 times a day
    for 10 days, then
      Iodoquinol 650 mg orally 3 times a day
        for 20 days
- Invasive amebic rectocolitis:
  - Metronidazole 750 mg orally 3 times a day
    for 5 to 10 days
      (Pediatric: 35 to 50 mg/kg/day orally
        given 3 times a day for 10 days), or
      2.4 g orally daily for 2 to 3 days or
      50 mg/kg orally for 1 dose,
      FOLLOWED BY
      Diloxanide furoate or Paromomycin as
        above, or

- Dehydroemetine 1 to 1.5 mg/kg/day intramuscularly (max = 90 mg/day) for 5 days (highly cardio- and neurotoxic and rarely used; available only through Centers for Disease Control and Prevention [CDC]), or
- Tetracycline 250 mg orally 4 times a day for 15 days, and
    Chloroquine base 600 mg orally for 1 day, 300 mg orally for 1 day, then 150 mg orally 3 times a day for 14 days
- Amebic liver abscess:
  - Metronidazole 750 mg orally 3 times a day for 10 days, or 2.4 g daily for 1 to 2 days, FOLLOWED BY
      Diloxanide furoate or Paromomycin as above, or
  - Chloroquine base 600 mg orally for 2 days, then 300 mg orally daily for 2 to 3 weeks, or
  - Dehydroemetine 1 to 1.5 mg/kg/day intramuscularly (max = 90 mg/day) for up to 5 days
    —May add Diloxanide furoate or Paromomycin as above to Dehydroemetine to shorten exposure
    —Generally reserved for seriously ill patients who have developed peritonitis or have a ruptured amebic liver abscess

Follow-Up:

- Outpatient management is usually appropriate for most patients, except for those who are seriously ill with peritonitis or other life-threatening extraintestinal manifestations
- Careful nutritional, fluid and electrolyte management is mandatory

- Monitor patient signs and symptoms
- Repeat stool examination for ova and parasites after therapy
- Teach prevention
  - Boil water
  - Decontaminate fruits and vegetables with acetic acid or vinegar
  - Avoid sexual practices allowing oral-fecal contact
- **Watch for:** signs and symptoms of
  - Toxic megacolon
  - Rupture of liver abscess
    —Peritonitis
    —Lung abscess and empyema
  - Pericarditis with hemodynamic compromise
  - Brain abscess
  - Genitourinary involvement
  - Skin involvement

GIARDIASIS

Presenting Symptoms:

SUBJECTIVE	OBJECTIVE
Up to 50% of patients are asymptomatic	Elicit history of risk factor for oral ingestion of *Giardia lamblia*
Chronic diarrhea lasting several weeks	
Abdominal cramps and bloating exacerbated by eating	—Day care centers
	—Male homosexuality
Flatulence and sulfuric belching	—Wilderness camping with use of unpurified water
Greasy, foul-smelling stools that float	—Overseas travel where water supply is suspect
Nausea and vomiting	
Weight loss (more than 10 lb.)	—Persons in custodial institutions with

Urticaria
Malaise
Gross blood, pus, and
  mucus usually
  absent from stools

poor fecal-oral
  hygiene
Evidence of
  malabsorption
Mild abdominal
  discomfort on
  palpation
Suspicion is raised in
  patient with
  prolonged diarrhea
  and weight loss

Differential Diagnosis:

Other intestinal parasites
Bacterial colitis
Celiac sprue
Tropical sprue
Bacterial overgrowth syndrome
Crohn's disease
Irritable bowel syndrome

Suggested Workup:

- Microbiology:
  - Examination of stool for ova and parasites
    - Finding of either trophozoite or cyst form of *G. lamblia* confirms diagnosis
    - At least 3 separate stool specimens should be examined (50% to 70% sensitivity with 1 stool specimen; greater than 90% sensitivity with 3 specimens)
  - Culture of stool specimens to rule out bacterial pathogens
- Laboratory:
  - Immunofluorescence or ELISA tests for *Giardia* antigens
    - Sensitivity 85% to 98%; specificity 90% to 100%
    - Both are commercially available

- –Immunofluorescence: Merifluor, Meridian Diagnostics, Cincinnati, OH
- –ELISA: Giardia Assay, Alexon, Inc., Mountain View, CA
- Special tests in diagnostic dilemmas:
  - String test
    - —Entero-Test, HDC Corp., San Jose, CA
    - —Gelatin capsule on a string that is secured at the mouth is swallowed
    - —After 4 to 18 hours incubation, string is removed and coating is examined microscopically for trophozoites
    - —May be more sensitive than stool examination
  - Duodenal aspiration
  - Upper endoscopy with duodenal biopsy

Definitive Diagnosis:

Giardiasis   ICD-9-CM 007.1

Suggested Treatment:

- Traditional therapy (may not be available in the United States in the near future except through the CDC):
  - Quinacrine 100 mg orally 3 times a day for 5 to 7 days—90% efficacy
- Newer therapy:
  - Metronidazole 500 mg orally 3 times a day for 5 to 7 days—80% to 95% efficacy despite not being approved by the Food and Drug Administration (FDA) for treatment of giardiasis
- Pediatric giardiasis:
  - Furazolidone suspension 8 mg/kg/day orally given 3 times a day, or 100 mg tablets orally 4 times a day for 7 to 10 days—80% efficacy

- Giardiasis in pregnancy:
  - If possible where symptoms are mild enough and dehydration or malnutrition are not too severe, therapy should be delayed after delivery or at least until after the first trimester of pregnancy
  - If treatment is necessary:
    Paromomycin 25 to 35 mg/kg/day orally 3 times a day for 5 to 10 days, or Metronidazole as above (only after the first trimester of pregnancy)

Follow-Up:

- Outpatient care is usually appropriate
- Frequent monitoring of symptoms and weight
- Periodic re-examination of stools
- Patient education regarding risk factors
  - Proper handling and treatment of water
  - Good personal hygiene
  - Avoidance of oral-anal and oral-genital sex
- **Watch for:** signs and symptoms of
  - Malabsorption
  - Malnutrition

INTESTINAL SPORE-FORMING PROTOZOA (*CRYPTOSPORIDIUM*, MICROSPORIDIA, *ISOSPORA*, AND *CYCLOSPORA*)

Presenting Symptoms:

SUBJECTIVE	OBJECTIVE
Asymptomatic infection may be found with varying frequency	History of positive risk factor(s):
	—International travel (Asia, Africa)
Intermittent abdominal cramps	—Children and immunodeficient persons
Acute diarrhea;	

intermittent or
prolonged and
voluminous
Low-grade fever
General malaise
Weakness, fatigue
Anorexia
Nausea and vomiting
Cough
Arthritis

—Low socioeconomic
status with poor
sanitation
—Overcrowded living
conditions
—Clinical
manifestations
depend on whether
host is
immunodeficient
and whether there is
extraintestinal
disease:
—Abdominal
tenderness; may
localize to right
upper quadrant
(biliary infection
causing sclerosing
cholangitis in
normal hosts or
acalculous
cholecystitis in
patients with
acquired
immunodeficiency
syndrome
[AIDS])
—Borborygmi
—Upper and lower
respiratory tract
symptoms
—Reactive arthritis
of wrists, hands,
knees, ankles, and
feet

Differential Diagnosis:

Other gastrointestinal infections
—*Salmonella*
—*Shigella*
—*Campylobacter*
—*Clostridium difficile*
—*G. lamblia*
—*E. histolytica*
—Cytomegalovirus
—*Mycobacterium avium*
Food poisoning
Malabsorption syndrome
Inflammatory bowel disease

Suggested Workup:

- Laboratory: Stool examination for fecal leukocytes and red blood cells (RBCs) → negative
- Microbiology:
  - Stool examination for ova and parasites (in most laboratories, must specifically include request for stains for these four organisms)
    —Cryptosporidia—modified acid-fast stain or monoclonal antibody-based immunofluorescent stain
    —*Isospora*—wet preparation or modified acid-fast stain
    —*Cyclospora*—wet preparation
    —Microsporidia—modified trichrome or fluorescent stain
  - Duodenal aspirate with appropriate stain examination for these four organisms
- Small bowel biopsy: Especially useful for microsporidia

Definitive Diagnosis:

Cryptosporidiosis   ICD-9-CM 007.8
Microsporidiosis   ICD-9-CM 136.8
Isosporosis   ICD-9-CM 007.2
Unspecified protozoal   ICD-9-CM 007.9
    intestinal infection

Suggested Treatment:

- Cryptosporidia:
    - Infection is self-limited in immunocompetent hosts
    - Where therapy is required (immunocompromised or elderly patients):
      —Paromomycin 25 to 35 mg/kg/day orally 3 times a day , or
        Azithromycin 2 g/day orally [EXPERIMENTAL TREATMENT]
        –Duration of therapy depends on clinical response
      —Antidiarrheal or antimotility agents
        –Bismuth subsalicylate
        –Diphenoxylate
        –Loperamide
      —Parenteral hydration and nutrition may be necessary
- *Isospora* and Cyclospora:
    - Trimethoprim-sulfamethoxazole (TMP-SMX) DS 1 tablet orally 2 times a day for 10 days
- Microsporidia:
    - Albendazole 400 mg orally 2 times a day for 3 weeks (may be obtained on a compassionate use basis from SmithKline Beecham Labs, Philadelphia, PA)

- NOT USEFUL for infections with *Enterocytozoon bieneusi*

Follow-Up:

- Outpatient care is typically adequate, except where severe dehydration or nutritional compromise requires parenteral therapy
- Nutritional support in all cases
- Aggressive treatment of an underlying immunodeficiency
- Patient education to reduce risk of reinfection and transmission
  - Good personal hygiene habits
  - Enteric precautions
  - Water purification
  - Proper food preparation
- Re-examination of stool specimens 2 to 4 weeks after therapy is completed
- **Watch for:** signs and symptoms of
  - Recurrent infection
  - Irritable bowel syndrome after acute infection is successfully treated
  - Lactose intolerance
  - Dehydration and malnutrition
  - Extraintestinal complications
    —Hepatic and biliary infections
    —Pancreatitis
    —Pulmonary and upper respiratory tract infections (e.g., laryngotracheitis)
    —Reactive arthritides
  - Disseminated disease, especially in severely immunocompromised patients

MALARIA

Presenting Symptoms:

SUBJECTIVE	OBJECTIVE

Benign Tertian Malaria
(Plasmodium vivax, Plasmodium ovale)

Cyclical, paroxysmal fevers every 48 hours	During paroxyms —Tachycardia —Fever
—An initial stage where the patient feels cold and has true shaking chills, lasting 15 minutes to several hours	—Hypotension —Altered consciousness Hepatosplenomegaly may be present
—A second feverish stage where temperatures exceed 40°C, lasting several hours, and including –Cough –Headache –Backache –Nausea and vomiting –Abdominal pain –Diarrhea –Somnolence –Convulsions	Elicit history of risk factors —Travel to endemic areas of sub-Saharan Africa, India, Haiti, Papua New Guinea, the Solomon Islands, the Far East, and Latin America —Travel to these areas typically occurs 10 to 30 days before onset of symptoms, but may be as much as 9 months earlier
—A third sweating stage with resolution of fever, onset of generalized diaphoresis, and appearance of marked fatigue,	

usually occurring
within 2 to 6 hours
after onset of chilled
stage

Quartan Malaria **(Plasmodium malariae)**

Cyclical, paroxysmal
fevers every 72
hours
—Paroxysms are
generally
indistinguishable
from tertian malaria

Clinical findings and
epidemiology similar
to tertian malaria

Malignant Falciparum Malaria **(Plasmodium falciparum)**

Continuous fevers with
intermittent irregular
spikes
Symptoms
indistinguishable
from tertian or
quartan malaria
early on
Life-threatening
complications
develop
—Seizure activity
—Coma
—Manifestations of
uremia
–Anorexia
–Nausea and
vomiting
–Diarrhea
–Altered sensorium
–Encephalopathy
–Asterixis

Clinical findings
similar to other
forms of malaria
early on, except
periodicity of fever
is lacking
Complications will
develop if untreated
—Coma, seizures, and
other evidence of
central nervous
system (CNS)
disease
—Oliguric renal failure
with dark malarial
pigment in the urine
(blackwater fever)
—Pulmonary edema

–Dyspnea
–Weakness
–Peripheral edema
–Dark urine

Differential Diagnosis:

Typhoid fever
Bacterial meningitis
Rickettsial infection
Arbovirus infection
Acute hepatitis
Acute hemolytic anemia
Stroke
Pneumonia
Acute viral infection
Other parasitemias
Rheumatic fever
Congestive heart failure

Suggested Workup:

- Microbiology:
  - Microscopic examination of several sequential thin or thick peripheral blood smears
    —Obtain every 6 hours over a 72-hour period
    —Thick blood smears optimal for detecting parasites of unidentified species
    —Thin blood smears are best suited for identifying species and for estimating degree of parasitemia
- Serology:
  - HRP-2 ELISA for *P. falciparum*—rapid commercial kit available
  - Polymerase chain reaction (PCR)—cumbersome and not useful clinically

- Laboratory:
  - Complete blood count (CBC)
    - —Profound anemia
    - —Leukopenia
    - —Thrombocytopenia
  - Liver function tests
    - —Elevated alanine aminotransferase (ALT)/aspartate aminotransferase (AST)
    - —Hyperbilirubinemia
  - Depressed albumin

Definitive Diagnosis:

Malaria, unspecified	ICD-9-CM 084.6
Malaria, *P. falciparum*	ICD-9-CM 084.0
Malaria, *P. malariae*	ICD-9-CM 084.2
Malaria, *P. ovale*	ICD-9-CM 084.3
Malaria, *P. vivax*	ICD-9-CM 084.1
Mixed malarial infection	ICD-9-CM 084.5

Suggested Treatment:

- Chloroquine-susceptible malaria:
  - Oral treatment for uncomplicated disease
    - —Chloroquine base 600 mg (= 1 g chloroquine phosphate or 800 mg chloroquine sulfate) orally for 1 dose, then 300 mg orally 6 hours later, to be repeated for another 2 days
    - —Pediatric: Chloroquine base 10 mg/kg orally for 1 dose, then 5 mg/kg 6 hours later, to be repeated for another 2 days
  - Parenteral treatment for severe disease
    - —Chloroquine base 10 mg/kg intravenous infusion over 8 hours, then 15 mg/kg intravenous infusion over 24 hours, or Chloroquine base 3.5 mg/kg intramuscularly/subcutaneously (sq) every 6 hours until a total dose of 25 mg/kg is achieved

- Chloroquine-resistant malaria (if there is any doubt about the drug sensitivity of the parasite, the infection should be considered to be resistant):
  - Oral treatment for uncomplicated disease in adults
    - —Quinine sulfate 650 mg orally every 8 hours for 3 to 7 days, and
        - Pyrimethamine-sulfadoxine 3 tablets orally on the last day of quinine therapy, or
        - Tetracycline 250 mg orally 4 times a day for 7 days, or
        - Doxycycline 100 mg orally 2 times a day for 7 days, or
        - Clindamycin 900 mg orally 3 times a day for 3 days
        - (Tetracycline, doxycycline, or clindamycin should be started 2 to 3 days after quinine sulfate therapy), or
    - —Mefloquine 15 mg/kg orally for 1 dose, or
    - —Halofantrine 500 mg orally every 6 hours for 3 doses, repeated 1 week later (not yet approved by the FDA for use in the United States)
  - Oral treatment for uncomplicated disease in children under 14 years of age
    - —Quinine sulfate 25 mg/kg/day orally given 3 times a day , and
        - Pyrimethamine-sulfadoxine 0.5 tablet (1- to 3-year old), 1 tablet (4- to 8-year old), or 2 tablets (9- to 14-year old) on the last day of quinine therapy, or
        - Tetracycline 20 mg/kg/day orally given 4 times a day, or
        - Clindamycin 20 to 40 mg/kg/day orally given 3 times a day, or

— Mefloquine 25 mg/kg orally for 1
  dose, or
— Halofantrine 8 mg/kg orally every 6
  hours for 3 doses, repeated 1 week later
- Parenteral treatment for severe disease in
  adults and children
  — Quinidine gluconate 10 mg/kg (max
    600 mg) intravenous infusion over 1 to 2
    hours, then 0.02 mg/kg/minute
    continuous intravenous infusion until the
    patient is well enough to change to oral
    therapy, or
  — Quinine dihydrochloride 20 mg/kg
    intravenously (IV) infused over 4 hours,
    then 10 mg/kg IV infused over 2 to 4
    hours every 8 hours (max 1800 mg/day)
    until the patient is well enough to change
    to oral therapy; MAY ADD
  — Clindamycin 10 mg/kg IV for 1 dose,
    then 5 mg/kg IV 3 times a day
- Prevention of relapse caused by *P. vivax* or
  P. ovale:
  - Primaquine phosphate 26.3 mg (15.3 mg
    base)/day orally for 14 days, or 79 mg
    (45 mg base)/week for 8 weeks
  - Pediatric: Primaquine phosphate 0.5 mg
    (0.3 mg base)/day orally 14 days
- Ancillary therapy:
  - Exchange transfusion
    — Indicated for seriously ill patients with
      parasitemia greater than 15%, or patients
      with parasitemia of 5% to 15% and a
      poor prognosis because of:
      – Impaired consciousness
      – Repeated seizure activity
      – Respiratory distress
      – Substantial bleeding
      – Shock

> –Renal impairment (serum creatinine
>   greater than 3 mg/dL)
> –Acidosis (plasma bicarbonate less than
>   15 mmol/L)
> –Hyperbilirubinemia greater than
>   2.5 mg/dL
> –Hyperlactatemia greater than 45 mg/dL
> –Hypoglycemia (blood glucose less than
>   40 mg/dL)
> –Elevated aminotransferase levels
>   greater than 3 times normal

- Chemoprophylaxis:
  - Drugs used for chemoprophylaxis should be started 2 weeks before departure to endemic area, and continued for 4 weeks after leaving the endemic area
  - Chloroquine-susceptible malaria
    —Chloroquine base 300 mg (= 500 mg chloroquine phosphate)/week orally
    —Pediatric: Chloroquine base 5 mg/kg (= 8.3 mg/kg of chloroquine phosphate)/week orally
  - Chloroquine-resistant malaria
    —Mefloquine 250 mg/week orally (Pediatric: 5 mg/kg/week orally), or
    —Doxycycline 100 mg orally once daily, or
    —Chloroquine as above, and
      Proguanil 200 mg/day orally
        (Pediatric: 50 mg/day [under 2 years old], 100 mg/day [2 to 6 years old, 150 mg/day [7 to 10 years old], 200 mg/day [older than 10 years])

Follow-Up:

- Falciparum malaria requires inpatient treatment
- Other forms of malaria may be managed as outpatient except during the acute phase

- **Watch for:** signs and symptoms of
    - *P. falciparum:*
        - —Cerebral malaria, including seizures and coma
        - —Acute renal failure
        - —Severe anemia from massive hemolysis
        - —Hypoglycemia
        - —Acidosis
        - —Bacterial pneumonia
        - —Pulmonary edema
        - —Adult respiratory distress syndrome (ARDS)
        - —Respiratory arrest
        - —Chronic splenomegaly
        - —Splenic rupture
        - —Resistance to chloroquine
        - —Death
    - *P. vivax:*
        - —Late splenic rupture 2 to 3 months after the initial infection
        - —Drug resistance
    - *P. malariae:*
        - —Immune complex glomerulonephritis
        - —Nephrotic syndrome

TAPEWORM INFESTATION

Presenting Symptoms:

SUBJECTIVE	OBJECTIVE
Diphyllobothriasis (**Diphyllobothrium latum**)	
Abdominal cramps	History of exposure to
Weakness	uncooked or
Dizziness	undercooked fish:

Craving for salt

Intermittent mild diarrhea

Peripheral neuropathy[1]

CNS degeneration[1]

—Consumption of dried or smoked fish

—Consumption of "raw bar" foods (sushi, sashimi, or ceviche)

—Tasting uncooked flavored freshwater fish (gefilte fish)

—Travel to endemic areas (Siberia, Scandinavia, Baltic countries, Japan, Chile)

Patients with prolonged infection may demonstrate signs of megaloblastic anemia:

—Glossitis

—Neurologic deficits

Taeniasis (Taenia saginata and Taenia solium)

Mild abdominal cramps

Anal irritation

Moving segments in feces

CNS complaints[2]

—Headache

—Visual deterioration

History of exposure to uncooked or undercooked beef or pork:

—Consumption of rare steak, steak tartare, raw or undercooked pork

[1] After prolonged infection of over 3 to 4 years

[2] Only in patients with cysticercosis

—Seizure activity
—Altered mental state

—Travel to endemic areas (Central Asia, Near East, Central and Eastern Africa, Central and South America)

May find motile proglottids of *T. saginata* in clothing or perianal areas

Physical signs associated with *T. solium* infection found only in cysticercosis (tissue infection with larval cysts of parasite)

Neurocysticercosis is most common
—Intracranial hypertension
—Diminished vision
—Altered mental status and coma
—Seizures

Hymenolepiasis (Hymenolepsis nana)

Abdominal cramps
Diarrhea
Vomiting
Anorexia and weight loss
Dizziness

History of travel to endemic areas (Asia, Southern and Eastern Europe, Central and South America, Africa)

History of living among institutionalized

> populations or under
> poor sanitary
> conditions
> History of malnutrition
> and/or
> immunocompromise

Differential Diagnosis:

Schistosomiasis
Intestinal protozoal infections
Bacterial or viral diarrhea
Drugs
Poisoning with heavy metals or mushrooms
Irritable bowel syndrome
Inflammatory bowel diseases
Malabsorption syndromes
Secretory neoplastic disorders
(**NOTE:** because the majority of tapeworm
   intestinal infections are asymptomatic, and the
   patient becomes aware of the infection only
   upon passing a proglottid in the stool, the
   diagnosis is usually obvious)

Suggested Workup:

- Microbiology:
  - Examination of stool for ova and parasites
    and proglottids
  - Perianal cellophane test for proglottids and
    ova of *T. saginata*
- Laboratory: Megaloblastic anemia → *D. latum*
- Imaging studies:
  - Barium upper gastrointestinal series with
    small bowel follow through → ribbonlike
    filling defects (especially with *T. saginata*)
  - Skull radiographs may show calcified cysts
    in *T. solium* neurocysticercosis

- CT/MRI of head can detect calcified and noncalcified cysts of *T. solium*
- Serology: ELISA test for *T. solium* is commercially available

Definitive Diagnosis:

Diphyllobothriasis ICD-9-CM 123.4
Taeniasis ICD-9-CM 123.3
—*T. saginata* ICD-9-CM 123.2
—*T. solium* ICD-9-CM 123.0
Hymenolepiasis ICD-9-CM 123.6

Suggested Treatment:

- Diphyllobothriasis:
  - Praziquantel 10 mg/kg orally for 1 dose (adults and children), or
      Niclosamide 2 g orally for 1 dose (adults)
      1.5 g orally for 1 dose (children over
        34 kg)
      1 g orally for 1 dose (children 11 to
        34 kg)
  - Vitamin B_{12} injections may be needed in patients with prolonged or heavy infection and evidence of megaloblastic anemia
- Taeniasis:
  - As above for noncysticercotic infections
  - Mild laxative 1 to 2 hours after niclosamide treatment may reduce incidence of internal autoinfection with *T. solium* eggs
  - Neurocystecircosis (adults or children)
    —Praziquantel 50 mg/kg/day orally for 15 to 30 days, or
        Albendazole 10 to 15 mg/kg/day
          orally given 3 times a day for 8 to
          30 days (not FDA-approved; must
          be obtained on investigational basis

from SmithKline Beecham
laboratories, Philadelphia, PA)
—Dexamethasone given concomitantly has
been shown in some cases to reduce CNS
inflammation, but may lower serum
praziquantel levels

- Hymenolepiasis:
  - Praziquantel 25 mg/kg orally for 1 dose;
  may be repeated 1 week later if *H. nana*
  infection is heavy, or
    Niclosamide 2 g orally for 1 dose, then
      1 g orally daily for 6 days
      (similar dose adjustments for children,
        with maximum dose for 1 day, then
        50% maximum dose for 6 days)

Follow-Up:

- Outpatient therapy is appropriate
- Re-examine stool for ova and parasites 2
  weeks after treatment
- If unresponsive to medical treatment, consider
  surgical intervention for patients with
  cysticercosis
- Patient education regarding thorough cooking
  of fish, beef, and pork, and appropriate
  sanitation
- **Watch for:** signs and symptoms of
      - Cysticercosis with *T. solium*
        infection
        —Epilepsy
        —Meningoencephalitis
        —Myopathy
      - Megaloblastic anemia with
        D. latum infection
      - Recurrent infections requiring
        retreatment

HELMINTHIC INFECTIONS

Presenting Symptoms:

<u>SUBJECTIVE</u>   <u>OBJECTIVE</u>

Schistosomiasis

SUBJECTIVE		OBJECTIVE
Skin rash ("swimmer's itch")	*dermatitis stage*	History of travel to endemic areas (Africa, South America, Asia, the Caribbean) with water contact
Fever and chills Sweating Headache Cough	*Katayama fever stage (4 to 8 weeks later)*	
Fatigue Abdominal pain Intermittent diarrhea Paragenital lesions	*chronic disease*	Hepatospleno-megaly Lymphadeno-pathy Paragenital granulomas

Trichinosis

SUBJECTIVE	OBJECTIVE
Often asymptomatic Fever (90% of patients) Myalgia (90%) Weakness and malaise (80%) Periorbital edema (80%) Photophobia (50%) Headache (50%) Skin rash (20%) Nausea and vomiting (10%) Diarrhea (10%)	Periorbital edema Myositis (starts in extraocular muscles, then masseters, neck muscles, limb flexors, and lumbar muscles) Chemosis Subconjunctival or retinal hemorrhages Macular/petechial rash Risk factor: consumption of

Cough (less than 10%)	undercooked pork, bear or walrus meat, or wild game

Filariasis

Often asymptomatic	Lymphangitis and lymphadenitis
Fever	Chronic lymphadenopathy
Headache	Chronic hydrocele
Backache	Pitting pretibial edema that eventually becomes nonpitting to involve the whole limb and may progress to elephantiasis of the lower limbs and scrotum
Nausea	Genital lymph varices
Pretibial limb edema that may progress to elephantiasis of the entire lower limbs and scrotum	Chyluria
	Risk factor: travel to tropics or subtropics (especially southeast Asia and Indonesia)

Enterobiasis (Pinworm)

Often asymptomatic	Most common in children 5 to 14 years old
Perianal and perineal pruritus	Familial/institutional infections with no socioeconomic predilections
	Prevalence in whites much higher than in blacks
	Nonspecific perianal

and perineal
inflammation
observed

Differential Diagnosis:

Gastroenteritis
Influenza
Typhoid fever
Sinusitis
Dermatomyositis
Glomerulonephritis
Angioneurotic edema
Measles
Scarlet fever
Typhus
Acute rheumatic fever
Collagen vascular diseases
Encephalitis
Eosinophilic leukemia
Tuberculosis
Undulant fever

Suggested Workup:

- Schistosomiasis:
  - Travel history
  - History of water contact
  - Examine stools (Kato thick smear) for schistosome eggs
  - Examine urine (noon to 2 pm collection) for schistosome eggs by passing specimen through Nuclepore filter
  - Anoscopy with rectal biopsy for schistosome eggs
- Trichinosis:
  - Look for cardinal quartet of periorbital edema, myositis, fever, and eosinophilia

- History of consumption of poorly cooked pork products
  - ELISA for anti-*Trichinella* antibodies
- Filariasis:
  - History of tropical/subtropical travel
  - Blood sample taken around midnight (unless the patient is from the South Pacific) and stained for microfilariae
  - Sample hydrocele fluid for microfilariae
  - Collect chylous urine and examine for microfilariae
  - ELISA assay to detect filarial antigens
- Enterobiasis:
  - Cellophane test tape in perineal area early in the morning can detect up to 99% of infections if repeated at least 4 to 5 times; pinworms stuck to the tape are visible to the naked eye

Definitive Diagnosis:

Schistosomiasis	ICD-9-CM 120.9
Trichinosis	ICD-9-CM 124
Filariasis	ICD-9-CM 125.9
Enterobiasis	ICD-9-CM 127.4

Suggested Treatment:

- Schistosomiasis:
  - *Schistosoma mansoni* or *Schistosoma haematobium:*
    Praziquantel 20 mg/kg orally twice in 1 day
  - *Schistosoma japonica* or *Schistosoma mekongi:*
    Praziquantel 20 mg/kg orally 3 times in 1 day
- Trichinosis:
  - Thiabendazole 25 to 50 mg/kg/day orally for 7 days for early disease

- Salicylates, bedrest, and corticosteroids for established infections
- Filariasis:
  - Diethylcarbamazine citrate 6 mg/kg/day orally given 3 times a day for 2 to 3 weeks, or
    Ivermectin 200 mcg/kg orally for 1 dose
  - Anti-inflammatory agents
  - Elastic stockings for mild lymphedema
  - Surgical management of hydrocele
- Enterobiasis:
  - Pyrantel pamoate 11 mg/kg orally for 1 dose (can be repeated 2 weeks later), or
    Mebendazole 100 mg orally 2 times a day for 3 days, or
    Mebendazole 100 mg orally for 1 dose, repeated 2 weeks later

Follow-Up:

- Outpatient care is typically sufficient
- Patients should be monitored frequently for clinical improvement and development of complications
- Patient education regarding proper preparation of pork and game meats (trichinosis)
- Patient education for mosquito avoidance, i.e., screens, nets, insect repellents (filariasis)
- All members of families with pinworm-infected individuals should be treated
- **Watch for:** signs and symptoms of
  - Meningitis
  - Encephalitis
  - Myocarditis and cardiac failure
  - Glomerulonephritis and renal failure
  - Recurrent or resistant infections requiring repeated treatment

ROCKY MOUNTAIN SPOTTED FEVER

Presenting Symptoms:

SUBJECTIVE

Fever over 40°C (100% of patients)

Chills (100%)

Rash 3 to 5 days after the onset of fever, usually around wrists and ankles or on trunk (95%)

No pruritus with rash

Severe headache (65%)

Myalgias (less than 50%)

Nausea, vomiting (50%)

Abdominal pain (less than 50%)

Diarrhea (less than 50%)

Cough (less than 25%)

Confusion, stupor (25%)

OBJECTIVE

Macular, maculopapular, or petechial rash, typically occurring first on the extremities and then spreading toward the trunk

Pustules/vesicles not seen

Palm and sole distribution of rash is classic

Hepatosplenomegaly

Generalized lymphadenopathy

Abdominal tenderness

Neurologic defects may be present

—Ataxia

—Seizures

—Coma

—Focal defects

Arrhythmias

Peripheral edema

Conjunctivitis

Evidence of tick bite(s) may be present

Elicit risk factors

—History of known tick bite 3 to 12 days prior to onset of symptoms

—Outdoor activity
during warm
months (usually
May to September)
—Contact with dogs or
rabbits
—Travel in highly
endemic areas (e.g.,
North Carolina,
Missouri, Oklahoma,
Georgia, Montana,
South Dakota)

Differential Diagnosis:

Measles
Rubella
Typhoid fevers
Murine typhus
Respiratory tract infection
Gastroenteritis
Enteroviral infection
Disseminated gonococcal infection
Secondary syphilis
Rickettsialpox
Ehrlichiosis
Lyme disease
Leptospirosis
Meningococcemia
Boutonneuse fever
Dengue fever
Colorado tick fever
Tularemia
Immune complex vasculitis
Idiopathic thrombocytopenic purpura
Thrombotic thrombocytopenic
  purpura

Infectious mononucleosis
Drug reaction

Suggested Workup:

- Laboratory:
  - Nonspecific changes
    - —Hyponatremia more pronounced than in Colorado tick fever, Ehrlichiosis, typhus, tularemia, or dengue fever
    - —Elevated serum blood urea nitrogen (BUN) and creatinine
    - —Mildly elevated liver enzymes (especially ALT)
    - —Elevated alkaline phosphatase
    - —Thrombocytopenia
    - —Prolonged prothrombin time (PT)/partial thromboplastin time (PTT)
    - —Modestly elevated cerebrospinal fluid (CSF) protein and white blood cell (WBC) count with normal glucose
  - Blood cultures
    - —Can be used to rule out other bacterial etiologies
    - —Few labs undertake isolation of *Rickettsia rickettsii* because of the biohazard involved
- Serology:
  - Antibodies to *R. ricketsii* antigens
    - —Indirect hemagglutination
    - —Indirect immunofluorescence
    - —Latex agglutination
    - —ELISA
  - Skin biopsy of rash—direct immunofluorescence and immunoperoxidase tests are available

Definitive Diagnosis:

Rocky Mountain spotted fever   ICD-9-CM 082.0

Suggested Treatment:

- Adults:
  - Doxycycline 200 mg orally for 1 dose, then 100 mg orally 2 times a day for 7 to 10 days, or
    Tetracycline 500 mg orally every 6 hours for 7 to 10 days, or
    Chloramphenicol 500 to 750 mg orally every 6 hours for 7 to 10 days, or
    Ciprofloxacin 500 to 750 mg orally every 12 hours for 7 to 10 days
  - If hospitalized:
    Doxycycline 100 mg IV every 12 hours, or
    Chloramphenicol 20 mg/kg IV every 6 hours
- Children:
  - Chloramphenicol 20 mg/kg orally every 6 hours for 7 to 10 days, or
    Doxycycline 2.0 to 2.5 mg/kg orally every 12 hours for 7 to 10 days, or
    Tetracycline 10 mg/kg orally every 6 hours for 7 to 10 days
  - If hospitalized:
    Chloramphenicol 20 mg/kg IV every 6 hours, or
    Doxycycline 4.4 mg/kg IV once, then 2.2 mg/kg IV every 12 hours
    (NOTE: Oral or parenteral doxycycline or tetracycline should not be used in children under 9 years old)

Follow-Up:

- Patients with mild disease may be followed as outpatients

- Office visit every 2 to 3 days to follow symptoms
  - Monitor electrolytes, CBC, and renal function
- Moderately ill patients and those with multiple organ involvement should be hospitalized
  - May require intravenous hydration and nutrition
  - May require Swann-Ganz catheterization to monitor hemodynamics
    —Watch for increased vascular permeability and extravasation of fluid into pulmonary alveoli
- **Watch for:** signs and symptoms of
  - Azotemia and renal failure
  - Encephalopathy
  - Seizure activity
  - Hepatitis and hepatic failure
  - Congestive heart failure
  - Respiratory failure

TYPHUS FEVERS

Presenting Symptoms:

SUBJECTIVE	OBJECTIVE
Acute onset of fever	**Epidemic typhus**
Chills	(person to person
Severe headache	transmission by
Myalgia	body louse)
Malaise	(*Rickettsia prowazekii*)
Nausea and vomiting	History of body
Anorexia	contact with suspect
Skin rash	carrier 1 week before
Cough	onset of symptoms
Seizure activity	History of living in
(variable)	unclean

Confusion/stupor
(variable)

circumstances with
poor sanitation
Macular/
maculopapular rash
on trunk 3 to 5 days
after onset of illness
Nonproductive cough
with diffuse rales/
rhonchi
**Murine (endemic)
typhus** (transmission
by rodent flea bite)
(*Rickettsia typhi*)
History of flea bite 1 to
2 weeks before onset
of symptoms
Macular/
maculopapular rash
on trunk and
extremities
(including palms and
soles) 3 to 5 days
after onset of illness
Petechiae (fewer than
10% of cases)
Scrub typhus
(transmission by
chiggers) (*Rickettsia
tsutsugamushi*)
History of chigger bite
1 to 3 weeks before
onset of illness
History of travel to
endemic areas
(eastern Asia,
western Pacific)
Eschar at bite site

Generalized or regional (bite-site) tender lymphadenopathy

Conjunctival injection

Macular/maculopapular rash on trunk and extremities 5 days after onset of illness

Splenomegaly

Neurologic findings in less than 10% of cases (ataxia, slurred speech, tremor, delirium, nuchal rigidity, deafness)

Differential Diagnosis:

Rocky Mountain spotted fever
Brucellosis
Meningococcemia
Bacterial and viral meningitis
Measles
Rubella
Toxoplasmosis
Leptospirosis
Typhoid fever
Dengue fever
Flavivirus infection
Relapsing fever
Secondary syphilis
Infectious mononucleosis
Kawasaki's disease
Toxic shock syndrome

Suggested Workup:

- Serology:
  - Indirect fluorescent antibody test for *R. typhi* antigens

- Latex agglutination tests
- Solid phase immunoassay tests
- ELISA tests for *R. prowazekii* and *R. typhi*
- PCR for *R. tsutsugamushi* and *R. typhi*
- Weil-Felix serology has low sensitivity and specificity and is clinically of limited utility

Definitive Diagnosis:

Epidemic (louse-borne) typhus   ICD-9-CM 080
Murine or endemic (flea-   ICD-9-CM 081.0
  borne) typhus
Scrub typhus   ICD-9-CM 081.2

Suggested Treatment:

- Mild to moderate illness (treatment is for 5 to 10 days or at least for 2 to 3 days after defervescence):
  - Tetracycline 25 to 50 mg/kg/day orally given every 6 hours, or
    Doxycycline 100 mg orally 2 times a day, or
    Chloramphenicol 50 to 75 mg/kg/day orally given every 6 hours
- Severe illness with complications (treatment is for 7 to 10 days or at least for 2 to 3 days after defervescence and clinical improvement):
  - Tetracycline 10 to 20 mg/kg/day IV given every 6 hours, or
    Doxycycline 4 to 5 mg/kg/day IV given every 12 hours, or
    Chloramphenicol 50 mg/kg/day IV given every 6 hours
- Doxycycline or chloramphenicol is preferred in severely ill patients in renal failure
- Corticosteroids IV/orally can be used as adjuncts for patients with severe CNS disease

Follow-Up:

- Outpatient care is appropriate unless patient is severely ill
- Outpatients should be checked weekly until clinical improvement is evident
- Patient education for prevention, especially for travelers to endemic areas
  - Control of flea vectors
  - Improve sanitary conditions
  - Delousing procedures where necessary
  - Rodent-control practices
  - Travelers should be advised to wear protective clothing and use insect repellents to avoid chigger bites
- An effective vaccine is available for epidemic typhus; may consider for persons at high risk of exposure
- **Watch for:** signs and symptoms of
  - Renal insufficiency and azotemia
  - Meningoencephalitis and other CNS abnormalities
  - Seizure activity
  - Delirium and coma
  - Myocardial failure
  - Respiratory failure
  - Hematemesis (murine typhus)
  - Electrolyte disturbances
    —Severe hyponatremia
    —Hypocalcemia
    —Hypokalemia
  - Hypoalbuminemia
  - Hypovolemia and shock

Q FEVER

Presenting Symptoms:

SUBJECTIVE	OBJECTIVE
High fever greater than 40°C	Findings of pneumonitis (100% of patients)

Chills with rigors and
  sweats
Severe headaches
Retrobulbar pain
Malaise and myalgias
Pleuritic chest pain
Cough
Nausea and vomiting
Diarrhea
All symptoms are of
  abrupt onset
—Inspiratory crackles
—Signs of pulmonary
  consolidation may
  be present
Findings of
  endocarditis (1%)
—Chronic indolent
  symptoms
Findings of hepatitis
  (15%)
—May be acute
  infectious type or
  indolent and
  subclinical
  –Hepatomegaly
  –Right upper
    quadrant
    abdominal pain
  –Jaundice may be
    present
Neurologic
  manifestations
—Meningoencephalitic
  signs
  –Confusion
  –Dementia
  –Extrapyramidal
    symptoms
  –Manic
    psychosis
Elicit history of high-
  risk occupation
—Abattoir worker
—Veterinarian
—Medical researcher,
  especially using
  pregnant ewes

Differential Diagnosis:

Miliary tuberculosis
Sarcoidosis
Histoplasmosis
Brucellosis
Tularemia
Syphilitic granulomas
Subacute bacterial endocarditis
Viral hepatitis
Bacterial or viral meningoencephalitis
Atypical pneumonia
Acute bacterial pneumonia
Salmonellosis

Suggested Workup:

- History and clinical suspicion:
    - Abrupt onset of high fever, severe headache, chills, myalgias, and pleuritic chest pain should evoke clinical suspicion
    - History of contact with animals, animal products (e.g., infected placenta), or ticks 18 to 21 days before onset of symptoms reinforces suspicion
- Serology:
    - ELISA and immunofluorescent antibodies to *Coxiella burnetii* antigens
      —Anti-Phase II antibodies are present in primary acute Q fever
      —Anti-Phase I antibodies are present in high titers during the chronic form of the illness
- Microbiology:
    - Isolation and culture of *C. burnetii* from the blood is not recommended; it is hazardous and difficult
    - Blood cultures should be drawn to rule out other bacterial infectious etiologies

Definitive Diagnosis:

Q fever   ICD-9-CM 083.0

Suggested Treatment:

- Adults and children 8 years of age and older:
  - Tetracycline 500 mg 4 times a day for 14 days, or
    Doxycycline 100 mg orally 2 times a day for 14 days, or
    Ofloxacin 300 mg orally 2 times a day for 14 days
- Children under 8 years of age:
  - Chloramphenicol 50 to 75 mg/kg/day orally given every 6 hours for 14 days
- Q fever endocarditis:
  - Tetracycline 500 mg orally 4 times a day, and
    TMP-SMX DS 1 tablet orally 2 times a day for 2 years, or
  - Doxycyxline 100 mg orally 2 times a day, and
    Rifampin 600 mg orally 2 times a day for 2 years
  - Valve replacement should be considered for hemodynamic failure

Follow-Up:

- Outpatient care is usually appropriate
- Follow clinical symptoms and serology after treatment
- Patients with endocarditis should be followed closely and monitored for evidence of hemodynamic compromise
  - Antibody titers should be determined every 6 months during therapy and every 3 months for the first 2 years after cessation of therapy

- Repeat ESR every 6 months
- Consider vaccination of high risk personnel
- **Watch for:** signs and symptoms of
  - Chronic infection
  - Endocarditis
  - Osteomyelitis
  - Hepatitis
  - Interstitial pulmonary fibrosis
  - Radiculopathy in patients with neurologic manifestations

LYME DISEASE

Presenting Symptoms:

SUBJECTIVE

OBJECTIVE

Stage 1 (Localized Infection)

SUBJECTIVE	OBJECTIVE
Red macule or papule at site of a tick bite that expands over time, leaving a clear center with bright red border	History of tick bite 3 to 32 days before onset of erythema chronicum migrans (ECM)
—Thigh, groin, and axilla are most common sites	—Initially, a red macule or papule
—Within 3 to 5 days after patient notices primary lesion, other similar smaller annular lesions will appear	—Area of redness around the center expands to a final median diameter of 15 cm, leaving central clearing with bright red, occasionally indurated borders
—All lesions will usually fade within 3 to 4 weeks, but may last up to 14 months	—Centers of early lesions may become indurated, blue,

Flu-like symptoms
—Malaise and fatigue
—Headache
—Fever and chills
—Generalized arthralgias
—Sore throat
—Cough
Episodic migratory pain in joints, muscle, or bone without joint swelling

vesicular, necrotic, or may remain erythematous
—Lesions are warm to the touch, but not painful
Multiple secondary annular lesions develop within 3 to 5 days after appearance of ECM (50% of cases)
—Smaller
—More evanescent
—Less migratory
—Lack indurated centers
—Not associated with site of tick bite
Malar rash
Conjunctivitis
Diffuse urticaria
Regional lymphadenopathy
Signs of meningeal irritation
Mild encephalopathy
Abdominal tenderness
Testicular swelling or tenderness

Stage 2 (Disseminated Infection)

Intermittent episodes of frank arthritis, particularly affecting the knee, but can affect any large joint

Frank arthritis of almost exclusively large joints, generally mono- or oligoarticular, and

Shoulder, ankle, elbow, and hip may also be involved

Attacks are intermittent, lasting a few weeks to months

Headache and stiff neck

Facial palsy (unilateral or bilateral)

Muscle weakness

Sensory loss

Chest pain

Shortness of breath

Eye redness, pain, and/or diminished vision

Testicular swelling and pain

almost never symmetric
—Swelling
—Increased warmth of joint
—Effusions are common, especially in the knee
—Baker's cysts are common
—Erosive synovitis rare
—Occur within 2 weeks to months after onset of illness

Meningeal irritation or frank meningitis with neck stiffness but with negative Kernig and Brudzinski signs

Encephalitis

Chorea

Cranial neuritis

Bell's palsy (unilateral or bilateral)

Peripheral radiculoneuropathy

Motor and sensory radiculoneuritis

Reticular pain, paresthesias, and hyperesthesias (Garin-Bujadoux or Bannwarth's syndrome)

Relatively brief period of fluctuating

degrees of atrioventricular heart block (typically less than 10% of patients)
Acute myopericarditis (also usually transient)
Conjunctivitis
Iritis and panophthalmitis
Mild hepatitis (20% of patients)
Frank orchitis

Stage 3 (Chronic Infection)

Red or violaceous lesions on trunk or extremities
Chronic arthritis (more than 1 year of inflammation)
Memory loss
Sleep disorders
Language disturbances
Peripheral sensory loss
Spasticity and ataxia
Cognitive impairment
Bladder dysfunction
Dementia
Psychiatric symptoms
Extrapyramidal symptoms
Stroke symptoms

Acrodermatitis chronica atrophicans (ACA): red violaceous lesions that become sclerotic or atrophic may develop months or years after ECM
Large joint monoarthritis can become chronic
Chronic neurologic disturbances
—Encephalopathies
 –Distal paresthesias
 –Spinal or radicular pain with diffuse axonal polyneuropathy
—Encephalomyelitis (primarily in Europe)

> −Neurogenic bladder
> −Spastic parapareses
> −Ataxia
> −Cranial neuropathy, especially cranial nerve (CN) VII or CN VIII
>
> Chronic cardiomyopathy is rare
>
> Chronic hepatitis is rare

Differential Diagnosis:

Rheumatoid arthritis
Viral syndrome
Chronic fatigue syndrome
Fibromyalgia
Aseptic meningitis
Pericarditis
Hepatitis
Viral encephalopathy
Multiple sclerosis
Cerebrovascular accident
Cranial nerve neuropathies
Optic neuritis
Transverse myelitis
Parkinson's disease

Suggested Workup:

- History and classic clinical picture (especially ECM) is very helpful in making diagnosis
- Laboratory:
    - ELISA test for immunoglobulin (Ig)M and IgG antibodies to *Borrelia burgdorferi* (poor

  sensitivity early in the infection; antibodies develop slowly)
  —Thirty to 40% seropositive patients early in the disease
  —Sixty to 70% seropositive patients 2 to 4 weeks after infection
- Western blotting can be used to confirm indeterminate or positive ELISA results
- Antibody-capture immunoassay
  —Can be used to compare anti-*B. burgdorferi* antibodies in serum and CSF in patients with neuroborreliosis
  —CSF/serum ratio of specific antibody greater than 1.0 suggests intrathecal anti-burgdorferi antibody production
- PCR of blood, urine, CSF, skin biopsy material, or synovial fluid
  —Eighty-five percent sensitivity in synovial fluid
  —Poorer sensitivity in CSF, blood, or urine
- ESR—elevated (usually greater than 35 mm/hr)
- Serum IgM level—elevated (usually greater than 300 mg/dL)
- AST—elevated (usually greater than 70 units/mL)
- Rheumatoid factor—negative
- Antinuclear antibody (ANA)—negative

Definitive Diagnosis:

Lyme disease   ICD-9-CM 088.81

Suggested Treatment:

- Stage 1—Early Localized Disease:
  - Doxycycline 100 mg orally 2 times a day for 21 days
    (NOT for children younger than 12 years old or for pregnant women), or

> Amoxicillin 500 mg orally 3 times a day
> for 21 days
> (Pediatric: 25 to 100 mg/kg/day orally
> given 3 times a day), or
> Cefuroxime 500 mg orally 2 times a day
> for 21 days, or
> Clarithromycin 500 mg orally 2 times a
> day for 14 to 21 days, or
> Azithromycin 500 mg orally once daily
> for 14 to 21 days

- Stage 2—Disseminated Disease:
  - CNS disease/neuroborreliosis:
    - —Mild (Bell's palsy, other isolated facial nerve palsies):
      - –Doxycycline 100 mg orally 2 times a day for 21 to 30 days, or
        - Amoxicillin 500 mg orally 3 times a day for 21 to 30 days
    - —More severe neurologic abnormalities (Lyme meningitis, encephalitis, radiculoneuropathy, peripheral neuropathy, Bannwarth's syndrome [meningopolyneuritis]):
      - –Ceftriaxone 2 g/day IV for 21 to 28 days, or
        - Cefotaxime 2 g IV 3 times a day for 21 to 28 days, or
        - Penicillin (PCN)-G 5 million units IV 4 times a day for 21 to 28 days
  - Lyme arthritis:
    - —Doxycycline 100 mg orally 2 times a day for 30 days, or
      - Amoxicillin 500 mg + probenecid 500 mg orally 4 times a day for 30 days
    - —May be extended to 45 to 60 days in patients who fail initial course of therapy

  —In more serious cases, in patients who
    develop neuroborreliosis during oral
    therapy, or who fail after repeat oral
    therapy:
    –Ceftriaxone 2 g/day IV for 14 to 28
      days, or
        Cefotaxime 2 g IV 3 times a day for
          14 to 28 days, or
        PCN-G 5 million units IV 4 times a
          day for 14 to 28 days
- Lyme carditis:
  —First/second-degree heart block:
    –Doxycycline 100 mg orally 2 times a
      day for 21 days, or
        Amoxicillin 500 mg orally 3 times a
          day for 21 days
  —Third-degree heart block/PR interval
    greater than 0.5 second:
    –Ceftriaxone 2 g/day IV for 14 to 28
      days, or
        PCN-G 5 million units IV 4 times a
          day for 14 to 28 days
    –Cardiac monitoring
    –Addition of corticosteroids in patients
      with complete heart block or congestive
      heart failure may be of benefit if they
      do not improve clinically on
      antimicrobial therapy alone within 24
      hours
- Stage 3—Persistent Infection:
  - Treat or retreat with Ceftriaxone or
    Cefotaxime IV for 3 to 4 weeks
  - Up to 50% of patients treated with PCN-G
    develop Stage 3 disease; it is unclear
    whether this is because of persistent
    infection, immune hyperreactivity to the
    infection, or irreversible pathologic changes
    caused by the initial infection

- Lyme disease vaccine:
  - Phase III testing of SmithKline Beecham's vaccine should have been completed by early 1998
  - FDA approval may be imminent, but vaccine may be available from manufacturer on a compassionate-use basis
  - For high-risk patients, a regimen of two primary doses plus biannual boosters may be indicated

Follow-Up:

- Stage 1 patients may be managed on outpatient basis, but Stage 2 and 3 patients may require hospitalization depending on their symptoms
- Stage 2 and 3 patients should be monitored carefully for months or years to follow resolution of symptoms, especially arthritic and neurological sequelae
- Patient education in endemic areas for prevention
  - Protective clothing
  - Insect repellents
- **Watch for:** signs and symptoms of
  - Recurrent infection
  - Persistent infection
  - Chronic Stage 3 symptoms
    —Synovitis
    —Tendinitis and bursitis
    —Neuropsychiatric symptoms
    –Memory loss and dementia
    –Depression
    –Disordered sleep
    —Encephalopathic symptoms
    –Chronic headache
    –Fatigue

—Peripheral neuropathies
  –Bannwarth's syndrome
    —Intense reticular pain
    —Paresthesias
    —Hyperesthesias
    —Meningeal signs
  –Asymmetric paresis
  –Spastic paraparesis
  –Neurogenic bladder
  –Chronic cardiac symptoms
   are rare

Immuno-compromised Hosts

10

INFECTIONS COVERED

HUMAN IMMUNODEFICIENCY VIRUS (HIV) INFECTION

Presenting Symptoms:

SUBJECTIVE	OBJECTIVE
May be asymptomatic	**Skin**
Persistent fever	—Abnormal pigmentation
Fatigue	—Variety of skin rashes
Sore throat	—Nail pigmentation
Unexplained weight loss	**Lymph nodes**
Myalgias	—Small, symmetric, mobile nodes
Headache	—May be generalized lymphadenopathy
Nausea and anorexia	**Examination of Head, Ears, Eyes, Nose, & Throat (HEENT)**
Persistent swollen lymph nodes in the neck	—Cheilitis
Night sweats	—Stomatitis
Diarrhea	—Pharyngitis
Vomiting	—Oral hairy leukoplakia
Rash	—Aphthous ulcers
Fecal incontinence	—Gingival/ periodontal infections
Painful defecation	—Sinusitis with headache
	—Headache without sinusitis
	Cardiopulmonary
	—Dyspnea on exertion or at rest
	—Cough with or without sputum

—Chest pain
—Spontaneous
  pneumothorax
—Postural hypotension

Gastrointestinal (GI)

—Odynophagia
—Dysphagia
—Retrosternal
  chest pain
—Hepatosplenomegaly
—Evidence of hepatitis
  and/or pancreatitis
—Perirectal abscess
—Proctitis

Genitourinary

—Painful, frequent
  urination
—Vaginitis with
  discharge
—Vaginal pruritus

Neurologic

—Memory loss
—Poor concentration
—Focal neurologic
  deficits
—Sensory
  polyneuropathy
—Personality changes

Musculoskeletal

—Proximal muscle
  weakness
—Muscle tenderness
—Muscle wasting
—Persistent
  oligoarthritis
  especially in lower
  limbs
—Psoriatic arthritis

Differential Diagnosis:

- Many illnesses mimic HIV infection, especially where there is a prolonged illness without ready explanation

Suggested Workup:

- Careful medical history, including
  - Travel history
  - Sexual history, including
    —Orientation
    —Practices
    —Lifetime number of partners
    —Prostitution
    —History of sexually transmitted diseases (STDs)
  - History of drug use
  - Other risk factors for exposure to HIV—occupational exposure
  - Underlying illnesses
  - History of common infections
  - Past toxic reactions to drugs
  - Social situation and occupational history
  - State of mind
  - Medication history, including
    —Vitamins
    —Minerals
    —Herbal supplements
  - Allergies
  - Dietary habits
  - Exposure to animals
- Careful physical examination
- Baseline laboratory studies
  - Anti-HIV antibody enzyme-linked immunosorbent assay (ELISA) (may need to be confirmed with Western blot technology)

> —A new oral mucosal transudate (OMT) method of collecting oral specimens for anti-HIV ELISA and Western blot testing may obviate the need for repeated blood testing (OraSure, Epitope, Inc., Beaverton, OR)

- p24 Antigen testing
- Plasma HIV-RNA testing (by polymerase chain reaction [PCR], branched DNA assay [bDNA], or nucleic acid sequence-based amplification [NASBA])
- Complete blood count (CBC) with differential and platelets
- CD3, CD4, and CD8 T-cell subset counts
- Chemistry panel with liver function tests
- Hepatitis profile
- Rapid plasma reagin (RPR) test or Venereal Disease Research Laboratories (VDRL) test (confirmed with fluorescent treponemal antibody absorption [FTA-ABS] if positive)
- Purified protein derivative (PPD) skin testing with controls
- Antitoxoplasma antibody (immunoglobulin G, IgG)
- Imaging studies—Chest radiograph

Definitive Diagnosis:

Human immunodeficiency virus   ICD-9-CM 042 infection

Suggested Treatment:

- Initial antiretroviral therapy (**NOTE:** Antiretroviral therapy should be initiated for patients:
  - With symptomatic HIV disease
  - With CD4 counts less than $500/mm^3$
  - With plasma HIV-RNA concentrations greater than 5,000 to 10,000 copies/mL by

bDNA assay or greater than 20,000 copies/mL by PCR, regardless of CD4 count, or
- [Possibly, depending on physician's clinical judgment] with documented HIV infection and detectable plasma HIV RNA, who request treatment and are committed to lifelong adherence to treatment
- **Preferred Triple Therapy** (Two nucleoside reverse transcriptase inhibitors [NRTI] plus one HIV protease inhibitor [PI]):
  —Zidovudine (AZT) 200 mg orally 3 times a day, and
  > Lamivudine (3TC) 150 mg orally 2 times a day, or
  > Didanosine (ddI) 200 mg orally 2 times a day, or
  > Zalcitabine (ddC) 0.75 mg orally 3 times a day, or
  —Stavudine (d4T) 20 mg orally 2 times a day, and
  > Lamivudine (3TC) 150 mg orally 2 times a day, or
  > Didanosine (ddI) 200 mg orally 2 times a day, plus
  —Indinavir 800 mg orally every 8 hours, or
  > Ritonavir 600 mg orally every 12 hours, or
  > Nelfinavir 750 mg orally 3 times a day
- **Alternative Triple Therapy** (Two NRTIs plus one non-nucleoside reverse transcriptase inhibitor [NNRTI]):
  —Zidovudine (AZT) 200 mg orally 3 times a day, and
  > Didanosine (ddI) 200 mg orally 2 times a day, and
  > Nevirapine 200 mg orally 2 times a day

      —**NOTE:** This combination has been shown to be useful in patients who are naive to antiretroviral drugs

- **Double NRTI Therapy** (Two NRTIs for patients who are not candidates for Triple Therapy because of lack of commitment, poor adherence, no access, cost, etc.):
  —Zidovudine (AZT) 200 mg orally 3 times a day, and
      Didanosine (ddI) 200 mg orally 2 times a day, or
  —Zidovudine (AZT) 200 mg orally 3 times a day, and
      Zalcitabine (ddC) 0.75 mg orally 3 times a day, or
  —Zidovudine (AZT) 200 mg orally 3 times a day, and
      Lamivudine[1] (3TC) 150 mg orally 2 times a day, or
  —Stavudine (d4T) 20 mg orally 2 times a day, and
      Lamivudine[1] (3TC) 150 mg orally 2 times a day, or
  —Stavudine (d4T) 20 mg orally 2 times a day, and
      Didanosine (ddI) 200 mg orally 2 times a day

- Modifying antiretroviral therapy (**NOTE:** Antiretroviral therapy should be changed when there is:
  - Treatment failure [less than 10-fold log reduction in viral load within 4 weeks of treatment], failure to suppress viral load to

[1] Lamivudine should be used only where the goal of therapy is to reduce viral RNA to undetectable levels, primarily because of the rapid development of resistance to the drug

undetectable levels within 4 to 6 months of treatment, repeated detection of plasma HIV-RNA after initial suppression to undetectable levels [suggesting development of resistance], documented *significant* rise in HIV-RNA, persistently declining CD4 count, or clinical deterioration,
- Unacceptable toxicity or intolerance of treatment regimen,
- Inability or unwillingness to adhere to treatment regimen, or
- Current use of a suboptimal regimen (e.g., antiretroviral monotherapy)
- **Toxicity:**
  —If a result of PI, dose reduction is to be avoided; discontinue offending drug and replace with NNRTI
  —If a result of NRTI, discontinue offending drug and replace with NRTI with a different toxicity profile
  —If cause is unclear, discontinue entire regimen until toxic effects are resolved; clinical judgment and availability of alternative drugs should guide what regimen to restart
- **Failure of Initial Triple Therapy:**
  —Failed AZT + 3TC + PI →
    –Stavudine (d4T) 20 mg orally 2 times a day, and
      Didanosine (ddI) 200 mg orally 2 times a day, and
      A different PI, or Nevirapine 200 mg orally 2 times a day, or
    –Ritonavir 600 mg orally 2 times a day, and
      Saquinavir 600 mg orally 3 times a day, and
      An NRTI

—Failed d4T + 3TC + PI →
  –Zidovudine (AZT) 200 mg orally 3
   times a day, and
      Didanosine (ddI) 200 mg orally 2
      times a day, and
      A different PI, or Nevirapine 200 mg
      orally 2 times a day, or
  –Ritonavir 600 mg orally 2 times a
   day, and
      Saquinavir 600 mg orally 3 times a
      day, and
      An NRTI
—Failed AZT + ddI + PI →
  –Stavudine (d4T) 20 mg orally 2 times a
   day, and
      Lamivudine (3TC) 150 mg orally 2
      times a day, and
      A different PI, or Nevirapine 200 mg
      orally 2 times a day, or
  –Ritonavir 600 mg orally 2 times a
   day, and
      Saquinavir 600 mg orally 2 times a
      day, and
      An NRTI
—Failed d4T + ddI + PI →
  –Zidovudine (AZT) 200 mg orally 3
   times a day, and
      Lamivudine (3TC) 150 mg orally 2
      times a day, and
      A different PI, or Nevirapine 200 mg
      orally 2 times a day, or
  –Ritonavir 600 mg orally 2 times a
   day, and
      Saquinavir 600 mg orally 3 times a
      day, and
      An NRTI

—Failed AZT + ddI + Nevirapine →
-Stavudine (d4T) 20 mg orally 2 times a
day, or
Zidovudine (AZT)[2] 200 mg orally
3 times a day, and
Lamivudine (3TC) 150 mg orally 2
times a day, and
A PI
- **Failure of Initial Double Therapy**:
—Failed AZT + ddI →
-Zidovudine (AZT) 200 mg orally 3
times a day, or
Stavudine (d4T) 20 mg orally 2 times
a day, and
Lamivudine (3TC) 150 mg orally 2
times a day, and
A PI,[3] or
-Ritonavir 600 mg orally 2 times a
day, and
Saquinavir 600 mg orally 3 times a
day, and
An NRTI
—Failed AZT + ddC →
-Zidovudine (AZT) 200 mg orally 3
times a day, or
Stavudine (d4T) 20 mg orally 2 times
a day, and
Lamivudine (3TC) 150 mg orally 2
times a day, and
A PI,[3] or

[2] Generally, failure of a given therapeutic regimen
dictates a switch of all three drugs, where possible
[3] A PI with potent in vivo activity is recommended
here, including Indinavir, Ritonavir, and Nelfinavir.
Saquinavir in its present formulation is not
recommended because of its poor bioavailability.

-Stavudine (d4T) 20 mg orally 2 times a
day, and
    Didanosine (ddI) 200 mg orally 2
    times a day, and
    A PI,[3] or
-Ritonavir 600 mg orally 2 times a day, and
    Saquinavir 600 mg orally 3 times a
    day, and
    An NRTI
—Failed AZT + 3TC →
-Stavudine (d4T) 20 mg orally 2 times a
day, and
    Didanosine (ddI) 200 mg orally 2
    times a day, and
    A PI,[3] or
-Ritonavir 600 mg orally 2 times a day, and
    Saquinavir 600 mg orally 3 times a
    day, and
    An NRTI
—Failed d4T + ddI →
-Zidovudine (AZT) 200 mg orally 3
times a day, and
    Lamivudine (3TC) 150 mg orally 2
    times a day, and
    A PI,[3] or
-Ritonavir 600 mg orally 2 times a day, and
    Saquinavir 600 mg orally 3 times a
    day, and
    An NRTI
—Failed d4T + 3TC →
-Zidovudine (AZT) 200 mg orally 3
times a day, and
    Didanosine (ddI) 200 mg orally 2
    times a day, and
    A PI,[3] or
-Ritonavir 600 mg orally 2 times a day, and
    Saquinavir 600 mg orally 3 times a
    day, and
    An NRTI

—**NOTE:** Two new compounds and one new combination product have recently been approved by the Food and Drug Administration (FDA) for use in antiretroviral therapy:
  –Delavirdine, an NNRTI to be used in Triple Therapy with two NRTIs or with one NRTI and one PI (Pharmacia & Upjohn, Kalamazoo, MI); Delavirdine 400 mg orally 3 times a day
  –Nelfinavir, a PI to be used in Triple Therapy with two NRTIs (Agouron Pharmaceuticals, La Jolla, CA); Nelfinavir 750 mg orally 3 times a day
  –Combivir, a combination tablet consisting of Zidovudine 300 mg and Lamivudine 150 mg (Glaxo-Wellcome, Research Triangle Park, NC); Combivir 1 tablet orally 2 times a day
- Prophylaxis against opportunistic infections:
  - *Pneumocystis carinii* pneumonia (PCP) (for patients with CD4 less than 200) or toxoplasmosis (CD4 less than 100):
    —Trimethoprim-sulfamethoxazole (TMP-SMX) BID 1 tablet orally 3 times a week, or Dapsone 100 mg orally once daily, or Atovaquone 750 mg orally 2 times a day
  - *Mycobacterium avium* complex (MAC) (for patients with CD4 less than 100):
    —Rifabutin 300 mg orally once daily, or Clarithromycin 500 mg orally 2 times a day, or Azithromycin 1200 mg orally/week
  - Fungal infections (for patients with CD4 less than 100):
    —Clotrimazole troche 10 mg orally 5 times a day, or Nystatin suspension 5 ml orally 4 times a day, or

        Fluconazole 100 mg orally once daily, or
        Ketoconazole 200 mg orally once daily, or
        Itraconazole 200 mg orally once daily
- Cytomegalovirus (CMV) infections (for patients with CD4 less than 50):
  —Ganciclovir 1 g orally 3 times a day
- Nutritional maintenance (for anorexia and cachexia):
  - Dronabinol 2.5 mg orally 2 times a day, or
    Megestrol acetate 800 mg orally daily
- Vaccinations:
  - Pneumococcal vaccine—may need to give booster at 5 years
  - Hepatitis B vaccine series at 0, 1, and 6 months; may need to give booster at 5 years
    —For patients without serologic evidence of hepatitis B exposure or immunity
  - Influenza vaccine each autumn
  - *Hemophilus influenza* vaccine
  - Inactivated polio vaccine
  - Diphtheria and tetanus vaccine
  - Measles, mumps, and rubella (MMR) vaccine

Follow-Up:

- Stable asymptomatic HIV-infected patients should be examined and re-evaluated every 3 to 6 months; pay close attention to signs and symptoms of:
  - Fever, chills
  - Diarrhea
  - Weight loss
  - Fatigue
  - Lymphadenopathy
  - Oral sores
  - Cough

- Dyspnea
- Visual changes
- Headaches
- Skin rashes
- Neurologic changes
- Sinusitis
- Odynophagia/dysphagia
- As degree of immunosuppression worsens, follow-ups should be more frequent and tailored to the patient's needs
- Psychosocial needs of the patient and the patient's family must be addressed as early as possible
- Educate patient regarding routes of HIV transmission (unprotected sex, needle sharing); provide educational resources:
  - National AIDS Hotline (800-342-2437; Spanish—800-342-7432)
  - NIH AIDS Clinical Trials Group (800-874-2572)
  - HIV Exposure/Centers for Disease Control (CDC) and Prevention Hotline (888-737-4448)
  - HIV Pregnancy Registry/CDC (800-722-9292, ext. 38465)
- Laboratory monitoring should include at least: CBC and chemistry profile, CD4 cell count, and HIV-RNA measurement every 3 months
- Give careful consideration to the overall clinical picture before changing antiretroviral therapy:
  - If patient is nonadherent to regimen because of low-grade toxic effects, modification of the toxic component may be advisable
  - If the regimen is too complex for the patient to follow, modification to a simpler regimen may be effective

- If drug toxicity early in the course of therapy prompts change, identify the offending drug and substitute a new drug rather than change the entire regimen
- **Watch for:** signs and symptoms of
    - Disease progression
      —Clinical deterioration
      —Falling CD4 counts
      —Rising plasma HIV-RNA
      —Especially important for patients on double NRTI therapy
    - Development of resistance to therapy (repeated detection of plasma HIV-RNA after initial suppression to undetectable levels)—especially with use of Lamivudine or Delavirdine
    - Development of AIDS-defining opportunistic infections
      —PCP
      —Cerebral toxoplasmosis
      —MAC
      —CMV disease
      —Cryptococcal meningitis
      —Herpes simplex virus (HSV) and varicella-zoster virus (VZV) infections
      —*Candida* esophagitis
  - Kaposi's sarcoma
  - AIDS meningoencephalitis
  - Neuropsychiatric symptoms
  - Hematologic dysfunction (drug- or disease-induced)
  - Drug intolerance requiring at least temporary discontinuation of antiretroviral therapy and

subsequent modification of
regimen

OPPORTUNISTIC INFECTIONS ASSOCIATED WITH ACQUIRED IMMUNODEFICIENCY SYNDROME (AIDS)

Presenting Symptoms:

SUBJECTIVE	OBJECTIVE
P. carinii *pneumonia (PCP)*	
May be asymptomatic or insidious	Immunodeficiency state —HIV infection
Dyspnea on exertion progressing to resting dyspnea	—Premature infant —Neoplasm —Congenital or acquired immunodeficiency
Fatigue, weakness	
Fever, chills	
Nonproductive cough	—Drug-induced immunodeficiency (e.g., chronic therapy with steroids)
	CD4 count less than 200 cells/mm^3
	Fever
	Tachypnea
	Diffuse bilateral rales and rhonchi with no wheezing
Cerebral toxoplasmosis	
Headache	Immunodeficiency state, especially HIV infection
Fever	
Mental status changes with impaired cognition	CD4 count less than 100 cells/mm^3
Seizures	Focal neurologic signs Frank meningismus is rare

M. avium *complex (MAC)*

Fever	Immunodeficiency state,
Night sweats	especially HIV
Anorexia	infection
Diarrhea	CD4 count less than 50
Weight loss/wasting	to 75 cells/mm^3
Abdominal pain	Hepatosplenomegaly

CMV Disease (Retinitis, Esophagitis, Colitis, Pneumonitis)

Visual impairment	Immunodeficiency state,
Dysphagia/	especially HIV
odynophagia	infection
Diarrhea	CD4 count less than
Abdominal pain	50 cells/mm^3
Weight loss/wasting	Characteristic white
Rectal ulcers	retinal infiltrates with
Nonproductive cough	associated retinal
Dyspnea	hemorrhage and
	possible retinal
	detachment per
	ophthalmoscopy
	Characteristic lesions on
	esophagoduodenoscopy
	and/or colonoscopy
	Bilateral rales and
	rhonchi with no
	wheezing

Cryptococcal Meningitis

Frontal or temporal	Immunodeficiency state
headache	Focal neurologic signs
Fever	are rare
Impaired mentation	Meningismus usually
(confusion,	absent
lethargy)	Mental status changes
Seizures	may range from mild

confusion to
obtundation with
cranial nerve deficits
Increased intracranial
pressure
Photophobia may
be present (less
than 30% of cases)

HSV and VZV Infections

Orolabial, genital,
and/or anorectal
vesicular rash
Dermatomal vesicular
rash with a
prodrome of
local pain

Immunodeficiency state
is an increased risk
factor
Erythematous-based
vesicular lesions that
become chronic and
nonhealing
Distribution may be
oral, genital, anorectal
(HSV); or in a
dermatomal
distribution, most
typically on the trunk
or face and scalp
(VZV)

Candida Infection

Recurrent oral thrush
Recurrent vaginal
yeast infections,
usually with
intense pruritus
Dysphagia/
odynophagia

Immunodeficiency state
—CD4 count less than
200 to 300/mm^3
White, raised, painless
oral patches, some
with deep fissures
Erythematous
vulvovaginal patches
with thick, cheesy
discharge

Differential Diagnosis:

PCP
—Bacterial pneumonia
—Tuberculosis
—*M. avium* intracellulare
—Viral pneumonia
—Fungal pneumonia
—Lymphoid interstitial pneumonitis (pediatric patients)

Cerebral toxoplasmosis
—Lymphoma
—Brain abscess
—Fungal infection
—Viral encephalitis
  –CMV
  –Herpes simplex
—Mycobacterial infection
—Progressive multifocal leukoencephalopathy (involves white matter only)
—Syphilis
—Vasculitis

MAC
—Tuberculosis
—Infection with enteric pathogen (*Salmonella, Shigella, Campylobacter, Entamoeba histolytica, Giardia lamblia*)
—Liver abscess

CMV retinitis
—*Toxoplasmosis* retinochoroiditis
—Herpes zoster retinitis
—Retinal hemorrhage cause by trauma
—Protozoan retinal infection
—Diabetic retinopathy
—Idiopathic retinal neovascularization

CMV esophagitis/colitis
—*Candida* esophagitis

—Herpes esophagitis
—Hepatitis
—Ulcerative colitis
—Crohn's disease
—Enteric pathogen (as for MAC above)
—Neoplasm
—Metastatic Kaposi's sarcoma
CMV pneumonitis (more common in bone
  marrow transplant patients)
—PCP
—Bacterial pneumonia
—Atypical pneumonia
—Disseminated MAC
Cryptococcal meningitis
—Tuberculous meningitis
—Bacterial meningitis
—Neurosyphilis
—Toxoplasmosis
—Lymphoma
—AIDS dementia complex
—Progressive multifocal leukoencephalopathy
—Viral encephalitis (especially herpes)
—Fungal infection
HSV/VZV
—Impetigo
—Aphthous stomatitis
—Syphilitic chancre
—Herpangina
—Stevens-Johnson syndrome
—Varicella
—Coxsackievirus A16 infection
—Contact dermatitis
—Superficial pyoderma
Candidiasis
—Hairy leukoplakia
—Other oral/vulvovaginal yeast infections

Suggested Workup:

- PCP:
  - Chest radiograph: bilateral interstitial or perihilar infiltrates
  - Saline nebulizer-induced sputum: identify *Pneumocystis* organism
  - Fiberoptic bronchoscopy
    —Bronchoalveolar lavage
    —Transbronchial biopsy
      –Both identify *Pneumocystis* organisms when sputum is negative
  - Open lung biopsy: reserved for cases where sputum and results of bronchoscopy are negative and patient is not improving on empiric anti-*Pneumocystis* therapy
  - Arterial blood gas analysis to stage disease
    —Mild to moderate disease = PaO_2 greater than 70 mm Hg and $P(A\text{-}a)O_2$ less than 35 mm Hg
    —Moderate to severe disease = PaO_2 less than 70 mm Hg and $P(A\text{-}a)O_2$ greater than 35 mm Hg
- Cerebral toxoplasmosis:
  - Serology: anti-*Toxoplasma* IgG antibodies
  - Imaging: Computed tomography (CT) or magnetic resonance imaging (MRI) of brain → multifocal, ring-enhancing hypodense lesions in the gray matter
  - Invasive: Brain biopsy typically reserved for patients with negative serology, atypical findings on CT/MRI, and failure to respond clinically to empiric anti-*Toxoplasma* therapy
- MAC:
  - CBC: pancytopenia
  - Blood cultures: positive for *M. avium*

- CMV:
  - Careful retinal examination: characteristic retinal lesions of CMV retinitis
  - Esophagoduodenoscopy with tissue biopsies of lesions: CMV inclusion bodies
  - Colonoscopy with tissue biopsies of lesions: CMV inclusion bodies
  - Bronchoscopy with tissue biopsies: CMV inclusion bodies
  - Microbiology: CMV culture from buffy coat (peripheral leukocytes), urine, or nebulizer-induced pulmonary secretions
- Cryptococcal meningitis:
  - Lumbar puncture
    - —Cerebrospinal fluid (CSF): positive cryptococcal antigen (titer greater than 1:1024 → poor prognosis)
    - —White blood cell (WBC) count mildly increased (lymphocytic) (if fewer than 20 cells/mm^3 → poor prognosis)
    - —Protein normal or mildly increased
  - Serology—positive cryptococcal antigen in blood
  - Microbiology
    - —India ink examination of CSF
    - —Culture *Cryptococcus neoformans* from blood, CSF, tissue specimens
  - Imaging: CT/MRI of brain rarely show mass lesions
- HSV/VZV:
  - Tzanck test of base of unroofed vesicle (will not distinguish HSV from VZV, which may be done clinically)
- Candidiasis:
  - Potassium hydroxide (KOH) preparation of oral lesion or vaginal discharge
  - Upper endoscopy with biopsy for patient with or without oral lesions and dysphagia

Definitive Diagnosis:

Pneumocystis carinii pneumonia	ICD-9-CM 136.3
Toxoplasmosis, unspecified site	ICD-9-CM 130.9
Toxoplasmosis, disseminated	ICD-9-CM 130.8
Mycobacterium avium infection	ICD-9-CM 031.0
Cytomegalovirus disease	ICD-9-CM 078.5
Cryptococcal meningitis	ICD-9-CM 117.5
Herpes simplex virus infection	ICD-9-CM 054.9
Varicella-zoster virus infection	ICD-9-CM 053.9
Candidiasis, oral	ICD-9-CM 112.0
Candidiasis, vulvovaginal	ICD-9-CM 112.1

Suggested Treatment:

- Mild to moderate PCP: Figure 10-1
- Moderate to severe PCP: Figure 10-2
- Cerebral toxoplasmosis:
  - Pyrimethamine 100 to 200 mg oral load, then 50 to 100 mg orally once daily, and
    Sulfadiazine 1 to 2 g orally 4 times a day for 6 weeks, then
    Pyrimethamine 25 mg orally once daily + sulfadiazine 2 g orally daily for life as suppressive therapy
  - Patients intolerant of sulfadiazine:
    Clindamycin 600 mg orally 4 times a day, and

Figure 10.1 Treatment for mild to moderate *Pneumocystis carinii* pneumonia (PCP).

TMP-SMX = trimethoprim-sulfamethoxazole; G6PD = glucose-6 phosphate dehydrogenase.

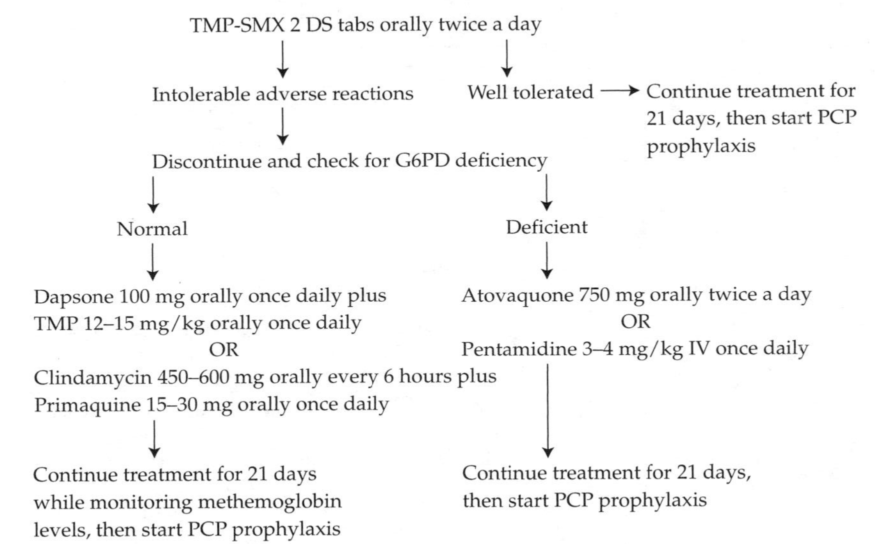

TMP-SMX 2 DS tabs orally twice a day
Intolerable adverse reactions
Well tolerated → Continue treatment for 21 days, then start PCP prophylaxis
Discontinue and check for G6PD deficiency
Normal
Deficient
Dapsone 100 mg orally once daily plus TMP 12–15 mg/kg orally once daily
OR
Clindamycin 450–600 mg orally every 6 hours plus Primaquine 15–30 mg orally once daily
Atovaquone 750 mg orally twice a day
OR
Pentamidine 3–4 mg/kg IV once daily
Continue treatment for 21 days while monitoring methemoglobin levels, then start PCP prophylaxis
Continue treatment for 21 days, then start PCP prophylaxis

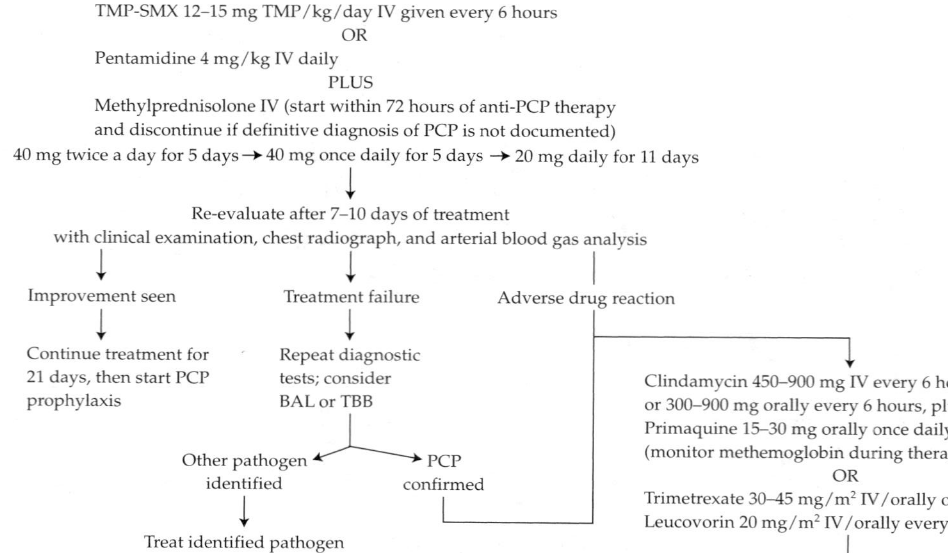

TMP-SMX 12–15 mg TMP/kg/day IV given every 6 hours
OR
Pentamidine 4 mg/kg IV daily
PLUS
Methylprednisolone IV (start within 72 hours of anti-PCP therapy
and discontinue if definitive diagnosis of PCP is not documented)
40 mg twice a day for 5 days → 40 mg once daily for 5 days → 20 mg daily for 11 days
Re-evaluate after 7–10 days of treatment
with clinical examination, chest radiograph, and arterial blood gas analysis
Improvement seen
Treatment failure
Adverse drug reaction
Continue treatment for 21 days, then start PCP prophylaxis
Repeat diagnostic tests; consider BAL or TBB
Clindamycin 450–900 mg IV every 6 hours or 300–900 mg orally every 6 hours, plus
Primaquine 15–30 mg orally once daily (monitor methemoglobin during therapy)
OR
Trimetrexate 30–45 mg/m² IV/orally once daily plus
Leucovorin 20 mg/m² IV/orally every 6 hours
Other pathogen identified
PCP confirmed
Treat identified pathogen
Continue treatment for 21 days, then start PCP prophylaxis

Pyrimethamine 100 mg oral load, then
100 mg orally once daily for 6 weeks, then
Dapsone 50 mg orally daily +
Pyrimethamine 25 mg orally once daily
for life as prophylactic therapy
- Third line agents, or for treatment failures:
Atovaquone 750 mg orally 4 times a day
for 6 weeks, then
Dapsone + Pyrimethamine as above
- MAC:
  - Clarithromycin 500 mg orally 2 times a
day, or
Azithromycin 500 mg orally once daily, and
Ethambutol 15 to 25 mg/kg orally once
daily
  - One or more of the following may be
added if the patient's clinical response is
unsatisfactory or there is relapse after a
positive initial response:
—Rifabutin 300 to 600 mg orally daily,
and/or
Clofazimine 100 to 200 mg orally daily,
and/or
Ciprofloxacin 750 mg orally daily,
and/or
Amikacin 7.5 mg/kg intravenously
(IV) daily or 2 times a day
  - MAC therapy is life-long because
disseminated infection can never be
completely eradicated

Figure 10.2 Treatment for moderate to severe
Pneumocystis carinii pneumonia (PCP).

TMP-SMX = trimethoprim-sulfamethoxazole; BAL = bronchoalveolar lavage; TBB = transbronchial biopsy.

- CMV (Systemic):
  - Induction therapy (for 14 to 21 days for retinitis; for 21 to 42 days for GI or pulmonary disease)
  - **NOTE:** Concurrent use of other myelotoxic drugs, including antiretrovirals, should be discontinued temporarily during induction therapy
    —Ganciclovir 5 mg/kg IV infused over 1 hour every 12 hours (check CBC daily and reduce dose if absolute neutrophil count (ANC) is less than $1000/mm^3$, and discontinue if ANC is less than $500/mm^3$ and platelet count is under $25,000/mm^3$; may restart when ANC is over $750/mm^3$), and
    —Granulocyte colony-stimulating factor (G-CSF) 300 mg subcutaneously (sq) 3 times a week or granulocyte-macrophage colony-stimulating factor (GM-CSF) 1 to 8 μg/kg/day sq 3 times a week (to reverse neutropenia), or
  - Induction therapy for patients exhibiting Ganciclovir resistance or intolerance (ANC always less than $750/mm^3$, platelets always less than $25,000/mm^3$, and intolerable central nervous system (CNS) effects [confusion, psychosis, seizures])
    —Foscarnet 60 mg/kg IV infused over 2 hours every 8 hours (check serum creatinine [Cr] 3 times a week and discontinue if Cr is higher than 2.9; restart when Cr is less than 2), and
    —Hydration with normal saline 1 to 2 L/day concurrent with therapy (to minimize nephrotoxicity), then

- Maintenance therapy (lifelong)
  - —Ganciclovir 5 mg/kg IV over 1 hour daily, or 6 mg/kg IV daily 5 times a week, and
    - G-CSF or GM-CSF as needed (check CBC weekly), or
  - —Foscarnet 120 mg/kg/day infused over 2 hours, and
    - Hydration with normal saline 1L/day (check Cr weekly)
    - (**NOTE:** This may be the drug of choice for maintenance therapy because there is less toxicity and lower incidence of resistant CMV)
- Combination maintenance therapy for treatment failures or recurrent disease
  - —Ganciclovir 3.75 mg/kg IV over 1 hour, followed by
    - Foscarnet 60 mg/kg IV over 1 hour daily, or
  - —Alternate days of Ganciclovir 6 mg/kg IV over 1 hour daily and
    - Foscarnet 120 mg/kg IV over 2 hours daily
- CMV (Alternatives for disease limited to retinitis):
  - Induction therapy
    - —Ganciclovir Mark II ocular insert (releases 1 to 2 μg/hour and has reservoir that can last up to 8 months; requires surgical implantation), and
      - Ganciclovir 1 g orally 3 times a day before or with food, or
    - —Foscarnet 1200 μg in 0.1 ml by intraocular injection 2 to 3 times a week, or

—Cidofovir 5 mg/kg IV once a week for 2
weeks
(Given with Probenecid 3 g orally), or
—Cidofovir 20 μg in 0.1 mL by
intravitreous injection every 5 to 6 weeks
(given with Probenecid 2 g orally 3 hours
before injection, and 1 g orally 1 hour
and 8 hours after injection)
- Maintenance therapy
As on pg. 529 above, or
Ganciclovir 1 g orally 3 times a
day before or with food, or
Cidofovir intravitreous injections (as
above)
- Cryptococcal meningitis:
- Moderate to severe case (altered mental
status, cranial nerve deficit, CSF
cryptococcal antigen titer greater than
1:1024; CSF WBC count less than 20/mm^3):
Amphotericin B 0.7 mg/kg/day slow
intravenous infusion
—Re-evaluate after 1 to 2 weeks
–Clear clinical improvement:
—Switch to Fluconazole 400 mg orally
daily for 8 to 10 weeks, then
—Maintenance therapy with
Fluconazole 200 mg orally daily
given indefinitely
–No definite clinical improvement:
—Continue Amphotericin B to a total
dose of 1.5 to 2.5 g over 6 to 8 weeks,
or add
5-Flucytosine 100 mg/kg/day IV
given 4 times a day for 6 to
8 weeks, then
—Maintenance therapy with
Fluconazole 200 mg orally daily
given indefinitely

—(**NOTE:** serum Cr must be monitored and amphotericin B discontinued if Cr is greater than 2.5; it can be restarted when Cr is less than 1.5)

- Worsening clinical status despite treatment as above may be from increased intracranial pressure, which may require repeated therapeutic lumbar punctures or placement of ventriculoperitoneal (VP) shunt
- Mild case (normal mental status, CSF cryptococcal antigen titer less than 1:1024, CSF WBC count over 20/mm^3):
  Fluconazole 400 mg orally once daily for
    8 to 10 weeks, then
  Fluconazole 200 mg orally once daily
    given indefinitely
- HSV:
  - Mild mucocutaneous infection:
    Acyclovir 200 to 400 mg orally 5 times a
      day for 10 days
  - Severe mucocutaneous infection:
    Acyclovir 5 mg/kg IV infused over 1
      hour every 8 hours for 10 days
  - Visceral organ infection:
    Acyclovir 10 mg/kg IV infused over
      1 hour every 8 hours for 10 to
      14 days
  - Suspected acyclovir-resistant infection:
    Acyclovir 800 mg orally 5 times a day for
      3 to 5 days; if no improvement or
      new lesions are still forming →
    Trifluridine topically with occlusive
      dressing every 8 hours until healed, or
    Foscarnet 60 mg/kg IV 2 times a day, or
      40 mg/kg IV 3 times a day for 10 to
      21 days

- Chronic suppressive therapy:
    Acyclovir 200 to 400 mg orally 3 times a
      day, or
    Foscarnet 40 mg/kg/day IV
- VZV:
  - Shingles:
      Acyclovir 800 mg orally 5 times a day for
        10 days
  - Disseminated infection:
      Acyclovir 10 mg/kg IV every 8 hours for
        10 days
  - Primary infection (high risk for
    disseminated visceral disease):
      Acyclovir 10 mg/kg IV every 8 hours for
        10 days
  - Suspected acyclovir-resistant infection:
      Acyclovir 10 mg/kg IV every 8 hours for
        7 to 10 days; if no improvement →
      Foscarnet 40 mg/kg IV 3 times a day or
        60 mg/kg IV 2 times a day
- Candidiasis:
  - Oropharyngeal disease:
      Clotrimazole 10 mg troche dissolved over
        20 minutes 5 times a day for 7 to 14
        days (for at least 48 hours after
        disappearance of thrush), or
      Nystatin oral suspension 10 mL swish
        and swallow 4 to 5 times a day for
        10 to 14 days
  - Chronic suppressive therapy for
    oropharyngeal disease:
      Clotrimazole or Nystatin as above 2 to
        3 times a day
  - Esophagitis:
      Ketoconazole 200 to 400 mg orally daily
        for 14 to 21 days, or
      Fluconazole 200 mg orally daily for 14 to
        21 days

—If there is no clinical improvement after 7
days, repeat endoscopy with biopsy
—If *Candida* infection is confirmed,
Amphotericin B 10 to 20 mg/kg/day IV
for 10 to 14 days
- Chronic suppressive therapy for *Candida*
esophagitis:
Ketoconazole 200 mg orally daily, or
Fluconazole 100 mg orally daily
- Vulvovaginal disease:
Miconazole 2% cream or 100 mg vaginal
suppository every night at bedtime for
7 days, or
Clotrimazole 100 mg vaginal suppository
every night at bedtime for 7 days, or
200 mg vaginal suppository every
night at bedtime for 3 days, or
Nystatin cream (100,000 units [U]/g) or
vaginal tablet (100,000 U/tablet) 2
times a day for 7 days, or
Fluconazole 150 mg orally for 1 dose

Follow-Up:

- Outpatient care is usually appropriate except
where there is evidence of impending
respiratory failure, dehydration, obtundation,
or other compelling reason for hospitalization
(e.g., intensive care unit (ICU) care or isolation
during infection with disseminated form of
disease)
- Frequent monitoring and treatment of
underlying immunodeficiency state (see AIDS
treatment section)
- Patients with cerebral toxoplasmosis and
cryptococcal meningitis may need chronic
anticonvulsant drug therapy
- CBC, serum electrolytes and Cr, and liver
function tests should be monitored frequently

- Chest radiograph, CT/MRI of brain, arterial blood gases, and pulmonary function tests should be repeated as needed based on patient responses to the respective therapies
- Repeat microbiologic tests should be performed with each recurrence of infection
- **Watch for:** signs and symptoms of
    - Respiratory failure
    - Pneumothorax
    - Disseminated infection
    - Septicemia
    - Multiple CNS complications
      —Recurrent seizures
      —Focal neurologic deficits
      —Partial or complete blindness
      —Mental retardation
      —Deafness
      —Encephalitis
      —Myelitis
  - Postherpetic neuralgia
  - Hepatitis
  - Renal failure
  - Recurrent infections

INFECTIONS IN CANCER PATIENTS

Presenting Symptoms:

SUBJECTIVE	OBJECTIVE
Fever	Neutropenic cancer
Other constitutional complaints will vary depending on location of infection and may involve symptoms affecting:	patient (neutrophils less than 500/mm^3)
	Unexplained fever (e.g., not from administration of pyrogenic drug or
—Oropharynx	biologic product

—Esophagus
—Lungs
—Skin
—Genitalia
—Perianal region
—Fingernails
—Perinasal sinuses
—Intravascular catheter entry sites

such as blood or platelet transfusion) A temperature of at least 38.3°C persisting for more than 2 hours is suggestive of infection

Differential Diagnosis:

Fever caused by drug
Fever caused by treatment with blood product or biological agent
Fever caused by malignancy
Collagen vascular disease
Granulomatous disease
Pulmonary emboli
Thermoregulatory disorder
Endocrine dysfunction (e.g., thyroiditis)
Factitious fever

Suggested Workup:

- Thorough physical examination, with special attention to oropharynx, lungs, skin and nails, genitalia, perianal area, paranasal sinuses, intravascular catheter sites
- Laboratory
  - CBC and platelets
  - Blood urea nitrogen (BUN) and serum Cr
  - Liver function tests
  - Antinuclear antibody (ANA) and rheumatoid factor
  - Thyroid function tests
  - Serum protein electrophoresis
- Microbiology (all materials for culture should be collected before initiating empiric antimicrobial therapy)

- Blood cultures (at least two sets; should be repeated daily while patient is still febrile)
  - Urine culture
  - Stool culture
  - Throat culture
  - Central venous catheter tip culture
  - Sputum culture
- Tuberculin skin test
- Imaging studies
  - Chest radiograph
  - CT or radiograph of paranasal sinuses
  - Bone scan (if osteomyelitis or metastatic disease is suspected)
  - Ultrasound of abdomen/pelvis (if mass lesions, renal obstruction, or biliary pathology are suspected)
  - Echocardiogram (if cardiac valvular lesions are suspected)
  - Perfusion-ventilation (V/Q) scan (if pulmonary emboli are suspected)
  - Gallium (^{67}Ga) scan or technetium-99m (Tc^{-99m}) scan in cases where infectious focus is still not apparent
- Invasive procedures (as indicated by clinical picture)
  - Bronchoscopy with bronchoalveolar lavage or transbronchial biopsy
  - Upper endoscopy with biopsy
  - Liver biopsy
  - Skin biopsy

Definitive Diagnosis:

Neutropenic fever   ICD-9-CM 780.6
(a more specific definitive diagnosis and ICD-9-CM code can be used when the exact nature of the infection is determined)

Suggested Treatment:

- Initial empiric therapy that may need to be altered after results of culture and antibiotic susceptibility testing become available (all therapy should be continued for a minimum of 7 days, and until all sites of infection have resolved and the patient has remained afebrile for at least 4 days):
  - Mezlocillin or Piperacillin 6 to 24 g/day IV given every 4 hours, and
    - Amikacin 15 mg/kg/day IV given every 8 hours, or
    - Tobramycin 3 to 5 mg/kg/day IV given every 8 hours, or
  - Ceftazidime 3 to 6 g/day IV given every 8 hours, or
    - Cefoperazone 2 to 8 g/day IV given every 12 hours, and
    - Amikacin 15 mg/kg/day IV given every 8 hours, or
    - Tobramycin 3 to 5 mg/kg/day IV given every 8 hours, or
  - Aztreonam 1.5 to 6.0 g/day IV given every 8 hours, or
    - Imipenem 1 to 4 g/day IV given every 6 hours, and
    - Amikacin 15 mg/kg/day IV given every 8 hours, or
    - Tobramycin 3 to 5 mg/kg/day IV given every 8 hours,
  - Or where aminoglycoside toxicity is unacceptable:
    - Mezlocillin or Piperacillin 6 to 24 g/day IV given every 4 hours, and
    - Ceftazidime 3 to 6 g/day IV given every 8 hours, or

> Cefoperazone 2 to 8 g/day IV given
> every 12 hours,

- Or where Gram-positive infection is
  suspected:
  > Mezlocillin or Piperacillin 6 to 24 g/day
  > IV given every 4 hours , or
  > Ceftazidime 3 to 6 g/day IV given every
  > 8 hours, or
  > Cefoperazone 2 to 8 g/day IV given
  > every 12 hours, and
  > Vancomycin 1 to 2 g/day IV given every
  > 12 hours,
- Or where there is penicillin allergy:
  > Ciprofloxacin 400 to 800 mg/day IV
  > given every 12 hours, or
  > Ofloxacin 200 to 400 mg/day IV given
  > every 12 hours,
  > (**NOTE:** fluoroquinolones should not be
  > used as therapy where they had been
  > used as prophylactic agents), and
  > Vancomycin 1 to 2 g/day IV given every
  > 12 hours
- And/or where fungal infection is
  suspected:
  > Amphotericin B 0.5 mg/kg/day IV
  > infused over 4 to 8 hours
- Where there is refractory yeast infection or
  infection with filamentous fungi:
  > Amphotericin B 1.25 mg/kg/day IV
  > infused over 4 to 8 hours, and
  > 5-Flucytosine 25 mg/kg orally every
  > 6 hours
- Adjunctive therapy to improve host defenses:
  - Granulocyte transfusions
  - GM-CSF
  - G-CSF
  - Interleukin-3 (IL-3)

- Monocyte/macrophage colony stimulating factor (M-CSF)
- **EXPERIMENTAL:** polyclonal sera, monoclonal antibodies, and cytokines (These agents are associated with high toxicities; their role in potentiating host defenses has not yet been fully established)
- Prevention of neutropenic infections
  - May start when granulocytes fall to less than $500/mm^3$ and continue throughout period of granulocytopenia

    Norfloxacin 400 mg orally every 12 hours, and may start

    Acyclovir 200 to 800 mg orally 5 times a day (higher doses to prevent herpes simplex reactivation)

Follow-Up:

- Detailed history and careful physical examination are hallmarks of diagnosis and treatment
- Inpatient care while patient is neutropenic and febrile
- Daily physical examinations, appropriate cultures, and screening laboratory/imaging studies while febrile
- Repeat detailed workup if there is no response to therapy within 48 to 72 hours
- Consider biomodulation for improving host defenses where the patient is profoundly neutropenic and fails to respond to appropriate antimicrobial therapy (25% of cases)
- **Watch for:** signs and symptoms of
  - Development of resistant bacteria
  - Superinfections

- Sepsis/shock
- Systemic fungal infection
- Acute renal failure due to antibiotic usage

INFECTIONS IN TRANSPLANT RECIPIENTS

Presenting Symptoms:

SUBJECTIVE	OBJECTIVE
	Organ transplant patient receiving immunosuppressive therapy
	—Cyclosporine
	—FK506
	—Azathioprine
	—High-dose methylprednisolone
	—Antilymphocyte antibody

Cytomegalovirus

Onset of symptoms usually within 1 to 4 months after transplant	Physical findings of pneumonia/ pulmonary consolidation
Pneumonitis symptoms with cough, fever, chills, chest pain	Physical findings of enterocolitis and possible intestinal perforation
Lower GI symptoms with bloody diarrhea, abdominal pain, fever	Physical findings of esophagitis/ gastritis
Upper GI symptoms with dysphagia, odynophagia,	Physical findings of myocarditis/ unexplained cardiac arrhythmias

abdominal pain,
fever
Myocardial symptoms
with chest pain,
dyspnea,
palpitations, fever,
malaise
Onset of chorioretinitis
symptoms more than
6 months after
transplant with
"floaters," loss
of visual acuity
(either peripheral or
central)

Characteristic findings
of retinal lesions on
funduscopic
examination

Epstein-Barr Virus (EBV)-Associated Posttransplant Lymphoproliferative Disorder (PTLD)

Fever
Sore throat
Enlarged, tender
cervical and/or
axillary lymph nodes
Abdominal pain
Hematemesis
Hematochezia/melena
Focal weakness/
sensory loss

Oropharyngeal
hyperemia
Diffuse
lymphadenopathy
Hepatosplenomegaly
Transplant failure
Focal neurologic
deficits
Bell's palsy
Stigmata of GI
bleeding
Stigmata of intestinal
perforation

Bacterial Infections

Symptoms begin more
than 6 months after
transplant

Listeria monocytogenes

Fever, fatigue, and malaise

Complaints suggestive of gastroenteritis, including abdominal pain, diarrhea, nausea

Complaints suggestive of meningitis or cerebritis, including headache, nausea and vomiting, stiff neck, delirium, or coma

Complaints suggestive of sepsis, including very high fever and generalized severe illness without localizing signs

Physical signs of bacterial gastroenteritis

Physical signs of meningitis

Physical signs of bacteremia/sepsis

Nocardia asteroides

Complaints suggestive of pulmonary nocardiosis, including fever, cough, pleuritic chest pain, dyspnea, anorexia, hemoptysis

Skin lesions suggestive of cutaneous nocardiosis

Complaints suggestive of disseminated metastatic nocardiosis,

Physical signs of pneumonia

Skin abscesses with localized lymphadenopathy

Physical signs of CNS and disseminated disease, primarily mental status

<table>
<tr><td>

including confusion,
disorientation,
dizziness, headache,
nausea and/or
vomiting, seizures

</td><td>

changes and
seizures

</td></tr>
</table>

Fungal Infections
P. carinii

<table>
<tr><td>

Onset of symptoms 1
  to 6 months after
  transplant
Abrupt onset of
  dyspnea
Weakness
Fever and chills
Nonproductive cough
Tachypnea

</td><td>

Physical signs of
  pneumonia, with
  diffuse bilateral rales
  and rhonchi,
  involving
  predominantly both
  lower lung fields

</td></tr>
</table>

Invasive aspergillosis

<table>
<tr><td>

Fever
Complaints suggestive
  of pulmonary
  invasion, including
  cough, dyspnea,
  pleuritic chest pain
Complaints suggestive
  of CNS invasion,
  including focal
  weakness and/or
  sensory deficits,
  seizures, confusion,
  stupor, coma

Complaints suggestive
  of GI invasion,
  including abdominal
  pain, hematemesis,
  melena

</td><td>

Physical signs of
  pneumonia, with
  diffuse bilateral rales
  and rhonchi

Physical signs of brain
  abscess or
  encephalitis, with
  focal neurologic
  deficits, cranial nerve
  abnormalities,
  altered mental
  status, seizures
Stigmata of GI
  bleeding
Systemic toxicity

</td></tr>
</table>

Invasive candidiasis

Inflamamation at wound site	Obviously infected wound site of intravenous line
Fever	Signs of systemic toxicity
Malaise	
Altered mental status	Signs of ureteral obstruction (in renal transplant patients)
Skin rash	

Cryptococcus neoformans

Onset of symptoms more than 6 months after transplant	
Complaints suggestive of pulmonary infection, including cough with sputum, hemoptysis, fever	Signs of pneumonitis with hemoptysis
Complaints suggestive of CNS involvement, including frontal or temporal headache, fever, impaired mentation; seizures and focal neurologic deficits are rare	Signs of meningitis or cerebritis
	Focal neurologic deficits suggest granulomas in the brain
Painless skin nodules or ulcers	Disseminated disease may produce stigmata of disease in heart, bone, kidney, adrenals, eyes, skin, prostate, and lymph nodes with toxic constitutional signs

Differential Diagnosis:

Acute transplant rejection
Infectious mononucleosis

Lymphoma
Viral hepatitis
Hypersensitivity pneumonitis
Tuberculosis
Histoplasmosis
Lung abscess
Bacterial meningitis
Inflammatory bowel disease
Malignancy

Suggested Workup:

- CMV:
  - Virus culture from urine, blood, body fluids, tissues
  - Bronchoscopy in bone marrow transplant patients if suspicious for CMV pneumonia
  - Endoscopic biopsy of GI tract if suspicious of CMV esophagitis/gastritis
- EBV:
  - CBC: lymphocytosis
  - Peripheral blood smear: EBV-transformed B-lymphocytes
  - EBV serology
    —Antiviral capsid-specific (VCA) IgM indicates active recent infection
    —Anti-early antigen (EA) IgM or IgG indicates active viral replication
    —Antinuclear antigen complex (EBNA) antibodies indicate active infection of 1 to 6 months duration
  - Biopsy of affected lymph nodes: mononuclear aggregates with presence of EBV-transformed cells
- Listeriosis:
  - Blood cultures
  - Lumbar puncture: CSF for Gram stain and culture (CSF protein and glucose may be normal)

- Serology and serotyping by public health laboratory
- Nocardiosis:
  - Gram stain, modified Ziehl-Nielsen stain, and culture of pulmonary secretions, CSF, or skin lesions
  - Blood cultures
  - Imaging studies
    —Chest radiograph: confluent bronchopneumonia
    —CT/MRI of brain: single or multiple intracranial abscesses
  - Bronchoscopy for bronchoalveolar lavage or transbronchial biopsy
  - Percutaneous aspiration of lung lesion
- *P. carinii:*
  - Arterial blood gases: hypoxemia and increased $p(A-a)O_2$ gradient (varies with severity of illness)
  - Cytologic examination of saline nebulizer-induced sputum → *Pneumocystis* organisms may be identified
  - Fiberoptic bronchoscopy with bronchoalveolar lavage or transbronchial biopsy where sputum examination is negative
  - Imaging studies
    —Chest radiograph: bilateral interstitial or perihilar infiltrates (75% of cases)
    —Gallium scan of lungs: sensitive but not specific for *Pneumocystis* (use where sputum analysis is not revealing and bronchoscopy is not available)
- Aspergillosis:
  - Laboratory
    —Eosinophilia
    —Immediate skin reactivity to *Aspergillus* antigen

- Blood cultures
- Imaging studies
  - —Chest radiograph may reveal round intracavitary mass (aspergilloma), or diffuse consolidation and cavitation (invasive disease)
  - —CT/MRI of lungs and/or brain may reveal cavitary lesions
- Bronchoscopy with bronchoalveolar lavage
- Transthoracic needle aspiration in invasive disease
- Candidiasis:
  - Isolation of *Candida* from blood, urine, wound site
- Cryptococcosis:
  - Laboratory
    - —Latex agglutination assay of cryptococcal antigen in serum and urine
    - —Lumbar puncture
      - –India ink preparation of CSF
      - –Latex agglutination assay of cryptococcal antigen in CSF
      - –Elevated protein
      - –Decreased glucose
      - –Lymphocytic pleiocytosis
  - Culture of CSF, blood, urine, saline nebulizer-induced sputum
  - Biopsy skin nodules or lesions
  - Imaging studies
    - —Chest radiograph nonspecific unless nodules or masses with cavitation are present
    - —CT/MRI of brain generally nonspecific and unrevealing

Definitive Diagnosis:

Cytomegalovirus inclusion disease	ICD-9-CM 078.5
Epstein-Barr virus infection	ICD-9-CM 075
Listeriosis	ICD-9-CM 027.0
Nocardiosis	ICD-9-CM 039.9
P. carinii pneumonia	ICD-9-CM 136.3
Aspergillosis	ICD-9-CM 117.3
Candidiasis	ICD-9-CM 112.9
Cryptococcosis	ICD-9-CM 117.5

Suggested Treatment:

- CMV:
    - Ganciclovir 5 mg/kg IV every 12 hours during active CMV infection, and
        CMV hyperimmune globulin (CMV-IGIV) 50 to 150 mg/kg IV daily at 2 to 4 week intervals when severe disease is present
- EBV:
    - Reduction/cessation of immunosuppressive therapy may result in regression of PTLD in up to 20% of cases
        —Acyclovir 5 to 10 mg/kg IV every 8 hours, or
            Ganciclovir 5 mg/kg IV every 12 hours during active disease
            (**NOTE:** It is doubtful that antimicrobial therapy will have an effect on PTLD once the disease is established)
        —Conventional lymphoma chemotherapy/radiotherapy may be attempted
- Listeriosis:
    - Ampicillin 200 mg/kg/day IV given every 4 to 6 hours, (+ 4 mg intrathecal every 12 hours if CNS infection is suspected)

(Penicillin allergy: TMP-SMX 5 mg/kg [based on TMP] IV every 6 hours), and Gentamicin 3 to 5 mg/kg/day IV given every 8 hours for 14 days

- Nocardiosis:
  - TMP-SMX 640 mg/day (based on TMP) orally/IV, or
  - Imipenem 1 to 4 g/day IV given every 6 hours, or
  - Minocycline 100 mg orally/IV every 12 hours for 4 to 6 months
- PCP:
  - Mild to moderate disease [PaO_2 greater than 70 mm and $P(A-a)O_2$ less than 35 mm]
    —TMP-SMX DS 2 tablets orally 3 times a day for 21 days
    —If intolerable adverse reactions,
      –Dapsone 100 mg orally daily, and TMP 12 to 15 mg/kg orally daily, or
      –Clindamycin 450-600 mg orally every 6 hours, and Primaquine 15 to 30 mg orally daily for 21 days
    —If patient has a glucose-6-phosphate dehydrogenase deficiency, Atovaquone 750 mg orally 3 times a day, or Pentamidine 3 to 4 mg/kg IV daily for 21 days
  - Severe disease [PaO_2 less than 70 mm and $P(A-a)O_2$ greater than 35 mm]
    —TMP-SMX 12 to 15 mg TMP/kg/day IV given every 6 hours, or Pentamidine 4 mg/kg IV daily for 21 days, and Methylprednisolone 40 mg IV 2 times a day, then 40 mg IV daily for 5 days, then 20 mg IV daily for 11 days (started within 72 hours of antimicrobial therapy)

—If intolerable adverse reactions,
  –Clindamycin 450 to 900 mg IV every 6 hours or 300 to 900 mg orally every 6 hours, and
      Primaquine 15 to 30 mg orally daily for 21 days, or
  –Trimetrexate 30 to 45 mg/m^2 IV/orally daily, and
      Leucovorin 20 mg/m^2 IV/orally every 6 hours for 21 days
—Following successful treatment, PCP prophylaxis should be instituted:
  –TMP-SMX DS 1 tablet orally daily, or 1 SS tablet orally daily, or 1 DS tablet orally 3 times a week (for those unable to tolerate the higher doses), or
  –Dapsone 50 to 100 mg orally daily, or
  –Atovaquone 750 mg orally daily, or
  –Aerosolized pentamidine 300 mg by aerosol monthly (less effective in preventing recurrent disease)

- Invasive aspergillosis:
  - Amphotericin B 0.5 to 1.0 mg/kg/day IV given as slow infusion over 4 to 8 hours for 14 days (total dose not to exceed 1.5 to 2.0 g), then
      Fluconazole 400 mg orally daily or Itraconazole 200 mg orally daily for 4 to 6 weeks

- Candidiasis:
  - Fluconazole 400 mg IV daily for 7 days, then 400 mg orally daily for at least 14 days after there is no evidence of infection, or
  - Amphotericin B 0.3 to 0.7 mg/kg/day IV to a total dose not exceeding 2.0 g until there is no evidence of infection (this is the preferred therapy in severely neutropenic or otherwise immunocompromised patients)

- Cryptococcosis:
  - Amphotericin B 0.5 to 1.0 mg/kg/day IV for 3 weeks, then
    Fluconazole 400 mg orally daily for 5 weeks (patients with mild disease and normal mental status may respond to oral fluconazole for 8 weeks without use of Amphotericin B)

Follow-Up:

- Routine surveillance cultures every 2 to 4 weeks for CMV and HSV
- Consider post-treatment prophylactic measures
  - TMP or pyrimethamine for *Pneumocystis* and toxoplasmosis
  - Acyclovir for HSV
  - Ganciclovir for CMV
  - Fluconazole for fungal infections
  - TMP-SMX or PCN for bacterial infections
  - Isoniazid for tuberculosis
- Frequent physical examinations
- **Watch for:** signs and symptoms of
  - Transplant rejection
  - Septicemia
  - Infections without fever (e.g., multifocal leukoencephalopathy)
  - Multiorgan failure (heart, liver, kidney)

INFECTIONS IN INTRAVENOUS DRUG ABUSERS (IVDA)

Presenting Symptoms:

SUBJECTIVE	OBJECTIVE
	History of IVDA with high-risk behavior

(sharing needles,
using "shooting
galleries," etc.)
Evidence of depressed
cell-mediated
immunity (reduced
CD4 counts,
diminished delayed
hypersensitivity skin
test reactions, etc.)

Infective Endocarditis

Fever
Chills
Nausea, vomiting
Sweats
Arthralgias
Respiratory distress
and dyspnea
Pleuritic chest pain
Cough (nonproductive
or productive of
scant, blood-tinged
sputum)

Respiratory distress
with signs of
congestive heart
failure
Heart murmurs found
with variable
frequency
—When tricuspid
valve is involved
murmurs are found
in 35% to 40% of
cases
—Mitral and aortic
valve murmurs are
found in over 50%
of cases involving
those valves
Osler nodes/Janeway
lesions rarely found

Skin and Soft Tissue Infections

Red, hot, swollen area
of skin
Fever and chills
Malaise

Evidence of cellulitis or
abscess formation at
injection sites
—Arms

Skin ulcerations may be present	—Legs and feet —Groin —Neck —Penis —Mammary glands —Axillae Local ischemia or necrosis Evidence of local thrombophlebitis

Bone and Joint Infections

Local pain and tenderness over affected area Fever (65% of cases) Few systemic constitutional signs	Knee is most commonly involved joint, left side > right side Vertebral involvement is common (cervical and lumbosacral) Wrist, shoulder, hip, sternoclavicular, and sacroiliac joints also often involved

Noncardiac Vascular Infections

Local pain over peripheral blood vessels Swelling at affected site Fever	Thrombosis/sclerosis of veins in arm or leg Pulsatile mass overlying a deep vessel (femoral, axillary, neck vessels), with accompanying bruit and distal ischemia (mycotic aneurysm)

NOTE: IVDA display increased susceptibility to pneumonia and other pulmonary infections, meningitis and cerebral abscess, endophthalmitis, and STDs. Aggressive antimicrobial therapy with standard regimens is generally effective in these cases.

Differential Diagnosis:

Infective endocarditis
—Septic thrombophlebitis
—Collagen vascular disease
—Myocardial infarction
—Pericarditis
—Rheumatic fever
—Tuberculosis
—Pulmonary embolus
—Septic pulmonary infarct
Skin and soft tissue infections
—Cellulitis
—Fasciitis
—Myositis
—Impetigo
—Thrombophlebitis
—Erysipelas
—Pyomyositis
Bone and joint infections
—Reiter's syndrome
—Rheumatoid arthritis
—Osteoarthritis
—Rheumatic fever
—Lyme arthritis
—Sarcoidosis
—Trauma/foreign body
—Sickle cell crisis
—Mycobacterial infection
—Fungal infection
Noncardiac vascular infections
—Cellulitis
—Fasciitis
—Myositis

—Thrombophlebitis
—Dry gangrene

Suggested Workup:

- Infective endocarditis (also see section on infective endocarditis in Chapter 5)
  - Blood cultures: positive in 80% to 100% of cases
    —Sets of two cultures taken at different times
    —Should include bacterial and fungal cultures
  - Serology
    —If initial cultures are negative, may need to look for presence of antibodies to *Chlamydia trachomatis* and *Chlamydia psittaci*, *Coxiella burnetii*, and *Bartonella*, all of which can cause "culture-negative" endocarditis
  - Echocardiogram (two-dimensional or transesophageal for better sensitivity) → helps in visualizing vegetations on affected valves
  - Laboratory evaluation
    —CBC:
      –Elevated WBCs
      –Anemia
    —Erythrocyte sedimentation rate (ESR) elevated
    —Urinalysis: hematuria
  - Chest radiograph: parenchymal infiltrates and possible pleural effusion
  - V/Q lung scan or pulmonary angiogram if septic pulmonary embolism is suspected
- Skin and soft tissue infections
  - Aspirate point of maximum inflammation for Gram stain and culture →
    —50% beta-hemolytic *Streptococcus*

- —35% *Staphylococcus aureus*, alpha-hemolytic *Streptococcus*, and coagulase-negative *Staphylococcus*
- —10% anaerobes
- —Less than 5% Gram-negative organisms (mainly enteric pathogens: *Escherichia coli, Klebsiella, Proteus, Pseudomonas,* and *Enterobacter*)
- —Less than 1% *Candida*
  - Skin biopsy for difficult cases
- Bone and joint infections
  - Diagnostic needle aspiration of bone or joint for Gram stain and culture (bacteria and fungi)
  - Blood cultures: may be negative or grow different bacteria than found in joint aspirates
  - Radiologic examination
    - —Radiograph of affected joint(s) may be useful to rule out contiguous osteomyelitis
    - —CT/MRI of affected joint may be useful to detect soft tissue involvement and abscess formation
- Noncardiac vascular infections
  - Venography
  - Ultrasound for possible aneurysm formation
  - CT scan of affected area
  - Digital subtraction angiography for femoral and peripheral aneurysms
  - Fine needle aspiration for Gram stain and culture only for peripheral vessels

Definitive Diagnosis:

Drug abuse   ICD-9-CM 995.81
Infective endocarditis   ICD-9-CM 421.0

—Tricuspid valve   ICD-9-CM 397.0
—Aortic valve   ICD-9-CM 424.1
—Mitral valve   ICD-9-CM 394.9
—Pulmonary valve   ICD-9-CM 424.3
Cellulitis, diffuse   ICD-9-CM 682.9
Abscess, skin   ICD-9-CM 682.9
Arthritis, septic/   ICD-9-CM 711.0
   pyogenic
Thrombophlebitis   ICD-9-CM 451.9
Thrombosis   ICD-9-CM 453.9
Aneurysm, mycotic   ICD-9-CM 421.0
Fistula, arteriovenous   ICD-9-CM 447.0

Suggested Treatment:

- Infective endocarditis:
  - Empiric coverage is begun after blood cultures have been drawn, and coverage may be modified after results of culture and antibiotic sensitivity testing are available
  - Right-sided/*S. aureus* is most common
    —Nafcillin 2 g IV every 4 hours, and
        Gentamicin 1 mg/kg IV every 8 hours
          for 2 to 4 weeks, or
    —Nafcillin 2 g IV every 4 hours for 4 to 6 weeks, and
        Gentamicin 1 mg/kg IV every 8 hours
          for the first 5 to 7 days
  - Penicillin allergy
        Cefazolin 2 g IV every 8 hours for 4 to 6 weeks, and
          Gentamicin 1 mg/kg IV every 8 hours
          for first 5 to 7 days
  - Methicillin-resistant *S. aureus* or penicillin allergy
        Vancomycin 15 mg/kg every 12 hours
          for 2 to 6 weeks

- Indications for surgery are not significantly different from recommendations made for the general population (see section on Infective Endocarditis in Chapter 5)
- Skin and soft tissue infections:
  - Mild infection
    Nafcillin 500 mg orally every 6 hours, or
    Dicloxacillin 500 mg orally every 6 hours for 14 days
    Penicillin allergy: Erythromycin 500 mg orally every 6 hours for 14 days
  - Serious infection:
    Vancomycin 0.5 to 1.0 g IV every 12 hours, or
      Clindamycin 300 mg IV every 8 hours, and
    Gentamicin 3 to 5 mg/kg/day IV given every 8 hours for 10 to 21 days, and
    Aggressive surgical debridement
- Bone and joint infections:
  - Antibiotic treatment is based on culture and sensitivity results of bone/joint aspiration; intravenous therapy is typically required for 4 for 6 weeks (for specific recommendations, see Chapter 8)
  - Frequent arthrocentesis and/or debridement of nonviable bone are also recommended
- Noncardiac vascular infections:
  - Nafcillin 2 g IV every 4 hours, or
    Vancomycin 15 mg/kg IV every 12 hours, and
    Gentamicin 3 to 5 mg/kg/day IV given every 8 hours for 4 to 6 weeks
  - Aggressive surgical treatment

Follow-Up:

- IVDA with infective endocarditis who are stable and only moderately ill can be safely observed without antibiotic therapy while waiting for the results of blood cultures
- BUN and serum Cr should be monitored 1 to 2 times a week while the patient is taking gentamicin
- Follow-up blood cultures should be taken until negative (in IVDA, positive blood cultures may persist for 10 to 14 days after initiating therapy)
- Drug counseling and rehabilitation
- Work-up for HIV infection
- **Watch for:** signs and symptoms of
    - HIV infection
    - Septic emboli
    - Pulmonary embolism
    - Pericarditis
    - Pneumothorax
    - Congestive heart failure
    - Cardiac arrhythmia
    - Renal failure
    - Inflammatory myocarditis
    - Mycotic aneurysms
    - Empyema
    - Hepatitis
    - Tuberculosis
    - Splenic abscess
    - CNS infections
    - Endophthalmitis
    - STDs
    - Bacteremia/sepsis
    - Chronic reinfections

INFECTIONS IN ALCOHOLIC PATIENTS

Presenting Symptoms:

<u>SUBJECTIVE</u> | <u>OBJECTIVE</u>

Pneumonias

SUBJECTIVE	OBJECTIVE
Fever with sudden onset of shaking chills	History consistent with recent aspiration of oropharyngeal flora or gastric contents
Cough with dark, thick, or rusty sputum production	Bronchial breath sounds
Pleuritic chest pain	Chest dullness to percussion
Weight loss	Diffuse rales and rhonchi
	Egophony and whispered pectoriloquy
	Vocal fremitus
	Tachypnea
	Tachycardia
	Pleural friction rub
	Poor oral hygiene

Tuberculosis

SUBJECTIVE	OBJECTIVE
Cough with mucopurulent or blood-tinged sputum	History of independent risk factor:
Hemoptysis	—Homelessness
Fever and night sweats	—HIV Infection
Anorexia and weight loss	—Institutionalized
Malaise and fatigue	—Recent close contact with patient with tuberculosis
Pleuritic chest pain	Generalized lymphadenopathy
	Hepatosplenomegaly

Localized dullness to
percussion
Post-tussive rales

Spontaneous Bacterial Peritonitis

Fever

Vomiting

Abdominal pain
exacerbated by
movement

Symptoms of end-stage
liver disease

—Abdominal
distension

—Hematemesis

—Melena

—Stupor, confusion

—Tremor

Diffuse abdominal
rebound

Generalized abdominal
rigidity

Diminished bowel
sounds

Abdominal
hyperresonance to
percussion

Signs of end-stage liver
disease

—Ascites

—Encephalopathy

—Asterixis

Differential Diagnosis:

Pneumonias

Other causes of infectious pneumonitis

—Viral (respiratory syncytial virus [RSV],
adenovirus, EBV, influenzae A and B,
enterovirus)

—Nocardiosis

—Fungal (*Pneumocystis, Blastomyces, Cryptococcus,
Aspergillus, Histoplasma, Coccidioides*)

—Toxoplasmosis

—Chlamydial

—Rickettsial (Q fever, *Coxiella*)

Tuberculosis

Pulmonary embolism

Bronchiolitis obliterans

Pulmonary vasculitis

Hypersensitivity pneumonitis

Pneumothorax

Sarcoid

Tuberculosis
Bacterial, viral pneumonia
Lymphoma
Fungal infection
Atypical pneumonia (*Mycoplasma, Nocardia*)
Spontaneous Bacterial Peritonitis
Abdominal abscess
Volvulus
Intussusception
Mesenteric adenitis
Appendicitis
Pancreatitis
Cholecystitis
Peptic ulcer (with or without perforation)
Inflammatory bowel disease
Diverticulitis
Gangrene of the bowel

Suggested Workup:

- Pneumonias:
  - Collect sputum for Gram stain and culture (aerobic and anaerobic)
  - Blood cultures
  - Chest radiograph
  - Thoracentesis to collect pleural fluid for Gram stain and culture (aerobic and anaerobic)
  - Bronchoscopy with bronchoalveolar lavage for Gram stain and culture
  - Transthoracic fine needle aspiration for Gram stain and culture
- Tuberculosis:
  - Collect sputum (if necessary, may induce with saline nebulizer) for Ziehl-Neelsen or auramine-rhodamine staining for acid-fast bacilli, and culture on Bactec system
  - Check all cultures for drug sensitivities

- Chest radiograph: cavitary lesions and upper lobe disease with hilar adenopathy common
- Bronchoscopy with bronchoalveolar lavage or transbronchial biopsy: washings or biopsy specimen sent for acid-fast staining and culture (reserved for cases where sputum examination is inconclusive)
- Open lung biopsy rarely needed
- Tuberculin skin test (false-negatives are common in patients with active disease)
- Spontaneous bacterial peritonitis:
  - Paracentesis to collect ascitic fluid for Gram stain and culture, chemical analysis, and CBC
  - Abdominal radiograph: free air in peritoneal cavity
  - Upright chest radiograph: free air under elevated diaphragm indicates perforation of abdominal viscus
  - Blood cultures
  - Serum amylase: elevated
  - Abdominal ultrasound and/or CT of abdomen to demonstrate ascites and intra-abdominal mass

Definitive Diagnosis:

Pneumococcal pneumonia	ICD-9-CM 481
Anaerobic pneumonia	ICD-9-CM 482.81
Klebsiella pneumonia	ICD-9-CM 482.0
Haemophilus pneumonia	ICD-9-CM 482.2
Tuberculosis	ICD-9-CM 011.9
Bacterial peritonitis	ICD-9-CM 567.2

Suggested Treatment:

- Pneumococcal pneumonia:
  - PCN-G 8 to 12 million U/day IV given every 4 hours, or
    Penicillin allergy: Cefazolin 1 to 2 g IV every 8 hours, or

>   Erythromycin 1 g IV every 6 hours for
>   10 to 14 days
> - For penicillin-resistant pneumococcus:
>   Cefotaxime 1 g IV every 8 hours, or
>   Ceftriaxone 2 g IV/intramuscularly daily, or
>   Vancomycin 1 g IV every 12 hours (for
>   highly resistant isolates)
- Anaerobic pneumonia:
  - PCN-G 8 to 12 million U/day IV given
    every 4 hours , or
      Penicillin allergy: Clindamycin 900 mg IV
      every 8 hours for 10 to 14 days
- *Klebsiella* pneumonia:
  - Cefotaxime 1 g IV every 8 hours, or
    Piperacillin 4 g IV every 6 hours, and
    Gentamicin 3 to 5 mg/kg/day IV given
    every 8 hours, or
  - Ciprofloxacin or Ofloxacin 400 mg IV every
    12 hours for 10 to 14 days
- *Haemophilus* pneumonia:
  - Ampicillin 2 g IV every 6 hours, or
    Ampicillin + sulbactam 3 g IV every
      6 hours, or
      Cefuroxime 750 mg IV every 8 hours (for
      ampicillin-resistant strains)
  - Penicillin allergy: Ciprofloxacin or
    Ofloxacin 400 mg IV every 12 hours, or
      Clarithromycin 500 mg orally every 12
      hours for 10 to 14 days
- Tuberculosis:
  - Directly observed therapy regimen is
    prudent in this generally less complaint
    patient population, to reduce risk of
    treatment failure and emergence of drug-
    resistant strains:
  - Isoniazid 300 mg orally, and
    Rifampin 600 mg orally, and

Pyrazinamide 2.5 g orally, and
Ethambutol 800 mg or Streptomycin 1 g
orally daily for 2 weeks, then 2 times
a week for 6 weeks, then
Isoniazid 300 mg orally and Rifampin
600 mg orally 2 times a week for
16 weeks, or
- Isoniazid 300 mg orally, and
Rifampin 600 mg orally, and
Pyrazinamide 2.5 g orally, and
Ethambutol 800 mg or Streptomycin 1 g
orally 3 times a week for 6 months
- Empiric therapy for bacterial peritonitis:
  - May need to be altered when results of
culture and antibiotic sensitivity testing
become available:
  - Ampicillin + sulbactam 3 g IV every 6
hours, or
Cefotaxime 2 g IV every 8 hours, or
Ticarcillin + clavulanate 3 g IV every 6
hours for 14 days

Follow-Up:

- Inpatient care generally required
- Aggressive nutritional support required
- **Watch for:** signs and symptoms of
  - Delirium tremens
  - Bacteremia and sepsis
  - Infectious endocarditis
  - Pancreatic abscess
  - Erosive gastritis and GI
bleeding
  - Viral hepatitis
  - HIV infection

Bacteremia, Sepsis, and Shock

11

INFECTIONS COVERED

SEPTICEMIA AND SEPSIS SYNDROME (SYSTEMIC INFLAMMATORY RESPONSE SYNDROME—SIRS)

Presenting Symptoms:

SUBJECTIVE

Fever
Chills, rigors
Myalgias
Lethargy, confusion
Hyperventilation
Skin lesions
Cough with sputum (primary site = respiratory tract)
Dysuria, flank pain (primary site = urinary tract)
Abdominal pain, nausea, vomiting, diarrhea (primary site = gastrointestinal tract)
Stiff neck, headache, photophobia, focal neurologic deficits (primary site = central nervous system [CNS])

OBJECTIVE

Elicit risk factors in patient's history:
—Immunocompromised
  –Human immunodeficiency virus (HIV) infection
  –Neutropenia
  –Complement deficiency
  –Hypogammaglob-ulinemia
  –Splenectomy
  –Diabetes mellitus
—Cancer, lymphoma, leukemia
—Alcoholism
—Cirrhosis
—Intravenous drug abuse
—Malnutrition
—Burn/trauma patient
—Recent surgical procedure
—Intravascular devices
—Indwelling catheters (urinary, biliary)
—Altered mental status with possible aspiration

—Disseminated
infection
—Pancreatitis
—Age extremes
Tachypnea
Tachycardia
Hypotension
Fever (paradoxic
hypothermia may
develop in patients
who are elderly,
immunocompromised,
alcoholic, or in
renal/hepatic
failure)
Altered mental status
Bleeding (disseminated
intravascular
coagulation [DIC])
Petechiae, embolic
lesions
Ecthyma gangrenosum
(*Pseudomonas
aeruginosa* infection)
Localizing physical
findings indicative of
infection or tissue
injury
—Dyspnea, tachypnea,
chest pain, cyanosis,
adult respiratory
distress syndrome
(ARDS)
—Oliguria,
costovertebral
angle (CVA)
tenderness

—Abdominal tenderness
—Meningeal signs, focal neurologic deficits, altered mental status
—Diminished cardiac function, heart murmurs
—Area of cellulitis, decubitus ulcer, gangrene

Differential Diagnosis:

Systemic infection
—Bacterial
—Viral
—Fungal
—Rickettsial
—Protozoal
—Spirochetal
Collagen vascular disease
Vasculitis
Myocardial infarction
Pulmonary embolus
Thrombotic thrombocytopenic purpura and hemolytic uremic syndrome (TTP-HUS)
Endocrinologic emergency
—Thyrotoxicosis
—Adrenal insufficiency
—Addison's disease
Aortic aneurysm
SIRS initiated by noninfectious etiology
—Trauma
—Burns
—Pancreatitis

Suggested Workup:

- Sepsis is strongly suggested by the five cardinal signs:
  - Tachypnea
  - Tachycardia
  - Fever or hypothermia
  - Hypotension
  - Altered mental status
- Microbiology
  - Blood cultures usually positive (at least two)
  - Gram stain and culture of other fluids usually positive (at least two)
    —Urine
    —Cerebrospinal fluid (CSF)
    —Sputum
  - Culture of indwelling catheter tips or intravascular devices may be positive
- Laboratory
  - Complete blood count (CBC)
    —Anemia
    —Leukocytosis with left shift
    —Thrombocytopenia
  - Chemistry
    —Hyperglycemia
    —Hypocalcemia
    —Mild hyperbilirubinemia
    —Lactic acidosis
    —Serum transaminases elevated
    —Serum blood urea nitrogen (BUN)/ creatinine elevated
  - Coagulation assessment
    —Prothrombin time (PT) prolonged
    —Activated partial thromboplastin time (APTT) near normal
    —Serum fibrinogen decreased

- —Serum fibrin split products increased
- —Thrombocytopenia
- Urinalysis
  - —Proteinuria
- Arterial blood gas analysis
  - —Respiratory alkalosis
  - —Metabolic acidosis
  - —Hypoxia
  - —Hypercapnia
- Imaging studies
  - Chest radiograph may show:
    - —Pneumonia
    - —ARDS
  - Ultrasound, computed tomography (CT), magnetic resonance imaging (MRI) may be used to detect and define focus of infection
- Electrocardiogram (ECG) may be used to rule out myocardial infarction
- Invasive procedures
  - Aspiration of body fluids suspected of infection with subsequent analysis by Gram stain and culture
    - —Thoracentesis
    - —Peritoneocentesis
    - —Pericardiocentesis
  - Incision and drainage of abscess
  - Percutaneous biopsy and drainage
    - —Biliary tree

Definitive Diagnosis:

Sepsis or septicemia   ICD-9-CM 038.9
Septic shock   ICD-9-CM 785.59

Suggested Treatment:

- **NOTE:** Antimicrobial therapy should be started immediately, before the results of culture and antibiotic sensitivity testing are known. Empiric therapy should be targeted based on the characteristics of the host and the epidemiologic circumstances of the infection. Avoiding ultrabroad, nontargeted therapy may significantly reduce the patient's risk of superinfection, fungemia, and infection with antibiotic-resistant strains of infecting microbes. Thus, scrupulous history, epidemiologic evaluation and physical examination must precede initiation of antimicrobial therapy.

- Community-acquired infection in a non-neutropenic host
    - Suspected skin/soft tissue source:
      —Cellulitis
        Oxacillin or Nafcillin 1 to 2 g
            intravenously (IV) every 4 to
            6 hours, and
        Gentamicin or Tobramycin 3 to 5 mg/
            kg/day IV given every 8 hours, or
      —Penicillin allergy: Vancomycin 15 mg/kg
        IV every 12 hours
    - Decubitus ulcers/necrotic tissue
      —Cefazolin 1 g IV every 8 hours, or
        Cephalothin 1 g IV every 4 hours, and
        Gentamicin or Tobramycin 3 to 5 mg/
            kg/day IV given every 8 hours, and
        Metronidazole 0.5 g IV every 6 to
            8 hours, or
      —Piperacillin + tazobactam 3.375 g IV
        every 6 hours, or
      —Ticarcillin + clavulanate 3.1 g IV every 4
        hours
    - Suspected lung source:
      —Ampicillin + sulbactam 1.5 to 3.0 g IV
        every 6 hours, or
      —Cefuroxime 0.75 to 1.5 g IV every 8
        hours, or

  —Ceftriaxone 1 to 2 g IV every 12 to 24
    hours
- Suspected urinary tract source:
  —Ampicillin 1 to 2 g IV every 4 to 6
        hours, and
      Gentamicin or Tobramycin 3 to
        5 mg/kg/day IV given every 8
        hours, or
  —Ceftriaxone 1 to 2 g IV every 12 to 24
    hours, or
  —Mezlocillin, Piperacillin, or Ticarcillin 3 g
    IV every 4 hours
- Suspected intra-abdominal or nonsexually
  transmitted gynecologic source:
  —Ampicillin 1 to 2 g IV every 4 to
        6 hours, and
      Gentamicin or Tobramycin 3 to
        5 mg/kg/day IV given every 8
        hours, and
      Metronidazole 0.5 g IV every 6 to
        8 hours, or
  —Clindamycin 600 to 900 mg IV every 8
    hours, and
      Gentamicin or Tobramycin 3 to
        5 mg/kg/day IV given every 8
        hours, or
  —Cefoxitin 1 to 2 g IV every 4 to 6 hours
- Suspected CNS source:
  —Cefotaxime 2 g IV every 4 to 6 hours, or
  —Ceftriaxone 1 to 2 g IV every 12 to 24
    hours, or
  —Chloramphenicol 0.75 to 1.0 g IV every 6
    hours, or
  —Vancomycin 15 mg/kg IV every 12 hours
- No obvious source:
  —Cefotaxime 2 g IV every 4 to 6 hours, or
  —Ceftriaxone 1 to 2 g IV every 12 to 24
    hours, or

- —Ceftizoxime 2 to 4 g IV every 8 to 12
  hours, or
- —Ampicillin + sulbactam 1.5 to 3.0 g IV
  every 6 hours, or
- —Cefazolin 1 to 2 g IV every 8 hours, and
      Gentamicin or Tobramycin 3 to
          5 mg/kg/day IV given every
          8 hours

- Hospital-acquired, or patient recently
  hospitalized, or recently given antimicrobial
  therapy
  - Suspected skin/soft tissue source:
    —Same treatment as for outpatient
  - Suspected contaminated intravascular
    device:
    —Vancomycin 15 mg/kg IV every 12 hours
  - Suspected lung source:
    —Mezlocillin, Ticarcillin, or Piperacillin 3 g
      IV every 4 hours, and
          Gentamicin or Tobramycin 3 to
              5 mg/kg/day IV given every
              8 hours, or
    —Piperacillin + tazobactam 3.375 g IV
      every 6 hours, and
          Gentamicin or Tobramycin 3 to
              5 mg/kg/day IV given every
              8 hours, or
    —Imipenem + cilastatin 0.5 to 1.0 g IV
      every 6 hours
  - Suspected urinary tract source:
    —Same treatment as for outpatient
  - Suspected intra-abdominal or non-STD
    gynecologic source:
    —Mezlocillin, Ticarcillin, or Piperacillin 3 g
      IV every 4 hours, and
          Gentamicin or Tobramycin 3 to
              5 mg/kg/day IV given every
              8 hours, and

Metronidazole 0.5 g IV every 6 to 8
hours, or
—Piperacillin + tazobactam 3.375 g IV
every 6 hours, and
Gentamicin or Tobramycin 3 to
5 mg/kg/day IV given every
8 hours, or
—Imipenem + cilastatin 0.5 to 1.0 g IV
every 6 hours
- Suspected CNS source:
—Postneurosurgical
—Vancomycin 15 mg/kg IV every 12
hours, and
Ceftazidime 1 to 2 g IV every 8 to
12 hours
—Pregnancy or postpartum
—Cefotaxime 2 g IV every 4 to 6 hours, or
Ceftriaxone 1 to 2 g IV every 12 to
24 hours, and
Ampicillin 1 to 2 g IV every 4 to 6
hours, or
—Chloramphenicol 0.75 to 1.0 g IV every 6
hours, and
Trimethoprim-sulfamethoxazole (TMP-
SMX) 8/40 mg/kg/day IV given
every 6 to 8 hours
- No obvious source:
—Mezlocillin, Ticarcillin, or Piperacillin 3 g
IV every 4 hours, and
Gentamicin or Tobramycin 3 to
5 mg/kg/day IV given every
8 hours, or
—Piperacillin+ tazobactam 3.375 g IV
every 6 hours, and
Gentamicin or Tobramycin 3 to 5 mg/
kg/day IV given every 8 hours, or
—Imipenem + cilastatin 0.5 to 1.0 g IV
every 6 hours

- Immunocompromised host
  - Intravenous drug abuser:
    - —Oxacillin or nafcillin 1 to 2 g IV every 4
      to 6 hours, and
        Gentamicin or Tobramycin 3 to
          5 mg/kg/day IV given every
          8 hours, or
    - —Vancomycin 15 mg/kg IV every 12
      hours, and
        Gentamicin or Tobramycin 3 to
          5 mg/kg/day IV given every
          8 hours
  - Neutropenic patient:
    - —Mezlocillin, Ticarcillin, or Piperacillin 3 g
      IV every 4 hours, or
        Ceftazidime 1 to 2 g IV every 8 to 12
          hours, and
        Gentamicin or Tobramycin 3 to
          5 mg/kg/day IV given every 8
          hours, or
    - —Ceftriaxone 1 to 2 g IV every 12 to 24
      hours, or
        Piperacillin + tazobactam 3.375 g IV
          every 6 hours, and
        Gentamicin or Tobramycin 3 to 5 mg/
          kg/day IV given every 8 hours, or
    - —Vancomycin 15 mg/kg IV every 12
      hours, and
        Ceftazidime 1 to 2 g IV every 8 to 12
          hours, and
        Gentamicin or Tobramycin 3 to 5 mg/
          kg/day IV given every 8 hours
  - Neonate (younger than 7 days old):
    - —Ampicillin 200 mg/kg/day IV given
      every 6 hours, and
        Gentamicin 5.0 to 7.5 mg/kg/day IV
          given every 8 hours

- Nonimmunocompromised child
  - Cefotaxime 200 mg/kg/day IV given every 6 hours
- Adjunctive Measures:
  - Corticosteroids
    - —The most comprehensive well-controlled clinical trials have failed to demonstrate a beneficial effect of corticosteroids in septic shock
    - —Large doses of corticosteroids cannot be recommended as adjunctive therapy for sepsis or shock; replacement doses in suspected adrenal insufficiency are appropriate
  - Anticoagulation in patients with DIC
    - —Clinical experience has demonstrated no benefit in terms of survival of patients with Gram-negative sepsis and DIC who received heparin compared to those who did not
    - —Transfusion of platelets in patients with severe thrombocytopenia or replacement of a specific clotting factor where indicated are appropriate measures to control hemorrhage; patients with refractory shock and coagulopathy who do not respond to these measures may be treated with heparin in an attempt to terminate DIC, but there is no evidence that this measure will prolong life
  - Recombinant colony stimulating factors (r-CSFs)
    - —To date, there is no firm evidence that r-CSFs (granulocyte or monocyte/ macrophage) improve patient outcome or survival in cases of sepsis or septic shock

- Other pharmacologic agents that block mediators of inflammation
  - —Naloxone, an antagonist of beta-endorphins
  - —Antihistamines
  - —Nonsteroidal anti-inflammatory agents
  - —Glucagon
  - —Cyclo-oxygenase inhibitors
  - —Alpha-adrenergic blockers
  - —Pentoxifylline
  - —No compelling data suggesting that using any of these agents improves patient outcome or survival in sepsis or shock have been collected
- Newer adjunctive therapies
  - —Anti-endotoxin monoclonal antibodies
  - —Interleukin-1 receptor antagonists
  - —Anti-tumor necrosis factor (TNF)-alpha monoclonal antibodies
  - —Anti-interleukin-10 monoclonal antibodies
  - —These newer innovative adjunctive treatments are **EXPERIMENTAL** and in various stages of clinical development, but none is approved by the Food and Drug Administration (FDA); clinicians with appropriate patients may be able to participate in clinical trials where these agents are being tested

Follow-Up:

- Inpatient care is required, often with admission to intensive care unit (ICU)
- Immediate removal of septic foci
- Aggressive supportive medical care is essential
  - Volume resuscitation
  - Adequate tissue perfusion

- Use of inotropic agents
- Mechanical ventilation
- Renal dialysis
- Management of electrolyte and acid-base disturbances
- Transfusion of red blood cells (RBCs), platelets, fresh frozen plasma (FFP)
- Nutrition/intravenous hyperalimentation
- Treat any underlying medical problems
  - Gamma globulin for hypogammaglobulinemic patients
  - Diabetes control
  - HIV treatment
- **Watch for:** signs and symptoms of
    - ARDS
    - Respiratory failure
    - Acute renal failure
    - Acute hepatic failure
    - Hemodynamic compromise with cardiac ischemia
    - DIC and generalized hemorrhage
    - Gastrointestinal hemorrhage
    - Up to 50% mortality even with aggressive care

TOXIC SHOCK SYNDROME (TSS)

Presenting Symptoms:

SUBJECTIVE	OBJECTIVE
High fever (over 40°C) (90% of cases)	Elicit risk factors: **Menstrual TSS**
Nausea and vomiting (90%)	Woman 15 to 25 years old
Diarrhea (98%)	High absorbency

Rash followed by desquamation of skin several days later (80%)

Myalgia (95%)

Headache (80%)

Sore throat (80%)

Lightheadedness/near-syncope or syncope (50%)

Diminished sensorium, confusion, agitation (40%)

Mucosal hyperemia (especially eyes, mouth, vagina) (35%)

Vaginal discharge (30%)

tampon use during menstrual periods

Abrupt onset of symptoms during menses

Nonmenstrual TSS

Prior vaginal infection treated with antibiotics

Use of contraceptive devices (especially intrauterine device [IUD] or sponge)

Postpartum period (especially after Caesarean section or episiotomy)

Postabortion

Postoperative (especially herniorrhaphy, mammoplasty, arthroscopy, or nasal surgery with packing)

Patient is listless and confused, but with no focal neurologic signs

Meningeal signs usually absent

Severe hypotension and signs of hypovolemic shock

Erythematous, deep red ("sunburn") rash, followed by extensive

desquamation,
especially on palms
of hands and soles
of feet
Conjunctival
inflammation
Erythematous mucosal
surfaces
Vaginal hyperemia and
discharge

Differential Diagnosis:

Scarlet fever
Rocky Mountain spotted fever
Drug reaction
Leptospirosis
Kawasaki's disease
Staphylococcal scalded skin syndrome
Gram-negative sepsis
Septicemia of other causes
Measles

Suggested Workup:

- Criteria for diagnosis of TSS (probable when three or more major criteria are present along with desquamation, or more than five major criteria are present without desquamation):
  - Temperature greater than 38.9°C
  - Systolic blood pressure (SBP) less than 90 mm Hg
  - Involvement of at least three of the following organ systems:
    —Gastrointestinal: vomiting, diarrhea
    —Muscular: severe myalgias and/or creatine phosphokinase (CPK) greater than 5 times normal

- -Mucous membranes (vagina, conjunctiva, pharynx): frank hyperemia
- —Renal:
  - -Serum BUN and creatinine greater than 2 times normal
  - -Abnormal urinary sediment
  - -Pyuria in the absence of urinary tract infection
- —Hepatic: serum bilirubin, aspartate aminotransferase (AST), alanine aminotransferase (ALT) greater than 2 times normal
- —Hematologic: platelets fewer than 100,000/mm^3
- —CNS: disorientation without focal neurologic signs
- Serology:
- —Negative for Rocky Mountain spotted fever
- —Negative for leptospirosis
- —Negative for measles
- Microbiology:
  - Gram stain and culture vaginal and cervical secretions (or surgical wound in nonmenstrual TSS): positive for *Staphylococcus aureus*
  - Blood cultures: rarely positive for *S. aureus*
  - Gram stain and culture CSF: rarely positive for *S. aureus*

Definitive Diagnosis:

Toxic shock syndrome   ICD-9-CM 040.89

Suggested Treatment:

- Removal of source of infection:
  - Removal of tampon or other vaginal foreign body (e.g., IUD)

- Surgical drainage of infected site (nonmenstrual TSS)
- Supportive care:
  - Fluid resuscitation with colloid and/or saline
  - Dopamine
  - Management of renal, hepatic, or pulmonary insufficiency
  - Cardiac monitoring
- Antimicrobial therapy:
  - Nafcillin 1.5 g IV every 4 hours, or Oxacillin 2.0 g IV every 4 hours
  - Penicillin allergy: Clindamycin 25 mg/kg/day IV given every 8 hours, or Vancomycin 30 mg/kg/day IV given every 6 hours
  - Therapy need not be continued for longer than 10 to 15 days as long as there is no evidence of bacteremic spread or of a primary focus (e.g., osteomyelitis)

Follow-Up:

- Inpatient care is appropriate, with admission to ICU for monitoring if shock is present
- Aggressive fluid replacement and supportive measures
- May consider intravenous immunoglobulin (IVIG) in severely ill patients (0.4 gm/kg IV infused over 6 hours)
- Patient education for prevention
  - Avoid continuous tampon use during menses, especially super absorbency tampons
  - Frequent tampon changes
  - Use of sanitary napkins at night
- **Watch for:** signs and symptoms of
  - Acute renal failure
  - ARDS

- DIC
- Encephalopathic changes
- Cardiomyopathy
- Bacteremic spread and/or septicemia
    - —Endocarditis
    - —Osteomyelitis and/or septic arthritis/bursitis
    - —Pericarditis
    - —Pyomyositis
- Recurrent infection (10% to 15%)
    - —Pulmonary infection

Nosocomial Infections and Fevers of Unknown Origin

12

INFECTIONS COVERED

NOSOCOMIAL INFECTIONS DUE TO PERCUTANEOUS INTRAVASCULAR DEVICES

Presenting Symptoms:

SUBJECTIVE	OBJECTIVE
Patient with an intravascular catheter in place	Fever
	Rigors
Pain and redness at catheter insertion site	Inflammation and/or exudate at catheter insertion site
	Signs of infection caused by metastatic emboli
	Signs of venous obstruction distal to central venous catheter

Differential Diagnosis:

Pyrexia of undetermined etiology
Bacteremia/sepsis of unrelated etiology

Suggested Workup:

- Evaluate risk factors for catheter-acquired infection
  - Type of catheter (infection rate of plastic > steel)
  - Location of catheter (central > peripheral or femoral > jugular or subclavian)
  - Method of placement (cutdown > percutaneous; emergent > elective; aseptic conditions > sterile conditions in operating room)
  - Duration of placement (longer than 72 hours increases risk of infection)
  - Skill of person placing catheter (risk of infection increases if catheter placed by anyone other than licensed venipuncturist, or surgeon in operating room)

- • Catheter management and care (the more
    frequently the catheter is entered, the
    higher the infection rate)
  • Catheter composition/construction (stiff
    polyvinyl chloride [PVC] catheter > flexible
    silicone elastomer or polyurethane catheter;
    larger catheter with increased number of
    lumens > smaller catheter with single
    lumen)
  • Catheter use (total parenteral nutrition
    [TPN] $\gg$ other uses; flow-directed, balloon-
    tipped arterial catheters and arterial lines >
    venous access)
  • Patient age under 1 year or over 60 years old
  • Immunosuppressed patient
  • Patient with disrupted skin integrity (e.g.,
    burns, psoriasis)
  • Patient with already established underlying
    distant infection can result in
    hematogenous seeding of catheter
  • Patient predisposed to thrombus formation
    can increase catheter thrombogenicity and
    lead to increased infection rate
- Careful examination of all catheter entry
  sites
- Collect exudate from catheter entry site for
  Gram stain and culture
- Catheter should be removed and the tip and
  intracutaneous sections cultured separately
  (Maki techniques)
  • If catheter cannot be removed, Gram stain
    or quantitative culture of skin insertion site
    should be performed
- Blood cultures
  • Drawn through catheter (these cultures
    may become easily contaminated in up to
    5% of cases)
  • Drawn from a different venous site

- Ultrasound to evaluate for perivenous abscess
- Ultrasonic duplex venous Doppler study to find intraluminal catheter obstruction or thrombosis

Definitive Diagnosis:

Infection due to arterial/   ICD-9-CM 996.62
  venous catheter

Suggested Treatment:

- Peripheral intravenous catheters:
  - Exit site infection (7-day treatment):
    —Dicloxacillin 250 to 500 mg orally every 6 hours
    —Penicillin allergy: Cephalexin 250 to 500 mg orally every 6 hours, or Cefadroxil 500 mg orally every 12 hours
    —Suspect systemic infection with fever: Vancomycin 1 g intravenously (IV) every 12 hours
    —Alter antibiotics according to culture results
  - Bacteremia (14 day treatment [up to 4 weeks if suspect metastatic infection, infective endocarditis]):
    —Remove catheter
    —Empiric antibiotic therapy until culture results are available (more than 90% of these infections are coagulase-negative *Staphylococcus*)
    –Nafcillin or Oxacillin 2 g IV every 6 hours
    –Penicillin allergy: Cefazolin 1 g IV every 8 hours, or Cephradine 1g IV every 6 hours, or Vancomycin 1 g IV every 12 hours

- Septic thrombophlebitis (14-day treatment [up to 4 weeks if suspect metastatic infection]):
  —Remove catheter
  —Empiric antibiotic therapy until culture results are available (>90% of these infections are coagulase-negative *Staphylococcus*): Vancomycin 1 g IV every 12 hours
  —Surgical excision may be required for perivenous abscess or refractory infections
- Central percutaneous catheters (14-day treatment [up to 4 weeks if metastatic infection is suspected or there is prolonged bacteremia despite use of appropriate antibiotics]):
  - Remove catheter
  - Empiric antibiotic therapy until culture results are available (usually a mixture of *Staphylococcus* and Gram-negative infections, with up to 25% prevalence of *Candida*)
    —Vancomycin 1 g IV every 12 hours, and
      Penicillin (PCN)-G 5 million units (U) IV every 6 hours, or
      Erythromycin 1 g IV every 6 hours, or
      Clindamycin 900 mg IV every 8 hours
      MAY ADD
      Amphotericin B 0.3 to 1.0 mg/kg/day IV
  - Concomitant full-dose anticoagulation with Heparin where there is evidence of septic thrombophlebitis
  - Surgical excision may be required for refractory infections

- Tunneled catheters and infusion ports:
    - Exit site infection (14-day treatment):
        —No systemic signs of infection in non-neutropenic patient:
          –Dicloxacillin 250 to 500 mg orally every 6 hours
          –Penicillin allergy: Cephalexin 250 to 500 mg orally every 6 hours, or Cefadroxil 500 mg orally every 12 hours
        —Suspect systemic infection with fever: Vancomycin 1 g IV every 12 hours
        —Alter antibiotics according to culture results
        —Remove catheter if there is:
          –Bacteremia with *Staphylococcus aureus, Candida,* or *Aspergillus*
          –Failure of antibiotic therapy to reduce signs of infection within 48 hours
          –Signs of metastatic infection or embolic events
          –Hemodynamic instability
    - Tunnel infection (14 days of treatment past resolution of local inflammatory signs):
        —Remove catheter
        —Vancomycin 1 g IV every 12 hours, and PCN-G 5 million U IV every 6 hours, or Erythromycin 1 g IV every 6 hours, or Clindamycin 900 mg IV every 8 hours
        —Alter antibiotics according to culture results
    - Bacteremia:
        —Vancomycin 1 g IV every 12 hours for 14 days
        —Alter antibiotics according to culture results

  —Remove catheter if there is:
    –Bacteremia with *Staphylococcus aureus,
      Candida,* or *Aspergillus*
    –Failure of antibiotic therapy to reduce
      signs of infection within 48 hours
    –Signs of metastatic infection or embolic
      events
    –Hemodynamic instability
- Septic thrombophlebitis (14 days of
  therapy):
  —Remove catheter
  —Vancomycin 1 g IV every 12 hours, and
        PCN-G 5 million U IV every 6
            hours, or
        Erythromycin 1 g IV every 6 hours, or
        Clindamycin 900 mg IV every 8 hours
  —Alter antibiotics according to culture
    results
  —Concomitant full-dose anticoagulation
    with Heparin
  —May need to treat for up to 4 weeks if
    there are signs of metastatic infection
    (e.g., infective endocarditis)
  —Surgical excision may be needed for
    refractory infections
- Arterial catheters:
  - Catheter should be removed regardless of
    whether there is bacteremia or simple exit
    site infection
  - Vancomycin 1 g IV every 12 hours for 14
    days may be used as empiric therapy
    pending culture results
  - Treatment for up to 4 weeks may be
    needed for
    —Metastatic infection
    —Infective endocarditis
    —Prolonged bacteremia

- Mild infections may be treated empirically
  with Vancomycin 0.5 g orally every 6 hours
  for 14 days

Follow-Up:

- Follow closely by clinical evaluation and
  microbiologic screening until there is clear
  improvement
- Patient should be kept in isolation until there
  is no evidence of bacteremia
- Prevention of reinfection
  - Place all lines and catheters using sterile
    technique with chlorhexidine or iodine
    preparation of the skin site
  - Place catheters percutaneously and anchor
    well to avoid catheter movement
  - Replace all continuous flow devices every
    48 to 72 hours
  - Replace all arterial lines every 96 hours (a
    changed line/catheter is NOT an exchange
    over an existing guidewire)
  - Minimize unnecessary junctions in the
    apparatus connected to the catheter
  - Mimimize manipulation of the system
  - **Watch for:** signs and symptoms of
    - Bacteremia, sepsis, and shock
    - Metastatic infections
      —Infective endocarditis
      —*Candida* endophthalmitis
    - Recurrent infections

NOSOCOMIAL RESPIRATORY INFECTIONS

Presenting Symptoms:

SUBJECTIVE	OBJECTIVE
Hospitalized patient with hospital-acquired lower	Hospitalized patient with nosocomial pneumonitis

respiratory tract infection

Consider risk factors:
—Intubation
—Patient with tracheostomy
—Patient in the intensive care unit (ICU)
—Patient receiving chronic nebulizer treatments
—Previous antibiotic use
—Postsurgical patient
—Patient with chronic lung disease
—Older patient (over age 60)
—Obese patient
—Immunosuppression
Variable clinical findings
—New fever
—New cough with sputum (may be purulent)
—New infiltrate on chest radiograph
—New hypoxemia

Differential Diagnosis:

Tracheobronchitis
Atypical pneumonia
Pulmonary embolus
Myocardial infarction
Pulmonary edema
Fungal infection
Bronchiectasis

Pulmonary vasculitis
Pneumothorax
Lung abscess
Pulmonary sarcoid

Suggested Workup:

- Initial evaluation by history and physical examination
- Collect respiratory secretions for Gram stain and culture (must take care not to contaminate specimens with upper airway flora)
  - Endotracheal aspiration
  - Transtracheal aspiration (not for intubated patients) (high rate of complications)
  - Bronchoscopy with shielded-tip sampling
  - Bronchoscopy with bronchoalveolar lavage
- Open lung biopsy (reserved for cases where a microbiologic diagnosis is essential and all other tests have yielded equivocal or misleading results)
- Blood cultures
- Serial chest radiographs
- Arterial blood gas analyses
- Serology
  - Herpes simplex
  - Cytomegalovirus (CMV)
  - *Chlamydia*
  - *Legionella*
  - *Mycoplasma pneumoniae*
  - *Coxiella* spp.

Definitive Diagnosis:

Acute bacterial pneumonia   ICD-9-CM 482.9
Anaerobic pneumonia   ICD-9-CM 482.81
Aspiration pneumonia   ICD-9-CM 507.0
Pseudomonas pneumonia   ICD-9-CM 482.1

Staphylococcal pneumonia   ICD-9-CM 482.4
Klebsiella pneumonia   ICD-9-CM 482.0
Escherichia coli pneumonia   ICD-9-CM 482.82
Haemophilus influenzae   ICD-9-CM 482.2
  pneumonia
Respiratory syncytial virus   ICD-9-CM 480.1
  (RSV) pneumonia

Suggested Treatment:

- Empiric anaerobic therapy (pending results of cultures):
  - Recommended for patients with:
    —Dense infiltrates in dependent portions of their lungs
    —Endotracheal intubation
    —High risk of aspiration (seizures, coma, esophageal obstruction, emesis, oropharyngeal disease that impairs swallowing)
      –Imipenem 0.5 to 0.75 g IV every 6 hours, or
      –Ticarcillin-clavulanate 1 to 4 g (ticarcillin) IV every 6 hours, or
      –Clindamycin 1.8 to 2.7 g/day IV given every 6 hours, and
        Ceftazidime 1 to 2 g IV every 8 hours
  - If *Pseudomonas aeruginosa* is suspected:
    —Ceftazidime 1 to 2 g IV every 8 hours, and
        Gentamicin 3 to 5 mg/kg/day IV given every 8 hours, or
    —Clindamycin 1.8 to 2.7 g/day IV given every 6 hours, and
        Aztreonam 1 to 2 g IV every 8 hours, or
        Ciprofloxacin 400 mg IV every 12 hours, or

> Gentamicin 3 to 5 mg/kg/day IV
> given every 8 hours,
> —May add Tobramycin 40 mg instilled into
> endotracheal tube every 8 hours (**NOTE:**
> This is an experimental treatment, the
> results of which are based on a limited
> number of patients)

- Empiric therapy for Gram-negative infections
  (*E. coli, Klebsiella, H. influenzae*):
  - Ceftazidime 1 to 2 g IV every 8 hours, and
    Gentamicin 3 to 5 mg/kg/day IV given
    every 8 hours, or
  - Imipenem 1 to 4 g/day IV given every 6
    hours, or
  - Piperacillin + tazobactam 3 g piperacillin
    IV every 6 hours for 14 to 21 days
- Fungal infections:
  - Amphotericin B 0.3 to 1.0 mg/kg/day slow
    intravenous infusion

Follow-Up:

- Inpatient therapy appropriate with daily
  assessment of patient's progress until there is
  significant clinical improvement
- Repeat chest radiographs every 2 to 3 days
  until there is clinical improvement, then
  weekly; repeat chest radiographs 6 weeks after
  complete recovery to exclude obstructing
  endobronchial lesion, especially in patients at
  high risk for malignancy
- Chest physical therapy and incentive spirometry
- Institute prophylactic measures to prevent
  recurrence of nosocomial pneumonia
  - Appropriate isolation procedures for
    intubated patients
  - Monitoring of respiratory equipment for
    bacterial contamination
  - H-2 blockers to prevent gastro-esophageal
    reflux disease (GERD)

- Consider organism-specific immunization for highly virulent respiratory pathogens (e.g., *Pseudomonas* lipopolysaccharide vaccine)
- **Watch for:** signs and symptoms of
    - Empyema
    - Pulmonary abscess
    - Purulent pericarditis
    - Pleurisy
    - Respiratory failure
    - Pneumothorax

NOSOCOMIAL URINARY TRACT INFECTIONS (UTIs)

Presenting Symptoms:

SUBJECTIVE	OBJECTIVE
Patient in hospital or nursing home	Elicit risk factors for nosocomial UTIs
Patient with indwelling urinary catheter (80% of infections) or after genitourinary manipulation or procedure (10% of infections)	—Prolonged urinary catheterization (daily increase in prevalence of bacteriuria is 3% to 10%)
Patient may be asymptomatic	—Lack of systemic antibiotics
Patient may complain of dysuria, flank pain, frequency, urgency (despite presence of catheter)	—Lack of urinemeter drainage
	—Being female
	—Diabetes mellitus
	—Microbial colonization of drainage bag
	—Serum creatinine greater than 2 mg/dL

—Indication for catheter is other than drainage during surgery or output measurement (e.g., urine retention, urinary incontinence, neurogenic bladder)
—Catheter with sealed collection junction
—Periurethral bacterial colonization

Fever
Suprapubic discomfort
Dysuria
Flank pain
May develop bacteremia and symptoms of sepsis

Differential Diagnosis:

Obstructive uropathy
Urethritis
Epididymitis
Vaginitis
Tumors (bladder, ureter, prostate, urethra)
Urinary calculi
Anatomic abnormality of urinary tract
Prostatitis
Nephrolithiasis
Perinephric abscess
Acute glomerulonephritis

Suggested Workup:

- Urinalysis
- Urine Gram stain and culture
  - Bacterial

- Fungal (especially if patient is on long-term antibiotic therapy)
- Blood cultures (especially if bacteremia is suspected)
- Renal ultrasound to evaluate for obstruction, calculi, parenchymal swelling suggestive of pyelonephritis, perirenal abscess
- Cystoscopy may be needed to evaluate for ureteral obstruction

Definitive Diagnosis:

Infection due to indwelling urinary catheter	ICD-9-CM 996.64
Infection due to other genitourinary device	ICD-9-CM 996.65
Other complication due to genitourinary device	ICD-9-CM 996.76

Suggested Treatment:

- Asymptomatic bacteriuria:
  - Long-term catheterization (LTC) patients:
    - —If asymptomatic, patient need not be treated nor the catheter removed
    - —Antimicrobial therapy may be instituted if urine culture shows presence of bacteria known to cause a high incidence of bacteremia (e.g., *Serratia marcescens*), or to control outbreaks of resistant organisms
      - –Treat according to culture and sensitivity results
  - Short-term catheterization (STC) patients:
    - —Remove catheter
    - —Reculture urine after catheter removal; if bacteriuria persists, treat with oral antibiotics according to culture and sensitivity results

- Symptomatic bacteriuria:
    - Remove or replace catheter
    - Evaluate patient for obstruction
    - Antimicrobial therapy (may be modified as results of urine and blood cultures and sensitivity testing are obtained):
      —Lower UTI:
        –Trimethoprim-sulfamethoxazole (TMP-SMX) DS 1 tablet orally 2 times a day, or
          Ciprofloxacin 500 mg orally 2 times a day for 3 to 7 days
      —Upper UTI, Urosepsis:
        –Ceftazidime 3 to 6 g/day IV given every 8 to 12 hours, or
          Ciprofloxacin 400 mg IV every 12 hours, or
          Ticarcillin + clavulanate 4 to 24 g/day (based on ticarcillin) IV given every 4 to 6 hours, or
          Aztreonam 1 to 2 g IV every 6 hours for 10 to 14 days
- Candiduria:
    - If uncomplicated, remove catheter in STC patients or change catheter in LTC patients
    - If infection persists despite removal or change of catheter, treat with antimicrobial therapy:
      —Amphotericin B 50 mg/L of sterile water
        –Irrigate bladder intermittently (200 to 300 mL instilled with clamping of catheter for 1 to 2 hours), or
        –Continuous irrigation at 40 mL/hour for 3 to 5 days, or
        –Fluconazole 200 mg orally for 1 dose, then 100 mg orally every day for 3 to 5 days

Follow-Up:

- May need to follow routine surveillance cultures (probably not necessary for asymptomatic LTC patients)
- Make certain other sources of infection are ruled out
- Make certain catheter obstruction, urinary calculi, and periurethral infection are ruled out
- If candiduria persists despite appropriate antimicrobial therapy, make certain fungus ball and invasive renal infection are ruled out
- Institute measures to prevent recurrence of infection
    - Use urinary catheters only when absolutely necessary and minimize the duration of their use
    - Try external collection devices (e.g., condom catheters)
    - Try intermittent catheterization, suprapubic catheterization, urinary diversions, or intraurethral catheters
    - If indwelling catheter is to be used, maintain a closed system

Watch for: signs and symptoms of
- Acute pyelonephritis
- Bacteremia and urosepsis
- Acute renal failure
- Urinary obstruction
- Perirenal abscess

FEVER OF UNKNOWN ORIGIN (FUO)

Presenting Symptoms:

SUBJECTIVE	OBJECTIVE
Fever of a type and pattern that is of	Fever over 38.3°C with no other tangible

little help in making a diagnosis

Constitutional symptoms may accompany fever
—Headache
—Myalgia
—Malaise

No localizing symptoms

manifestations of disease, on at least four occasions over a 14- to 21-day period

No obvious cause for the fever

Differential Diagnosis:

Infection

Lymphoma

Leukemia

Solid tumors (e.g., hypernephroma, hepatoma, atrial myxoma, colon cancer)

Collagen vascular disease

Granulomatous disease

Pulmonary emboli

Drug fever

Thermoregulatory disorder

Endocrine disorders (especially thyroid dysfunction)

Factitious fevers

Transient ischemic events

Alcoholic hepatitis

Suggested Workup:

- Exhaustive history
  - Recent travel
  - Exposure to biologic or chemical agents
  - Acquired immunodeficiency syndrome (AIDS) risk factors
  - Drug abuse
  - Recent immigration
- Careful physical examination

- Laboratory
  - Complete blood count (CBC)
    —Leukopenia, leukocytosis
    —Anemia
    —Thrombocytopenia, thrombocytosis
  - C-reactive protein
  - Erythrocyte sedimentation rate (ESR)
  - Liver function tests—Elevated alkaline phosphatase?
- Tuberculosis skin test
- Blood cultures (three sets of two each, taken at different times)
- Urinalysis and urine culture
- Sputum Gram stain and culture
- Serology
  - Human immunodeficiency virus (HIV)
  - Epstein-Barr virus (EBV)
  - Hepatitis
  - Syphilis
  - CMV
  - Amebiasis
  - Coccidiomycoses
  - Q fever
  - Lyme disease
- Thyroid function tests
- Collagen vascular tests
  - Rheumatoid factor
  - Antinuclear antibody
  - Serum protein electrophoresis
- Imaging studies
  - Chest radiograph
  - Abdominal/pelvic ultrasound (if suspect mass lesions, renal obstruction, or gallbladder/biliary tree pathology)
  - Sinus radiographs (if clinically indicated)
  - Panorex dental radiographs to rule out cryptic dental abscess
  - Bone scan (if suspect osteomyelitis or metastatic disease)

- Computed tomography (CT)/magnetic resonance imaging (MRI) of abdomen/pelvis (if infectious process or mass lesions are suspected)
- Gallium (^{67}Ga) or technetium-99m (Tc^{99m}) colloid scan (if suspect infectious or neoplastic process that is not detected by other techniques)
- Echocardiogram (if cardiac valve lesions or atrial myxoma are suspected)
- Perfusion-ventilation (V/Q) scan or pulmonary angiogram (if pulmonary emboli is suspected)
- Indium (^{111}In)-labeled leukocyte scan (if inflammatory process is suspected and all other tests are inconclusive)
- Invasive testing
  - Bone marrow aspirate and biopsy (if granulomatous disease, infection, or malignancy are suspected)
  - Liver biopsy (if granulomatous disease is suspected)
  - Temporal artery biopsy (if temporal arteritis is suspected)
  - Biopsy lymph node, muscle, or skin (if clinically indicated)
  - Lumbar puncture (if clinically indicated)
  - Exploratory laparotomy (if all other tests are inconclusive and there is reasonable suspicion of a peritoneal or intra-abdominal process)

Definitive Diagnosis:

Fever of unknown origin   ICD-9-CM 780.6
  (until a definite etiology is
  established)
Specific ICD-9-CM code once a specific etiology is established

Suggested Treatment:

- Specific diagnosis established:
  - Treatment as appropriate for diagnosis
- Specific diagnosis not established (20% of FUO patients):
  - Antipyretics
    —Acetaminophen
    —Indomethacin
    —Naproxen
  - Steroid trial
  - Antibiotic trial based on patient's history and clinical suspicion (should be delayed until diagnostic workup is completed)
  - Psychiatry consultation if factitious fever is a possibility
  - Re-evaluate patient with history, physical examination, and screening laboratory studies
    —Target:
      –Pediatric:
        –Collagen vascular disease
        –Inflammatory bowel disease
      –Geriatric:
        –Acute leukemia
        –Hodgkin's lymphoma
        –Intra-abdominal infections
        –Tuberculosis
        –Temporal arteritis
        –Drug fever

Follow-Up:

- Outpatient workup is acceptable except for patients who are debilitated or where an invasive procedure is necessary
- Attempt to determine etiology before initiating any therapeutic measure
- Avoid "shotgun" antibiotics or other therapies

- **Watch for:** signs and symptoms of
    - Factitious fevers
    - Münchausen syndrome
    - Abrupt clinical worsening requiring immediate diagnostic re-examination

FEVER IN THE INTENSIVE CARE UNIT (ICU)

Presenting Symptoms:

SUBJECTIVE

Fever in ICU patient that develops more than 48 hours after entry into ICU

OBJECTIVE

Fever in ICU patient that develops more than 48 hours after entry into ICU

No or low grade fever prior to ICU admission, now reaching as high as 39° to 40° C

Clinical signs vary according to organ system affected:

—Lung: worsening hypoxemia; increased ventilator dependence

—Skin: bleb formation, gangrenous discoloration, crepitus, erythematous decubiti with/without black eschars

—Urine: history of

long-standing
indwelling urinary
catheter
—Thrombosis: few
revealing physical
signs; higher
probability in
patients with
congestive heart
failure, prolonged
immobility,
malignancy
—Vascular: difficulty
withdrawing blood
through
intravascular
catheter; erythema at
catheter site
—Drugs: history of
administration of
pyrogenic substances
(e.g., atropine,
phenothiazine
derivatives,
amphotericin B,
hydralazine,
procainamide)
—Gastrointestinal:
abdominal rigidity,
tenderness, loss of
bowel sounds,
palpable mass,
melena,
hematochezia
—Blood products:
history of
transfusion of blood,

platelets, fresh
frozen plasma (FFP);
leukoagglutinin
reaction

Differential Diagnosis:

Pneumonia (especially in ventilator-dependent
  patients)
Adult respiratory distress syndrome (ARDS)
Tracheobronchitis
Atelectasis
Empyema
Parapneumonic effusion
Surgical wound infection
Cellulitis
Infected decubitus ulcer
UTI
Deep-vein thrombosis
Catheter sepsis
Infected thrombophlebitis
Infective endocarditis
Drug fever
Pulmonary emboli
Pseudomembranous colitis
Ischemic colitis
Cholecystitis
Hepatitis
Pancreatitis
Transfusion reaction
Sinusitis (especially if there is nasal intubation,
  nasogastric tube, or posterior nasal packing in
  place)

Suggested Workup:

- Careful history and chart review to
  differentiate fever present on admission to
  ICU from fever that developed 48 hours later

- Careful review of medications, especially those added in the preceding 7 to 10 days
- Careful physical examination
- Laboratory
  - CBC
  - Liver function tests
  - ESR
  - C-reactive protein
- Microbiology
  - Sputum Gram stain and culture
  - Blood cultures (three sets of two each at different times)
  - Urinalysis and urine culture
  - Culture indwelling intravascular catheter tips with blood cultures through tips prior to catheter removal
- Serology
  - HIV
  - EBV
  - Hepatitis viruses
  - CMV
  - Coccidiomycoses
- Thyroid function tests
- Collagen vascular studies
  - Rheumatoid factor
  - Antinuclear antibody
  - Serum protein electrophoresis
- Imaging studies
  - Chest radiograph
  - Sinus radiographs
  - Abdominal ultrasound/CT scan
  - Pelvic ultrasound/CT scan
  - Doppler venography
  - Contrast/digital subtraction venography
  - V/Q scan or pulmonary angiogram
  - Bone scan

- Echocardiogram
- ^{67}Ga scan
- Invasive testing
  - Bronchoscopy with bronchoalveolar lavage, transbronchial biopsy, or protected specimen brushing technique
  - Biopsy local wounds or affected skin
  - Remove decubitus eschars and culture wound
  - Lumbar puncture

Definitive Diagnosis:

Pyrexia, undetermined   ICD-9-CM 780.6
Once specific etiology is determined, use appropriate ICD-9-CM code

Suggested Treatment:

- Once the specific diagnosis is established, treat accordingly
- Remove all possible sources of infections:
  - Change endotracheal tube and all ventilator fittings that are possible sources of infection
  - Institute aggressive skin care and wound management
  - Remove indwelling urinary catheter and replace with external collection devices (e.g., condom catheters); consider intermittent catheterization, suprapubic catheterization, or intraurethral catheters
  - Heparin IV in therapeutic dosages for thromboembolic disease
  - Remove all intravascular catheters and replace with new devices at different sites under sterile conditions
  - Discontinue all nonessential drugs
  - Re-evaluate need for biologic products including blood, platelets, FFP

Follow-Up:

- Determine etiology of fever before initiating therapy
- Avoid "shotgun" antibiotics
- Re-evaluate via screening tests frequently until a differential diagnosis is established
- **Watch for:** signs and symptoms of
    - Overwhelming sepsis and shock

Immunization 13

NORMAL ADULTS

Presenting Symptoms:

SUBJECTIVE

Adult patient (25 to 64 years of age) presenting for immunization

OBJECTIVE

Adult patient (25 to 64 years old) presenting for immunization

Suggested Workup:

- Careful medical and social history

Definitive Diagnosis:

Immunization
—Hepatitis A   ICD-9-CM 99.4
—Hepatitis B   ICD-9-CM 99.4
—Varicella   ICD-9-CM 99.4
—Tetanus and diphtheria (Td)   ICD-9-CM 99.39
—Measles, mumps, rubella (MMR)   ICD-9-CM 99.48
—Influenza   ICD-9-CM 99.52
—Pneumococcal vaccine   ICD-9-CM 99.3
—Typhoid   ICD-9-CM 99.32
—Rabies   ICD-9-CM 99.44

Suggested Treatment:

- Td:
  - Traditional recommendation: Td booster every 10 years throughout life
    —0.5 mL intramuscularly (deltoid muscle), or
  - For persons having completed the full pediatric series including a booster as a teenager, 1 Td booster may be given at age 50

- MMR:
  - Not necessary for adults born before 1957
  - For adults born after 1957, a documented physician's diagnosis of measles and mumps, or laboratory evidence of infection, obviates need for immunization
  - Persons vaccinated against measles between 1963 and 1967 should receive a single dose of measles vaccine 0.5 mL subcutaneously (deltoid area)
  - Immunity against rubella requires proof of immunization or serologic confirmation
  - Susceptible women who are pregnant should receive rubella vaccine **AFTER DELIVERY**
- Influenza:
  - Healthy adults younger than 65 years old generally do not require influenza virus immunization
  - Approximately 35% of persons 50 to 64 years of age have conditions for which they should receive influenza vaccine
  - Health care personnel or those who provide community services and come into contact with a large number of people should receive immunization
    —0.5 mL intramuscularly (deltoid muscle)
    —Optimal time is mid-October to mid-November
- Pneumococcal vaccine:
  - Healthy adults under 65 years of age without risk factors for acquiring invasive pneumococcal disease do not require immunization
  - Approximately 35% of persons 50 to 64 years of age have conditions for which they should receive pneumococcal vaccine
    —Polyvalent vaccine 0.5 mL subcutaneously/ intramuscularly (deltoid area)

- Hepatitis A:
  - Risk factors that argue for immunization for normal adults include:
    - —Personal contact with a person who has hepatitis A
    - —Employment in or attendance at a day care center
    - —History of injection drug use
    - —Planned international travel, especially to an area endemic for hepatitis A infections
  - HAVRIX 1440 enzyme-linked immunosorbent assay (ELISA) units (1 mL) or VAQTA 50 units (1 mL) intramuscularly (deltoid muscle)
    - —Booster dose may be given over 6 months later (confers more than 99% immunity)
    - —Hepatitis A immune globulin may be administered concomitantly
- Varicella:
  - Approximately 10% of adults have neither contracted chickenpox nor been immunized against varicella
    - —Those who do contract the infection have an increased risk of pulmonary and central nervous system complications
  - VARIVAX 0.5 ml subcutaneously (deltoid area)
    - —Booster dose may be given 4 to 8 weeks later (confers more than 99% immunity)
- Typhoid:
  - Appropriate for adults traveling to countries in which typhoid is endemic
  - Purified typhoid Vi polysaccharide vaccine (Vi CPS) 25 μg intramuscularly (deltoid area)
- Rabies vaccine:
  - Preexposure vaccination is recommended for persons traveling for more than 1

month to areas where rabies is a constant threat, for animal care workers who may come into contact with rabid animals, and veterinarians

—Human diploid cell vaccine 1 mL intradermally (deltoid area) on days 0, 7, and 28, or

—0.1 mL intradermally on days 0, 7, 21, and 28

- Hepatitis B:
  - For health care workers who come into contact with blood, homosexual or bisexual men, institutionalized individuals, intravenous drug abusers, immunocompromised patients
  - Recombinant vaccine 10 μg intramuscularly (deltoid muscle) at 0, 1, and 6 months

Follow-Up:

- Consider special immunization needs for certain groups of adults
  - Pregnant women—Td
  - Nursing home residents—influenza, pneumococcal
  - Prison inmates or other institutionalized people—Hepatitis B
  - Homeless persons—all vaccinations must be reviewed
  - Immigrants and refugees—all vaccinations must be reviewed
  - Health care workers—Hepatitis B, influenza, MMR
  - Laboratory workers—Hepatitis B
  - Persons with recurrent sexually transmitted diseases—Hepatitis B
  - Homosexual or bisexual men—Hepatitis B
  - Intravenous drug users—Hepatitis B, Td
  - Prostitutes—Hepatitis B

- Monitor adverse reactions to immunizations; **NOT** contraindications to vaccination are:
  - Mild to moderate local tenderness, swelling, or fever less than 40.5°C to previous immunization
  - Current antimicrobial therapy
  - Convalescence from a recent illness
  - Recent exposure to an infectious disease
  - Breast feeding
  - Personal or family history of allergies to antibiotics
- **Watch for:** signs and symptoms of
  - Anaphylactic reactions

IMMUNOCOMPROMISED ADULTS

Presenting Symptoms:

SUBJECTIVE	OBJECTIVE
Immunocompromised patient	Immunocompromised patient in which altered host defenses requires special consideration for prevention of infection
—Human immunodeficiency virus (HIV) infection	
—Chronic immunosuppressive therapy	
—Congenital immunodeficiency state (antibody, cellular, phagocytic, complement deficiencies)	Elicit history of type and extent of immune deficiency
—Asplenia	
—Diabetes mellitus	
—Renal failure	
—Alcoholic	

—Malignancy
—Nutritional
  deficiency

Suggested Workup:

- Take careful history for risk factors
  - Family history
  - Drug abuse and parenteral blood exposure
  - Sexual lifestyle
  - Past medical history
- Careful physical examination
- Laboratory
  - Complete blood count (CBC) with differential
  - Immunoglobulin (Ig) levels, including IgG and subclasses, IgM, IgA, and IgE
  - Quantitate mononuclear cell populations
  - Total lymphocyte count and subsets
  - Complement levels
  - Phagocyte function tests
  - Skin testing battery
- Imaging studies may be needed to evaluate suspected acquired causes for immunodeficiency

Definitive Diagnosis:

Immunization
—Bacillus Calmette-Guérin   ICD-9-CM 99.33
  (BCG)
—Diphtheria-pertussis-   ICD-9-CM 99.39
  tetanus (DPT)
—*Haemophilus influenzae*   ICD-9-CM 99.52
—Measles   ICD-9-CM 99.45
—Meningococcus   ICD-9-CM 99.55
—Mumps   ICD-9-CM 99.46
—Pertussis   ICD-9-CM 99.37

—Poliomyelitis	ICD-9-CM 99.41
—*Staphylococcus/Streptococcus*	ICD-9-CM 99.55
—Tetanus	ICD-9-CM 99.38
—Viral	ICD-9-CM 99.55

Suggested Treatment:

- Td:
  - Tetanus and diphtheria toxoids adsorbed for adult use 0.5 mL intramuscularly (deltoid area)
- MMR:
  - Vaccine 0.5 mL subcutaneously (deltoid area)
  - **CONTRAINDICATED** in patients who are on chronic immunosuppressive therapy following organ transplantation, or who are severely immunocompromised for reasons other than HIV infection
  - **CONSIDER CAUTIOUSLY** in patients who have progressed to acquired immunodeficiency disease (AIDS) based on the likelihood they will come into contact with measles, mumps, or rubella
  - In HIV-infected patients with CD less than $200/mm^3$ exposed to measles, should give: Measles immune globulin 0.5 mL/kg intramuscularly within 6 days of exposure
- Hepatitis B:
  - Vaccine 10 μg (1.0 mL) intramuscularly (deltoid muscle) at 0, 1, and 6 months
- *H. influenzae* type b (Hib):
  - Conjugate vaccine 0.5 mL intramuscularly (deltoid muscle)

- Pneumococcal:
  - Polyvalent vaccine 0.5 mL subcutaneously/intramuscularly (deltoid area)
- Meningococcal:
  - Menomune A/C/Y/W-135 polysaccharide vaccine 0.5 mL subcutaneously (deltoid area)
- Influenza:
  - Multivalent vaccine 0.5 mL intramuscularly (deltoid muscle)
- BCG:
  - Vaccine 0.2 to 0.3 mL percutaneously with multipuncture disc (deltoid area)
  - May need to be repeated in 2 to 3 months if patient remains skin-test negative to 5 tuberculin units (TU) of purified protein derivative (PPD)
  - **CONTRAINDICATED** in patients with HIV infection, on chronic immunosuppressive therapy following organ transplantation, or otherwise severely immunosuppressed
  - **INDICATED** in patients with asplenia, renal failure, diabetes, alcoholism, or alcoholic cirrhosis
- Polio vaccine:
  - Inactivated vaccine 0.5 mL subcutaneously (deltoid area) in 3 doses at 0, 1 to 2, and 6 to 12 months
  - Live oral trivalent vaccine 0.5 mL orally in 3 doses at 0, 2 months, and 8 to 14 months (third dose may be given 6 to 8 weeks after the second dose if there is substantial risk of exposure to polio)
  - **LIVE ORAL POLIO VACCINE IS CONTRAINDICATED** in patients with HIV infection, on chronic

immunosuppressive therapy following organ transplantation, or who are otherwise severely immunocompromised
- Varicella-zoster virus (VZV):
  - Live Oka vaccine 0.5 mL subcutaneously (deltoid area) in 2 doses at 0 and 4 to 8 weeks
  - Immune globulin (VZIG)
    —125 to 150 units (U)/kg intramuscularly (deltoid area)
    —Modifies clinical illness, but does not provide complete protection
    —Half-life is approximately 3 weeks, so repeat exposures to VZV require repeat treatment in patients with no antibodies to VZV

Follow-Up:

- Monitor patient carefully for hypersensitivity reactions following immunization
- Avoid live attenuated vaccines in HIV-infected patients and patients with severe immunosuppression not caused by HIV (those with congenital immunodeficiency diseases, malignancy)
- Monitor for failure to develop cell-mediated and/or humoral immunity following immunization
- **Watch for:** signs and symptoms of
  - Steroid interference with vaccine efficacy
    —Patients who receive high doses of systemic steroids for 2 weeks or longer should not be vaccinated until at least 3 months after therapy is discontinued

- Hypersensitivity/anaphylactic reactions to vaccines

NORMAL INFANTS, CHILDREN, AND ADOLESCENTS

Presenting Symptoms:

SUBJECTIVE
Normal infant or child
  for immunization

OBJECTIVE
Normal infant or child
  for immunization

Suggested Workup:

- Verify past immunization history
- Determine that there are no intercurrent illnesses precluding immunization

Definitive Diagnosis:

Immunization
—Hepatitis B   ICD-9-CM 99.55
—DPT   ICD-9-CM 99.39
—*H. influenzae* type b ICD-9-CM 99.52
—Polio   ICD-9-CM 99.41
—MMR   ICD-9-CM 99.45-47
—Varicella   ICD-9-CM 99.55

Suggested Treatment:

- Recommended immunization schedule (infants): (Table 13-1)
- Recommended immunization schedule (children and adolescents): (Table 13-2)
- Specific recommendations:
  - Hepatitis B:
    - Infants born to hepatitis B surface antigen (HB_sAg)-negative mothers:
      -2.5 μg Recombivax HB or 10 μg Engerix-B at each dose

-The second dose should be at least 1
month after the first dose
-The third dose should be at least 2
months after the second dose but not
before age 6 months
—Infants born to HB_sAg-positive mothers:
-0.5 mL hepatitis B globulin within 12
hours of birth, and
-5 μg Recombivax HB or 10 μg Energix-
B (at a separate site)
-The second dose is recommended at 1
to 2 months of age and the third dose
at 6 months of age
—Infants born to mothers with unknown
HB_sAg status:
-5 μg Recombivax HB or 10 μg Energix-
B within 12 hours of birth
-The second dose is recommended at 1
month of age and the third dose at 6
months of age
-At time of delivery, mother's blood
should be tested for HB_sAg status;
if positive, infant should receive
hepatitis immune globulin as soon as
possible and no later than at 1 week
of age
- DTP or DTaP (diphtheria, tetanus, acellular
pertussis):
  - DTaP 0.5 mL intramuscularly (preferred,
even in children who have previously
received DTP vaccine), or
  - DTP 0.5 mL intramuscularly
  - Td is recommended at 11 to 12 years of age
if at least 5 years have elapsed since the
last dose of DTP, DTaP, or Td
—Subsequent routine boosters of Td are
recommended every 10 years

Table 13.1.

Recommended Immunization Schedule (Infants)

Hepatitis B
    First dose: birth to 2 months
    Second dose: 1 month to 6 months
    Third dose: 6 to 18 months
DTP or DTaP
    First dose: 2 months
    Second dose: 4 months
    Third dose: 6 months
    Fourth dose: 15 to 18 months
Hib
    First dose: 2 months
    Second dose: 4 months
    Third dose: 6 months
    Fourth dose: 12 to 15 months

(continued)

Polio virus
First dose: 2 months
Second dose: 4 months
Third dose: 12 to 18 months
MMR
First dose: 12 to 15 months
Varicella
First dose: 12 to 18 months

DTP = diphtheria, tetanus, pertussis; **DTaP** = diphtheria, tetanus, acellular pertussis; **Hib** = *H. influenzae* type b; **MMR** = measles, mumps, rubella.

Table 13.2.

Recommended Immunization Schedule (Children and Adolescents):

Vaccine	4–6		11–12	14–16
		Age (years)		
Hepatitis B			[<---------------- X----------------->]	
DTP or DTaP	5th dose			
Td			[<------- every 10 years -------->]	
Polio virus	4th dose			
MMR	2nd dose	or	#2	
Varicella			XX	

DTP = diphtheria, tetanus, pertussis; DTaP = diphtheria, tetanus, acellular pertussis; Td = tetanus and diphtheria toxoids; MMR = measles, mumps, rubella.

X = children and adolescents who were not vaccinated against hepatitis B in infancy may begin the series during this time; a series of 3 doses is given at 0, 1, and 4 months.

XX = susceptible children who lack a reliable history of chickenpox and who failed to receive Varicella vaccine in infancy may be vaccinated at this time; adolescents over 13 years of age should receive 2 doses, at least 1 month apart.

- Hib:
  - If PedvaxHIB was administered at 2 and 4 months of age, a third dose at 6 months is not required
- Polio:
  - Any of these three schedules is acceptable using inactivated polio virus vaccine (IPV) or oral polio virus vaccine (OPV):
    —IPV at 2 and 4 months; OPV at 12 to 18 months and 4 to 6 years (recommended by the Advisory Committee on Immunization Practices), or
    —IPV at 2, 4, and 12 to 18 months, and 4 to 6 years, or
    —OPV at 2, 4, 6 to 18 months, and 4 to 6 years
- MMR:
  - 0.5 mL subcutaneously (deltoid area or inner aspect of upper thigh)
  - **DO NOT GIVE** immune globulin concurrently with MMR
- Varicella:
  - 0.5 mL subcutaneously (deltoid area or inner aspect of upper thigh)
  - **DO NOT GIVE** immune globulin concurrently with Varicella vaccine

Follow-Up:

- Consider other vaccines for certain adolescents at high risk for other infections:
- Annual Influenza vaccine for children 10 to 18 years old with:
  - Asthma
  - Other chronic pulmonary disorders
  - Disorders of the cardiovascular system
  - Reside in chronic care facilities or institutional settings (e.g., dormitories)

- Have chronic metabolic diseases, renal dysfunction, hemoglobinopathy, or immunosuppression
- Receive long-term aspirin therapy
- Have close contact with persons with chronic respiratory, cardiovascular, or metabolic disorders
- Pneumovax 23 (with a booster 5 years after the first dose) for children and adolescents 2 to 18 years old with:
  - Anatomic or functional asplenia
  - Sickle cell disease
  - Nephrotic syndrome
  - Cerebrospinal fluid leaks
  - Immunosuppression
- Hepatitis A vaccine for children 5 to 14 years old who:
  - Travel or work in a country that has a high or intermediate endemicity of hepatitis A virus infection
  - Reside in a community with a high rate of hepatitis A infection
  - Have chronic liver disease
  - Receive clotting factors
  - Use illegal drugs (by injection or not)
  - Are homosexual males
- Keep careful records of all vaccinations administered
- Screen all adolescents ages 11 to 12 years to spot immunization deficiencies
- Educate parents and adolescents regarding value of immunizations
- **Watch for**: signs and symptoms of
  - Allergic reactions to vaccines
  - Excessive simultaneous administration of vaccines (try not to give more than three vaccines at any one visit)

Prophylaxis   14

INFECTIVE ENDOCARDITIS

Presenting Symptoms:

<u>SUBJECTIVE</u>	<u>OBJECTIVE</u>

Patient presenting as a candidate for receipt of prophylaxis against infective endocarditis prior to invasive procedure	Evaluate conditions for which prophylaxis against infective endocarditis is recommended (see Suggested Workup below for full text):
	—Prosthetic valve(s)
	—Previous case of infective endocarditis
	—Valvular abnormalities from rheumatic heart disease or other causes
	—Mitral valve prolapse with mitral regurgitation
	—Hypertrophic cardiomyopathy
	—Congenital cardiac malformations
	Patient scheduled for invasive procedure associated with a high incidence of bacteremia
	—Dental procedures
	  –Tooth extraction
	  –Peridontal procedures (e.g., surgery, scaling, planing, probing)
	  –Dental implant placement and reimplantation of avulsed teeth

- –Endodontic instrumentation or surgery (e.g., root canal)
- –Initial placement of orthodontic bands but not brackets
- –Intraligamentary local anesthetic injections
- –Prophylactic cleaning where bleeding is anticipated
- —Respiratory tract
  - –Tonsillectomy and/or adenoidectomy
  - –Bronchoscopy with a rigid bronchoscope
  - –Surgical operations that involve respiratory mucosa
- —Gastrointestinal tract
  - –Sclerotherapy (esophageal varices)
  - –Esophageal stricture dilation
  - –Endoscopic retrograde cholangiopancreatography (ERCP) with biliary obstruction
  - –Biliary tract surgery
  - –Surgical operations that involve intestinal mucosa
- —Genitourinary tract
  - –Prostatic surgery
  - –Cystoscopy
  - –Urethral dilation

Suggested Workup:

- Complete history and physical to verify presence of a risk factor for infective endocarditis
- High-risk factors include:
  - Prosthetic valves (biosynthetic and homograft)
  - Previous bacterial endocarditis
  - Complex cyanotic congenital heart disease (e.g., single ventricle states, transposition of the great vessels, tetralogy of Fallot)
  - Ventricular septal defect
  - Coarctation of the aorta
  - Aortic valve disease
  - Mitral regurgitation
  - Marfan syndrome
  - Arteriovenous fistulae
  - Surgically constructed systemic pulmonary shunts or conduits
- Intermediate-risk factors include:
  - Mitral valve prolapse with regurgitation
  - Tricuspid valve disease
  - Asymmetric septal hypertrophy
  - Mitral stenosis
  - Degenerative valvular disease
  - Rheumatic heart disease
  - Hypertrophic cardiomyopathy
- Low-risk factors include:
  - Mitral valve prolapse without regurgitation
  - Atrial septal defects
- Negligible-risk factors for which prophylaxis is not routinely recommended include:
  - Isolated secundum atrial septal defect
  - Prior coronary artery bypass graft (CABG) surgery
  - Physiologic murmurs without valvular structural abnormalities

- Presence of cardiac pacemaker or implanted defibrillator
- Coronary artery disease
- Arteriosclerotic plaques
- Previous rheumatic fever without valvular dysfunction

Definitive Diagnosis:

Anomaly, heart valve — ICD-9-CM 746.9
Rheumatic heart disease — ICD-9-CM 398.90
Mitral valve prolapse — ICD-9-CM 424.0
Hypertrophic cardiomyopathy — ICD-9-CM 425.4
Tetralogy of Fallot — ICD-9-CM 745.2
Ventricular septal defect — ICD-9-CM 745.4
Coarctation of the aorta — ICD-9-CM 747.10
Mitral regurgitation — ICD-9-CM 746.6
Marfan syndrome — ICD-9-CM 759.82
Arteriovenous fistula — ICD-9-CM 447.0

Suggested Treatment:

- Oral and upper respiratory procedures:
  - Amoxicillin 2.0 g orally 1 hour before procedure
  - Penicillin allergy: Clindamycin 600 mg orally 1 hour before procedure, or
    Cephalexin or cefadroxil 2.0 g orally 1 hour before procedure, or
    Azithromycin or Clarithromycin 500 mg orally 1 hour before procedure
  - Patient unable to take oral medication:
    Ampicillin 2 g intravenously (IV)/ intramuscularly 0.5 hour before procedure
    Penicillin allergy: Clindamycin 600 mg IV 0.5 hour before procedure

- Genitourinary and gastrointestinal procedures:
  - High-risk patients:
    Ampicillin 2.0 g IV/intramuscularly, and
    Gentamicin 1.5 mg/kg IV within 0.5
      hour before procedure, and
    Ampicillin 1.0 g intramuscularly /IV or
      Amoxicillin 1.0 g orally 6 hours later
    Penicillin allergy: Vancomycin 1.0 g IV
      over 1 to 2 hours, and
        Gentamicin 1.5 mg/kg IV, both to be
        completed within 0.5 hour of
        starting the procedure
  - Moderate-risk patients:
    Amoxicillin 2.0 g orally 1 hour before
      procedure, or
        Ampicillin 2.0 g intramuscularly /IV
        within 0.5 hour of starting the
        procedure
        Penicillin allergy: Vancomycin 1.0 g
        IV over 1 to 2 hours, to be
        completed within 0.5 hour before
        the procedure
- Surgical procedures involving infected tissues
  (e.g., cellulitis, pyogenic arthritis,
  osteomyelitis):
  - Dicloxacillin 500 mg orally 1 hour before
    procedure, or
      Cephalexin or Cefadroxil 2.0 g orally 1
      hour before procedure
  - Penicillin allergy: Clindamycin 600 mg
    orally 1 hour before procedure
  - Patient unable to take oral medication:
    Vancomycin 1.0 g IV given over 1 to 2
      hours, to be completed within 0.5 hour
      before the procedure
- Cardiac surgery and implantation of
  prosthetic valves:
  - Cefazolin 2.0 g IV at induction of anesthesia,
    repeated 8 and 16 hours later, or

> Vancomycin 1.0 g IV slowly over 1 hour starting at induction of anesthesia, and 0.5 g IV given 12 hours later

Follow-Up:

- Careful physical examination following procedure or instrumentation
- Echocardiogram to evaluate appearance of any new murmurs or change in cardiac status
- **Watch for:** signs and symptoms of
  - Infective endocarditis despite use of appropriate prophylactic measures

PROSTHETIC JOINTS

Presenting Symptoms:

SUBJECTIVE	OBJECTIVE
Patient with indwelling joint prostheses presenting for prophylactic antibiotic therapy in anticipation of bacteremic event	Patient with indwelling joint prostheses
	Patient scheduled for invasive procedure associated with a high incidence of bacteremia
	—Dental surgery
	—Cystoscopy
	—Indwelling urinary catheter
	—Colonoscopic biopsy
	—Surgical procedures on infected or contaminated tissues

Suggested Workup:

- Thorough history and physical examination
- Determine the cost effectiveness of prophylactic antibiotic therapy in these

patients (**NOTE:** At present, use of prophylactic antibiotics in these patients is controversial and decisions regarding prophylactic antimicrobial treatment for expected transient bacteremias in patients with prosthetic joints should be made on an individual basis)

Definitive Diagnosis:

Prophylactic antibiotics   ICD-9-CM V07.39

Suggested Treatment:

- Oral and upper respiratory procedures:
  - Amoxicillin 3.0 g orally 1 hour before procedure and 1.5 g orally 6 hours later
  - Penicillin allergy: Clindamycin 300 mg orally 1 hour before procedure and 150 mg orally 6 hours later, or
    Erythromycin 1 g orally 2 hours before procedure and 0.5 g orally 6 hours later
  - Patient unable to take oral medication:
    Ampicillin 2 g IV/intramuscularly 0.5 hour before procedure and 1 g IV/intramuscularly 6 hours later
    Penicillin allergy: Clindamycin 300 mg IV 0.5 hour before procedure and 150 mg IV 6 hours later
  - High risk patient:
    Ampicillin 2.0 g IV/intramuscularly, and Gentamicin 1.5 mg/kg IV 0.5 hour before procedure and repeated 8 hours later
    Penicillin allergy: Vancomycin 1.0 g intravenous infusion slowly over 1 hour given 1 hour before procedure
- Genitourinary and gastrointestinal procedures:
  - Ampicillin 2.0 g IV/intramuscularly, and Gentamicin 1.5 mg/kg IV 0.5 hour before procedure and repeated 8 hours later

- Penicillin allergy: Vancomycin 1.0 g intravenous infusion slowly over 1 hour, and
    Gentamicin 1.5 mg/kg IV 1 hour before procedure and repeated 8 hours later
- Low-risk patient:
    Amoxicillin 3.0 g orally 1 hour before procedure and 1.5 g orally 6 hours later
    Penicillin allergy: Clindamycin 300 mg orally 1 hour before procedure and 150 mg orally 6 hours later, or
        Erythromycin 1.0 g orally 2 hours before procedure and 0.5 g orally 6 hours later

Follow-Up:

- Careful physical examination following procedure or instrumentation
- **Watch for:** signs and symptoms of
    - Joint infection with hematogenous spread
    - Infective endocarditis
    - Bacteremia/sepsis

ACUTE RHEUMATIC FEVER (ARF)

Presenting Symptoms:

SUBJECTIVE	OBJECTIVE
Patient with documented or suspected streptococcal infection, especially of the upper respiratory tract	Elicit risk factors for ARF:
	—Children in 6 to 15-year-old group
	—Antecedent streptococcal infection primarily of the upper
May follow mild or	

subclinical streptococcal infection that never came to medical attention

respiratory tract (pharyngitis, tonsillitis)

—Lower socioeconomic status, with concomitant poor access to health care

—Overcrowded school, working, or living conditions

—Tendency toward upper respiratory infections

Suggested Workup:

- Need for primary prevention of ARF is determined by history (see examples above), and existence of antecedent upper respiratory infection with Group A *Streptococcus*

Definitive Diagnosis:

Antibiotic prophylaxis   ICD-9-CM V07.39

Suggested Treatment:

- Standard continuous prophylactic regimens:
  - Benzathine penicillin (PCN)-G 1.2 million units (U) intramuscularly administered every 4 weeks, or
    PCN-V 250 mg orally 2 times a day
  - Penicillin allergy: Sulfadiazine 1.0 g/day orally, or
    Erythromycin 250 mg orally 2 times a day
  - All regimens should be continued indefinitely until the physician believes that the risk of ARF to the patient has declined, the risk of acquiring a streptococcal

infection is low, and the patient has reached at least his or her early 20s

Follow-Up:

- Periodic reassessment of need for continued ARF prophylaxis is appropriate, with consideration of appropriate risk factors
  - Age
  - Presence of heart disease
  - Contact with school-age children
  - If rheumatic valvular disease is present, patient must be protected from bacterial endocarditis whenever they undergo dental or surgical procedures that consistently evoke bacteremia

CHEMOPROPHYLAXIS AFTER EXPOSURE TO COMMON PATHOGENS

Presenting Symptoms:

SUBJECTIVE

Patient presenting as having had close contact with person with meningitis

Patient presenting as having had sexual contact with person with a sexually transmitted disease

High-risk patient presenting as having had close contact with person with influenza or whooping cough

Patient presenting with

OBJECTIVE

Elicit history of family member, room-mate, or day-care contact of meningitis patient

Elicit history of sexual contact with exposure to syphilis, gonorrhea, or nongonococcal urethritis

Elicit history of exposure to influenza A or whooping cough by patient who is elderly,

history of human or animal bite	immunocompromised, or has chronic pulmonary disease
Patient presenting after a sexual assault	Elicit history of patient who was bitten by a human or animal
	Elicit history of patient presenting after a sexual assault

Suggested Workup:

Detailed history and physical examination

Definitive Diagnosis:

Contact with communicable disease	ICD-9-CM V01.9
Prophylactic antibiotics	ICD-9-CM V07.39

Suggested Treatment:

- Close contact of patient with meningococcal meningitis (*Neisseria meningitis*):
    - Adult:
        Rifampin 600 mg orally every 12 hours for 2 days, or
        Ciprofloxacin 500 mg orally 2 times a day for 5 days, or
        Ceftriaxone 250 mg intramuscularly for 1 dose
    - Pediatric: Rifampin 10 mg/kg orally every 12 hours for 2 days
- Children younger than 4 years old in close contact with patient with *Haemophilus influenzae* meningitis:
    - Rifampin 20 mg/kg/day orally for 4 days
- Within 90 days of exposure to syphilis (*Treponema pallidum*):
    - Benzathine PCN-G 2.4 million U intramuscularly for 1 dose

- Penicillin allergy: penicillin desensitization or
  - Ceftriaxone 250 mg intramuscularly for 1 dose, and
  - Doxycycline 100 mg orally every 12 hours for 7 days
- Sexual contact with trichomonas (*Trichomonas vaginalis*):
  - Metronidazole 2 g orally for 1 dose
- Sexual contacts with gonorrhea or chlamydia (*Neisseria gonorrhoeae, Chlamydia trachomatis*):
  - Ceftriaxone 250 mg intramuscularly for 1 dose, and
    - Doxycycline 100 mg orally every 12 hours for 7 days
- Unvaccinated high risk patients during outbreaks of influenza A:
  - Amantadine or rimantadine 100 mg orally 2 times a day for 2 weeks if given with vaccine, or for 5 to 7 weeks if given alone
  - Patients over 65 years old should receive 100 mg orally once a day
- Unvaccinated high risk patients during outbreaks of whooping cough (*Bordetella pertussis*):
  - Adult: Erythromycin 500 mg orally 4 times a day for 14 days
  - Pediatric: Erythromycin 50 mg/kg orally 4 times a day for 14 days
- Patient presenting after human bite (*Staphylococcus aureus, Streptococcus, Eikenella corrodens*):
  - Amoxicillin + clavulanate 250 mg orally 3 times a day for 3 to 5 days
  - Penicillin allergy: Clindamycin 300 mg orally 4 times a day for 3 to 5 days

- Patient presenting after dog or cat bite (*S. aureus, Streptococcus*, anaerobes, *Pasteurella multocida, Capnocytophaga canimorsus*):
  - PCN-V 500 mg orally 4 times a day for 3 to 5 days, or
    Amoxicillin + clavulanate 250 mg orally 3 times a day for 3 to 5 days
  - Penicillin allergy: Doxycycline 100 mg orally every 12 hours for 3 to 5 days
- Patient presenting after sexual assault:
  - Ceftriaxone 250 mg intramuscularly for 1 dose, and
    Doxycycline 100 mg orally every 12 hours for 7 days, or
    Azithromycin 2 g orally for 1 dose, or
    Erythromycin 500 mg orally 4 times a day for 7 days (choice for pregnant victim), and
    Metronidazole 2 g orally for 1 dose

Follow-Up:

- Directed physical examination 7 and 14 days after completion of prophylactic therapy
- **Watch for:** signs and symptoms of development of index infection despite prophylaxis

CHEMOPROPHYLAXIS AGAINST TUBERCULOSIS

Presenting Symptoms:

SUBJECTIVE
Patient presenting as having a risk factor for developing tuberculosis

OBJECTIVE
Patient has recently converted to a positive purified protein derivative (PPD) skin test (greater than 10 mm increase in induration) within

the previous 2
years[1]
Elicit history of risk
factor
—Human
immunodeficiency
virus (HIV) infection
—Immunocompromised
—Abnormal chest
radiograph
—Intravenous drug
abuser
—Silicosis
—Institutionalized
person
—Immigrant from area
where tuberculosis is
endemic
—Exposure to
tuberculosis

Suggested Workup:

- Detailed history and physical examination
- PPD skin test if not already done
- Chest radiograph
- Three sputum samples for acid-fast staining
  and Bactec culture to rule out active
  tuberculosis before starting prophylaxis, if
  chest radiograph is abnormal
- HIV serology
- Baseline liver function tests

Definitive Diagnosis:

Contact with or exposure   ICD-9-CM V01.1
  to tuberculosis

[1] See section on Mycobacterium tuberculosis (Chapter 4)
for full description of skin test conversion in a variety
of clinical situations.

Suggested Treatment:

- Conventional preventive therapy:
  - Adult: Isoniazid 300 mg orally once daily for 6 months
  - Pediatric: Isoniazid 10 mg/kg/day orally for 6 months
- HIV-infected patients:
  - Isoniazid 300 mg orally once daily, and Pyridoxine 50 mg orally once daily for 12 months
  - **NOTE:** Some authorities recommend life-long prophylaxis
- Exposure to suspected isoniazid-resistant tuberculosis:
  - Rifampin 600 mg orally once daily for 12 months, and Pyrazinamide 25 mg/kg/day for 2 months

Follow-Up:

- Periodic directed physical examinations
- Repeat PPD skin tests and chest radiograph after 2 months
- **Watch for:** signs and symptoms of
  - Drug-related liver dysfunction
  - Development of active tuberculosis

SURGICAL ANTIMICROBIAL PROPHYLAXIS

Presenting Symptoms:

SUBJECTIVE	OBJECTIVE
Patient presenting for surgical procedure	Preoperative patient to be considered for surgical antimicrobial prophylaxis

Suggested Workup:

History and physical examination:
- Identify treatable infections and/or colonizations that may promote postoperative infection
  - Urinary tract infection
  - Nasal carriers of *S. aureus*
  - Pustular dermatitis or cellulitis
  - Infection that may contaminate surgical site through direct extension or venous or lymphatic drainage

Definitive Diagnosis:

Prophylactic antibiotic   ICD-9-CM V07.39
  therapy

Suggested Treatment:

- Major head, neck, and oral surgery:
  - Clindamycin 600 mg IV preoperatively and every 8 hours for 2 doses postoperatively; MAY ADD
      Gentamicin 1.7 mg/kg IV preoperatively and every 8 hours for 2 doses postoperatively
- Ophthalmic surgery:
  - Tobramycin 2 to 3 drops instilled locally every 2 hours for 6 to 12 doses starting just preoperatively
- Cardiothoracic and vascular surgery:
  - Coronary artery bypass graft (CABG) and valvular surgery:
      —Cefazolin 2 g IV preoperatively, 1 g IV every 4 to 6 hours intraoperatively, and 2 g IV every 8 hours postoperatively
      —In hospitals where *S. aureus* wound infections persist despite prophylaxis:
        –Cefuroxime 1.5 g IV preoperatively, 750 mg IV every 4 hours

    intraoperatively, and every 4 hours
    postoperatively for 2 doses, or
    –Vancomycin 15 mg/kg IV
    preoperatively, 10 mg/kg IV
    intraoperatively, and every 8 hours
    postoperatively for 2 doses
- Reoperation of recently closed incision:
  —Cefotaxime 2 g IV, plus
    Metronidazole 1 g IV immediately
      postoperatively and every 12 hours
      for 2 to 4 doses
- Pacemaker insertion:
  —Cefazolin 1 g IV preoperatively and
    every 6 hours postoperatively for 24
    hours
- Thoracic surgery (e.g., lobectomy,
  pneumonectomy):
  —Cefazolin 1 g IV preoperatively and
    every 6 hours postoperatively for 24
    hours
- Peripheral vascular surgery:
  —Cefazolin 1 g IV preoperatively and
    every 6 hours postoperatively for 24
    hours, or
      Vancomycin 15 mg/kg IV
        preoperatively, and 10 mg/kg IV
        postoperatively every 8 hours for 24
        hours
- Abdominal surgery:
  - Simple appendectomy:
    —Cefoxitin 2 g IV preoperatively and every
      3 hours intraoperatively
  - Appendectomy of perforated appendix:
    —Add Metronidazole 500 mg IV
      preoperatively and every 8 hours for 3 to
      5 days

- Cholecystectomy:
  —Cefazolin 2 g IV preoperatively, or
      Gentamicin 80 mg IV preoperatively
        and every 8 hours for 3 doses
- Penetrating abdominal trauma with intact bowel:
  —Cefazolin 2 g IV preoperatively and
    every 8 hours for 3 doses
- Penetrating abdominal trauma with perforated bowel:
  —Cefotaxime 2 g IV preoperatively and
    every 8 hours for 3 doses, and
      Metronidazole 1 g IV every 12 hours
        for 24 hours, or
  —Cefoxitin 2 g IV every 6 hours for 5 days
- Gastric resection:
  —Cefazolin 1 g IV preoperatively, or
  —Gentamicin 120 mg plus Clindamycin
    600 mg IV preoperatively
- Elective colorectal surgery:
  —Neomycin 1 g plus Erythromycin 1 g
    orally at 1, 2, and 11 pm on day before
    surgery, and
      Cefazolin 2 g IV immediately
        preoperatively
  —**NOTE:** Where surgery is to begin after
    11 AM or extend past 12 noon, instead of
    Cefazolin, may use:
      Cefotaxime 2 g plus Metronidazole 1 g
        IV immediately preoperatively
- Emergency colorectal surgery:
  —Cefoxitin 2 g IV preoperatively and every
    4 hours for 3 doses, or
  —Metronidazole 500 mg IV plus
    Gentamicin 1.7 mg/kg IV preoperatively
    and every 8 hours postoperatively for 3
    doses, or

      —Cefotaxime 2 g IV plus Metronidazole
      1 g IV immediately preoperatively and
      12 hours later

- Gynecologic surgery:
  - Caesarean section:
    - —Cefazolin 1 g IV after clamping the cord and 12 hours later, or
    - —Metronidazole 500 mg IV after clamping the cord
  - Dilatation and curettage and abortion (recommended only for complicated cases and second trimester instillation abortions):
    - —Cefazolin 1 g IV preoperatively and every 6 hours postoperatively for 2 doses, or
    - —Metronidazole 400 mg orally preoperatively and every 4 hours postoperatively for 2 doses
  - Hysterectomy (abdominal or vaginal):
    - —Cefazolin 1 g IV preoperatively and 6 and 12 hours later, or
    - —Doxycycline 200 mg IV preoperatively (proven effective in vaginal hysterectomy only)
- Urologic surgery:
  - Prostatectomy (transurethral or peritoneal):
    - —Gentamicin 80 mg IV preoperatively
    - —Culture urine and give 1 dose of appropriate antimicrobial immediately preoperatively based on culture result
  - Penile prosthesis implantation:
    - —Cefotaxime 2 g IV plus Metronidazole 1 g IV immediately preoperatively and every 12 hours for 2 doses postoperatively
- Orthopedic surgery:
  - Arthroplasty of joints including replacement:
    - —Cefazolin 1 to 2 g IV preoperatively and every 6 hours for 3 doses

- Open reduction of fracture:
  —Cefazolin 1 g IV preoperatively and
    every 6 hours for 3 doses (extend to 1 g
    every 8 hours for 10 days if complex,
    open, or contaminated fractures are
    involved)
- Lower limb amputation:
  —Cefoxitin 2 g IV preoperatively and every
    6 hours for 4 doses
- Neurosurgery:
  - Cerebrospinal fluid (CSF) shunting
    procedures:
    —In institutions with infection rates of less
      than 10%, antibiotic prophylaxis is not
      indicated
    —Where infection rates are greater than
      20%:
      –Trimethoprim (TMP)160 mg-
        sulfamethoxazole (SMX) 800 mg IV
        preoperatively and every 12 hours for 3
        doses
  - Craniotomy:
    —Clindamycin 300 mg IV preoperatively
      and 4 hours later, or
    —Vancomycin 10 mg/kg (up to 500 mg)
      IV, plus
        Gentamicin 2 mg/kg (up to 120 mg)
          IV preoperatively, plus
        Gentamicin irrigating solution
- Other:
  - Hemodialysis vascular shunt implantation:
    —Mupirocin ointment intranasally for 7
      days before operation

Follow-Up:

- Institute surgical wound surveillance program
- Ensure proper postoperative nutrition

- Ensure proper postoperative isolation and antisepsis techniques by hospital staff
- **Watch for:** signs and symptoms of
    - Postoperative wound infections
    - Bacteremia
    - Pneumonia

Travel Medicine 15

CONDITIONS COVERED

REQUIRED PRETRAVEL VACCINATIONS AND MALARIA CHEMOPROPHYLAXIS

Presenting Symptoms:

SUBJECTIVE
Worldwide traveler
   presenting for
   immunizations

OBJECTIVE
Worldwide traveler
   presenting for
   immunizations

Suggested Workup:

- Take detailed immunization history and examine Certificate of Vaccination, if available
- Perform physical examination to determine if traveler has any special medical needs during travel

Definitive Diagnosis:

Vaccination, cholera	ICD-9-CM V03.0
Vaccination, bacterial, unspecified	ICD-9-CM V03.9
Vaccination, hepatitis, viral	ICD-9-CM V05.3
Vaccination, typhoid-paratyphoid	ICD-9-CM V03.1
Vaccination, diphtheria-pertussis-tetanus	ICD-9-CM V06.2
Vaccination, encephalitis, arthropod	ICD-9-CM V05.0
Vaccination, yellow fever	ICD-9-CM V04.4

Suggested Treatment:

- Immunizations of worldwide importance: (see chapter on Immunizations for specific recommendations)
  - Diphtheria-tetanus
  - Polio
  - Measles-mumps-rubella (MMR)
  - Pneumococcus

- Influenza
- Hepatitis B
- Immunizations especially important to the traveler
  - **NOTE:** Most vaccines may be administered simultaneously except that human diploid cell rabies vaccine (HDCV) intradermal [id] rabies prophylaxis may not be administered simultaneously with malaria chemoprophylaxis
  - Live attenuated yellow fever vaccine 0.5 mL subcutaneous within 10 days before travel (booster every 10 years)
    - —**For:** Endemic areas of Africa and South America
    - —**NOTE:** Contraindicated in travelers who are immunosuppressed, pregnant, or allergic to egg products
  - Live attenuated typhoid vaccine 1 enteric-coated capsule 1 hour before a meal every other day for 4 days (boosters every 5 years), or
    - Inactivated typhoid vaccine 0.5 mL intramuscularly 1 time (booster every 2 years)
    - —**For:** Endemic areas of Africa, Asia, and Central and South America
  - Inactivated cholera vaccine 0.5 mL sq/ intramuscularly for 2 doses, 7 to 30 days apart and at least 6 days before travel
    - —**For:** Only those who will be living and working in the midst of an epidemic, or travelers with achlorhydria or postgastrectomy; otherwise, not generally recommended
  - Adsorbed rabies vaccine 1.0 mL intramuscularly (in deltoid) for 3 doses, on

days 0, 7, and 21 or 28 (booster of 1 mL
intramuscularly 1 time every 2 years; in
travelers with a high and continuous risk,
should check serology every 6 months and
maintain antibody titer of greater than 1.5
per fluorescent focus inhibition test), or
> HDCV 0.1 mL intradermally for 3 doses,
> on days 0, 7, and 21 or 28 (booster
> 0.1 mL intradermally 1 time every
> 2 years)

—**For:** Travelers to endemic areas of
Mexico, Central and South America (e.g.,
El Salvador, Guatemala, Peru, Colombia,
Ecuador), India, Nepal, Philippines,
Sri Lanka, Thailand, Vietnam
* Meningococcal quadrivalent vaccine
(A/C/Y/W-135) 0.5 mL subcutaneously 1
time (booster every 3 years)
—**For:** Travelers to sub-Saharan Africa,
India, Nepal, Mecca, Chad, Burundi,
Kenya, Saudi Arabia, and Tanzania
* Japanese B encephalitis vaccine 1 mL
subcutaneously for 3 doses, on days 0, 7,
and 30 (booster every 3 years)
—**For:** Travelers to southeast Asia
* Hepatitis A vaccine 1 mL intramuscularly
(booster 6 to 12 months later), or
> Hepatitis A immunoglobulin 0.02 ml/kg
> intramuscularly for travel up to
> 3 months, or 0.04 ml/kg
> intramuscularly for travel lasting
> 4 to 6 months (booster every 4 to
> 6 months)

—**For:** Travel to any area with uncertain
water and sanitation conditions
* Malaria chemoprophylaxis
—For travel to areas where chloroquine-
resistant *Plasmodium falciparum* has NOT

been reported (e.g., Dominican Republic, Haiti, Central America west of the Panama Canal Zone), Egypt, and the Middle East):

- –Chloroquine phosphate 300 mg base (500 mg salt) orally once a week for 2 weeks before travel, weekly during travel, and for 4 weeks after departure from endemic area
- —For travel to areas where chloroquine-resistant *P. falciparum* exists:
    - –Mefloquine 228 mg base (250 mg salt) orally once a week for 2 weeks before travel, weekly during travel, and for 4 weeks after departure from endemic area
- —Where mefloquine is contraindicated (history of hypersensitivity to mefloquine, first trimester of pregnancy, history of neuropsychiatric problems, child weighing less than 15 kg):
    - –Doxycycline 100 mg orally once daily for 1 to 2 days before travel, daily during travel, and for 4 weeks after departure from endemic area, or
    - –Proguanil 200 mg orally once daily for 1 to 2 days before travel, daily during travel, and for 4 weeks after departure from endemic area, plus

        Chloroquine 500 mg orally once a week for 2 weeks before travel, weekly during travel, and for 4 weeks after departure from endemic area (especially useful for children less than 15 kg and women in first trimester of pregnancy traveling to area with known chloroquine-resistant *P. falciparum*)

—For terminal prophylaxis to prevent
relapses with persistent *Plasmodium vivax*
and *Plasmodium ovale:*
  –Primaquine 15 mg base (26.3 mg salt)
  orally once daily for 14 days during the last
  2 weeks of post-travel chemoprophylaxis
  –**For:** Travel to sub-Saharan Africa,
  Papua New Guinea, the Solomon
  Islands, India, Haiti, the Far East (e.g.,
  Thailand, Cambodia, Burma), and Latin
  America
  –Further information can be obtained
  from the Centers for Disease Control
  (CDC) and Prevention
  Malaria Hotline: 404-332-4555 or FAX
  404-332-4565

Follow-Up:

- Provide guidelines for travel health kit
  - Adequate supply of usual prescription drugs
  - Aspirin, Racetominophen (™Tylenol),
    nonsteroidal anti-inflammatory drugs
    (NSAIDs)
  - Bismuth subsalicylate, loperamide
  - Mild oral laxative
  - Antihistamine/decongestant
  - Insect repellent
  - Topical solution for athlete's foot
  - Hydrocortisone cream 0.5%
  - Antimotion sickness medication (may need
    to prescribe ™Scopolamine transdermal
    patches)
  - Rehydration solution or tablets
  - Water purification tablets
  - Adhesive bandages, gauze pads, tape,
    scissors, tweezers
  - Bactericidal solution, antiseptic soap

- Alcohol wipes
- Thermometer
- Insect repellent
- Sunscreen
- Flashlight
- Educate traveler as to malaria prevention
  - Wear protective clothing (long sleeves, pants) between dusk and dawn
  - Use mosquito repellents
  - Sleep under netting or in screened rooms
- Provide list of information resources for travelers
  - CDC Health Information for International Travel (202-783-3238 or voice information 404-332-4559)
  - International Association for Medical Assistance to Travelers (716-754-4883)
  - International Society of Travel Medicine (404-488-7679)

TRAVELER'S DIARRHEA

Presenting Symptoms:

SUBJECTIVE

Mild abdominal discomfort and diarrhea (mild to voluminous) that begins during or shortly after a trip

Few other constitutional symptoms

Dehydration is rare

OBJECTIVE

History of travel to area of the world presenting risk

—High-risk areas
  –Latin America
  –Africa
  –Middle East
  –Asia
—Intermediate-risk areas
  –Southern Europe
  –Far East

> –Former Soviet Union
> –Caribbean Islands
> History of ingestion of
> high-risk foods/
> beverages
> —Tap water or ice
> made from tap
> water
> —Fresh salads
> —Sauces
> —Raw seafood
> —Unpasteurized milk
> —Butter
> —Undercooked foods

Differential Diagnosis:

Amebic dysentery
Irritable bowel syndrome
Inflammatory bowel disease

Suggested Workup:

- Initial empiric therapy based on history and physical examination is generally warranted without diagnostic tests
- If antimicrobial therapy or symptomatic treatment does not sufficiently provide relief, diagnostic tests for enteric pathogens or parasites may be done (see Chapter 6 on Gastrointestinal Infections)

Definitive Diagnosis:

Traveler's diarrhea   ICD-9-CM 009.2

Suggested Treatment:

- Symptomatic relief for diarrhea:
  - Loperamide 4 mg orally for 1 dose, then 2 mg orally after each unformed stool up to 16 mg/day, or

Diphenoxylate 2 tablets or 10 mL liquid orally 4 times a day, or

Bismuth subsalicylate 2 tablets or 30 mL liquid orally every 1 hour as needed up to 8 doses/day

- Rehydration:
  - Electrolyte solutions
  - Water, tea, broth, carbonated beverages, and a salt source (consommé, salted crackers)
  - Bananas, oranges as a source of potassium
  - Bland diet, avoiding alcohol and fats
- Antimicrobial therapy:
  - Indicated when symptomatic relief alone is not effective or in high-risk groups:
    —Travelers with history of repeated bouts of traveler's diarrhea
    —Travelers with a diminished gastric barrier or preexisting gastrointestinal disease
    —Travelers with underlying medical conditions for whom volume depletion might be poorly tolerated
    —Travelers taking certain medications (e.g., diuretics, digitalis, lithium)
    —Travelers with immunodeficiency disorders
  - Trimethoprim-sulfamethoxazole (TMP-SMX) DS 1 tablet orally for 1 dose, up to 1 tablet orally 2 times a day for 2 to 3 days, or

    Ciprofloxacin 750 mg orally 1 time, up to 500 mg orally 2 times a day for 3 to 5 days (usually given with loperamide)
- Chemoprophylaxis:
  - Indicated for high-risk travelers:
    —Acquired immunodeficiency disease (AIDS) patients

—Diabetic patients
—Elderly travelers
—Travelers with heart disease
—Travelers taking chronic H-2 receptor antagonists
- Ciprofloxacin 500 mg orally once daily, or TMP-SMX DS 1 tablet orally once daily, or Bismuth salicylate 2 tablets orally 4 times a day (chewed)

Follow-Up:

- Outpatient, stepwise treatment is recommended
- Monitor hydration status
- Initiate antimicrobial therapy only if symptomatic treatment is not effective after 2 to 3 days
- Educate regarding safe travel habits
  - Avoid tap water and ice
  - Boil water or drink bottled water
  - Eat only food that is freshly prepared and served steaming hot
  - Eat only fruit that can be peeled
- **Watch for:** signs and symptoms of
  - Serious enteric/parasitic infection:
    —Fever, chills, severe cramps, blood or mucus in the stool
  - Dehydration
  - Electrolyte imbalances (especially potassium, sodium, calcium)

CHOLERA

Presenting Symptoms:

SUBJECTIVE	OBJECTIVE
Symptoms may range from mild, self-	Symptoms may range from mild abdominal

limited diarrhea to
life-threatening
illness
Abdominal discomfort
Anorexia
Apathy and lethargy
Profuse diarrhea
Fever
Malaise and listlessness
Seizures
Vomiting
Weakness and muscle
cramps
Overwhelming thirst

tenderness to life-
threatening
hypovolemic shock
History of travel/living
in endemic area:
—India, Southeast
Asia, Africa, Middle
East, Southern
Europe, Oceania,
South and Central
America, Gulf Coast
of the United States
History of exposure to
contaminated food
or water
Abdominal discomfort
Decreased skin turgor
and other indicia of
dehydration
Distant heart sounds
Hypotension and
tachycardia
Weak peripheral pulses
Oliguria or anuria

Differential Diagnosis:

Infection by other enteric pathogens that cause
diarrhea and dehydration
—*Salmonella*
—*Shigella*
—Viruses
—*Escherichia coli*

Suggested Workup:

- Collect stool for dark field microscopy →
characteristic *Vibrio cholerae* motility
- Collect stool for culture on selective media
(TCBS)

- Collect stool for ova and parasites
- Serology with typed antisera-agglutination tests
- Laboratory abnormalities consistent with severe dehydration

Definitive Diagnosis:

Cholera   ICD-9-CM 001.9

Suggested Treatment:

- Antimicrobial therapy:
  - Tetracycline 500 mg orally 4 times a day for 3 days, or
  - Ciprofloxacin 500 mg orally 2 times a day for 3 days, or
  - Erythromycin 500 mg orally 4 times a day for 3 days, or
  - Furazolidone 100 mg orally 4 times a day for 3 days
  - Pediatric: Tetracycline 12.5 mg/kg (up to 500 mg) orally 4 times a day for 3 days
  - Pregnant women: Ampicillin 500 mg orally every 6 hours for 3 days
- Oral or intravenous rehydration therapy:
  - Ringer's lactate is recommended for intravenous rehydration
  - Rate and volume must be tailored to patient's needs
  - Oral Rehydration Solution (ORS) from World Health Organization can be used for oral rehydration

Follow-Up:

- Most patients can be treated on outpatient basis
- Close contacts of patient should be treated with Tetracycline 500 mg orally 4 times a day

for 3 days or Doxycycline 300 mg orally for
1 dose
- Enteric precautions must be taken with patient
- Patient education for cholera prevention if
  travel to or living in endemic area is necessary
  - Water purification
  - Proper food selection: no raw unpeeled
    fruits or vegetables, and no undercooked
    seafood
- **Watch for:** signs and symptoms of
  - Hypovolemic shock
  - Chronic biliary infection
  - Invasive disease and septicemia

SCHISTOSOMIASIS

Presenting Symptoms:

SUBJECTIVE	OBJECTIVE
Intensely pruritic skin rash	Papular dermatitis within 24 to 72 hours after contact with schistosomes
Symptoms of Katayama fever 4 to 6 weeks later	Katayama fever phase
—Fever, chills	—Hepatosplenomegaly
—Sweating	—Diffuse lymphadenopathy
—Headache	—Marked eosinophilia
—Nonproductive cough	Elicit appropriate travel history
—Abdominal pain	
—Arthralgia	—Arabia, Africa, South America, Caribbean (*Schistosoma mansoni*)
—Malaise	—Japan, China, Philippines (*Schistosoma japonicum*)

—Southeast Asia (*Schistosoma mekongi*)

—Africa, Middle East (*Schistosoma haematobium*)

—West and Central Africa (*Schistosoma intercalatum*)

Differential Diagnosis:

Other trematode infections
—Clonorchiasis (liver)
—Opisthorchiasis (liver)
—Fascioliasis (liver)
—Fasciolopsiasis (intestinal)
—Paragonimiasis (lung)
Tapeworm infection
Helminth infections
Early trypanosomiasis

Suggested Workup:

- Examine stool for schistosome eggs:
  - Kato thick smear technique can be used to quantify infection from stool sample to estimate the intensity of infectivity
- Examine urine for schistosome eggs:
  - Collection is best between noon and 2 PM
- Rectal biopsy examination for schistosome eggs:
  - Four small mucosal samples should be collected
- Serology:
  - Falcon assay screening test-ELISA (FAST-ELISA) (enzyme-linked immunosorbent assay) for antischistosomal antibodies cannot distinguish between past and present infections (available at Centers for Disease Control [CDC] & Prevention)

- Abdominal ultrasound (especially important for patients with *S. haematobium* infection) to evaluate for possible complications of infection
  - Hydronephrosis
  - Renal polyps or stones
  - Carcinoma of the bladder
  - Periportal fibrosis
  - Evidence of portal hypertension

Definitive Diagnosis:

Schistosomiasis   ICD-9-CM 120.9

Suggested Treatment:

- Standard drug management:
  - Praziquantel 20 mg/kg orally 2 times a day (*S. mansoni or S. haematobium*) or 3 times a day (*S. japonica or S. mekongi*) for 1 day
- Alternate therapies:
  - Metrifonate 7.5 mg/kg orally for 3 doses at 2-week intervals (effective against *S. haematobium* only)
  - Oxamniquine 15 to 20 mg/kg orally for 1 dose (effective against *S. mansoni* only; patients who acquired their infection in Egypt or East Africa may need 20 mg/kg/day orally for 3 days)
- Corticosteroids:
  - May be given to severely ill patients concomitantly with antischistosomal therapy

Follow-Up:

- Outpatient therapy is generally appropriate
- Re-examine stool and urine for eggs 3 and 6 months after completion of therapy
- Eosinophilia persisting beyond 6 months after treatment should trigger repeated

parasitologic workup for etiologies other than schistosomiasis
- **Watch for:** signs and symptoms of
  - Recurrent disease from delayed egg laying during antimicrobial therapy
  - Invasive disease leading to
    —Urinary tract pathology
    —Intestinal invasion
    —Hepatocellular disease, including periportal fibrosis, portal hypertension, and esophageal varices

POST-TRAVEL DIARRHEA

Presenting Symptoms:

SUBJECTIVE

Traveller returning from exotic parts of the world

Acute diarrhea (for 5 to 10 days) or persistent diarrhea (longer than 10 days) after return from a trip

Crampy abdominal pain

Vomiting

Tenesmus

Flatulence

Diarrhea may be watery or bloody

OBJECTIVE

Returning traveler

Diffuse abdominal tenderness

History of acute onset of watery or bloody diarrhea

Focal neurologic signs (in cases of neurotoxin ingestion)

Differential Diagnosis:

Acute diarrhea (for less than 10 days)
—Viral illness
—*Campylobacter*

—*Salmonella*
—Enterotoxigenic *E. coli*
—*Staphylococcus aureus* (less than 12-hour incubation period)
—*Bacillus cereus* (less than 12-hour incubation)
—*Cryptosporidium*
—*Entamoeba histolyticum*
—*Giardia lamblia*
—*Shigella* spp. (especially after travel in Mexico)
—*Vibrio parahaemolyticus* (especially after travel in Japan)
—Malaria
—Appendicitis

Persistent diarrhea (for longer than 10 to 14 days)
—Enterotoxigenic *E. coli*
—*G. lamblia*
—*Cryptosporidium*
—*E. histolyticum*
—*Campylobacter jejuni*
—*Shigella* spp.
—*Strongyloides*
—*Dientamoeba*
—*Isospora belli*
—*Clostridium difficile* toxins
—*Yersinia*
—Malaria
—Appendicitis

Suggested Workup:

- Detailed history of travel, including:
  - Areas visited and travel calendar
  - Types of accommodations used
  - Traveler's lifestyles and activities
  - Traveler's immunizations
  - Traveler's medical history and use of medications

- Traveler's adherence to preventive measures
- Known exposures to infectious agents
- Illness among fellow travelers
- Temporal relationship between possible exposure and onset of traveler's symptoms
- Evaluation of symptom patterns:
  - Sudden onset of diarrhea (less than 12 hour-incubation) with vomiting: consider *S. aureus, B. cereus*
  - Acute onset of watery diarrhea with low-grade fever: consider enterotoxigenic *E. coli*
  - Fever, abdominal cramps, bloody diarrhea, tenesmus: consider *Shigella* spp., *E. histolytica*
  - Chronic watery diarrhea with or without abdominal bloating, flatulence, foul-smelling stool, and weight loss: consider *G. lamblia, Cryptosporidium* spp.
  - Chronic inflammatory (bloody) diarrhea: consider *E. histolytica, C. jejuni, Yersinia enterocolitica*
  - Abdominal pain mimicking appendicitis: consider *Y. enterocolitica*
  - Watery diarrhea with focal neurologic symptoms: consider *Clostridium botulinum*, neurotoxins from fish or shellfish
- History of possible exposures during travel:
  - Consumption of shellfish: consider *Vibrio* spp., Norwalk-like viruses, Hepatitis A
  - Chronic antibiotic use: consider *C. difficile*
  - Homosexual contact: consider *Chlamydia, Neisseria gonorrhoeae, Treponema pallidum*
  - Travel in under-developed countries: suspect enterotoxigenic *E. coli, Shigella* spp., *Salmonella* spp., *C. jejuni, E. histolytica, G. lamblia, Cryptosporidium* spp.

- Travel in developed countries: suspect
  S. aureus, B. cereus, Salmonella spp.,
  G. lamblia, C. jejuni
- Travel to Russia: suspect *G. lamblia*
- Travel to Mexico: suspect *Shigella* spp.
- Travel to Thailand: suspect *Aeromonas hydrophila*
- Travel to mountain resorts, on camping trips, or after drinking unboiled well water: suspect *G. lamblia*
- Collect three separate stool samples for:
  - Fecal leukocytes
  - Fecal blood
  - Culture, ova, and parasites
  - *C. difficile* toxin
  - Acid-fast stain for *Cryptosporidium* and *I. belli*
  - Modified trichrome stain for *E. histolytica* and *G. lamblia*
- Complete blood count
- Peripheral blood smear for malaria
- Blood cultures
- Serology:
  - Hepatitis
  - Human immunodeficiency virus (HIV)
  - Indirect hemagglutination assay for antiamebic antibodies
- Imaging:
  - Abdominal ultrasound
  - Computed tomography (CT) of abdomen if abscess is suspected
- Invasive:
  - Biopsy of mucosa of involved areas of bowel for diagnosis of invasive amebic colitis
  - Small bowel aspiration with mucosal biopsy

Definitive Diagnosis:

Acute diarrhea   ICD-9-CM 787.91
Inflammatory diarrhea   ICD-9-CM 008.8
Chronic diarrhea   ICD-9-CM 558.9

Suggested Treatment:

- Acute diarrhea in the returning traveler
  - Incubation period less than 6 to 12 hours (most likely an enterotoxin-mediated illness caused by *S. aureus, B. cereus, Clostridium perfringens, C. botulinum,* or poisoning from fish [Ciguatera or Scombroid] or shellfish):
    —Initially, oral rehydration alone
    —May add Bismuth subsalicylate
    —If symptoms persist for longer than 3 days, there is clinical worsening, or diarrhea becomes inflammatory (with blood, mucus, and fecal leukocytes), but ova and parasites (O & P) evaluation is negative:
    –Ciprofloxacin 500 to 750 mg orally every 12 hours for 5 to 7 days
    —If *C. difficile* toxin-positive, discontinue other antibiotics and consider
    –Metronidazole 500 mg orally every 12 hours, or
    –Vancomycin 500 mg orally every 12 hours for 10 to 14 days
  - Incubation period for longer than 12 to 24 hours with more severe symptoms:
    —Inflammatory diarrhea (fecal blood, mucus, and leukocytes; patient with fever and tenesmus):
    –Stool exam for O & P negative:
    —Ciprofloxacin 500 to 750 mg orally every 12 hours, and
    Oral rehydration therapy until there is resolution of symptoms

-Stool exam for O & P positive:
—Treat with antimicrobial specific for parasite found (see Chapter 9 on Parasites for specific treatment recommendations), and
Oral rehydration therapy
—Noninflammatory diarrhea (watery stool with no blood or fecal leukocytes; patient with no or low-grade fever):
-Stool exam for O & P negative:
Ciprofloxacin 500 mg orally every 12 hours, or
TMP-SMX DS 1 tablet orally 2 times a day, and
Oral rehydration therapy until symptoms resolve
-Stool exam for O & P positive:
Treat with antimicrobial specific for parasite found (see Chapter 9 on Parasites for specific treatment recommendations), and
Oral rehydration therapy
- Chronic diarrhea in the returning traveler:
  - Treatment based on results of tests:
  —C. *difficile* toxin-positive:
  -Stop all antibiotics
  -Vancomycin 0.5 g orally every 6 hours for 7 to 14 days
  —Fecal leukocytes positive/O & P negative:
  -Culture stool for common pathogens
  -Ciprofloxacin 500 mg orally every 12 hours for 7 to 10 days
  —Fecal leukocytes negative/O & P negative:
  -Ciprofloxacin 500 mg orally every 12 hours, or

      –Metronidazole 500 mg orally every 12
       hours for 7 to 10 days
     —Stool O & P positive:
      –Specific antiparasite therapy (see
       Chapter 9 on Parasites for specific
       treatment recommendations)
- Oral rehydration therapy

Follow-Up:

- Outpatient care is generally sufficient unless hospitalization is required for severe dehydration
- **Watch for:** signs and symptoms of
  - Serious enteric or parasitic infection
  - Dehydration
  - Electrolyte imbalances

POST-TRAVEL FEVER

Presenting Symptoms:

SUBJECTIVE	OBJECTIVE
Traveler returning from exotic parts of the world	Returning traveler
	Fever with no localizing signs
Fever with no other signs	

Differential Diagnosis:

Fever occurring less than 21 days after travel
—Arboviral infection (e.g., dengue fever, yellow
  fever)
—Typhus fever
—Typhoid and paratyphoid fevers
—Malaria (should be at least 8 days after
  exposure to mosquitoes)

—Hemorrhagic fever (e.g., Lassa fever, Ebola
virus, Marburg virus)
—African trypanosomiasis
—Brucellosis
—Leptospirosis
—HIV infection
—Hepatitis A

Fever occurring more than 21 days after travel
—Hepatitis A, B, C, or E
—HIV infection
—Tuberculosis
—Malaria
—Visceral leishmaniasis
—Amebic liver abscess
—Filariasis
—Typhoid and paratyphoid
—Brucellosis

Suggested Workup:

- Detailed history of travel including:
  - Areas visited and travel schedule
  - Accommodations used
  - Lifestyle and activities while traveling
  - Immunizations received before travel
  - Medications used during travel
  - Adherence to recommended preventive
    measures during travel
  - Illness among fellow travelers
  - Known exposures to communicable
    diseases
  - Temporal relationship between known
    exposure to communicable illness and
    onset of traveler's symptoms
    —1 to 3 days: consider bacterial diarrhea
    —5 to 8 days: consider arboviral infections
    (e.g., dengue fever, yellow fever)
    —7 to 14 days: consider leptospirosis and
    rickettsial diseases (e.g., scrub typhus)

> —8 to 17 days: consider *P. falciparum* malaria
> —9 to 15 days: consider *P. vivax* malaria
> —10 to 20 days: consider giardiasis, hepatitis A, hemorrhagic fever agents (Lassa, Ebola, Marburg), African trypanosomiasis
> —21 to 60 days: consider hepatitis E, tuberculosis, HIV infection, leishmaniasis, filariasis, brucellosis

- Traveler's health history
- Evaluation of fever pattern:
  - Periodic intermittent fevers at intervals of 48 to 72 hours: consider malaria (*P. vivax* or *Plasmodium malariae*)
  - Relapsing fevers lasting a few days, separated by afebrile periods of several days: consider borreliosis, African trypanosomiasis, brucellosis
  - Persistent fever with continuously abnormal temperatures: consider typhoid and *P. malariae*
  - Double-hump fevers that lasts a few days, followed by an afebrile period of 1 to 2 days, then a return of the fever: consider dengue fever or other viral infection
  - Intermittent but persistent fever: consider pyrogenic infection, miliary tuberculosis, lymphoma
  - Two fever spikes each day (double quotidian fever): consider kala-azar, early malaria, infective endocarditis (*N. gonorrhoeae*)
- Urinalysis and urine culture
- Liver function tests
- Tuberculin skin test
- Complete blood count with platelets

- Peripheral blood smears (thick and thin) for malaria
- Blood cultures
- Collection of three separate stool specimens
  - Saline smear
  - Concentration examination
  - Stained slide examination
  - Culture
- Serologic tests
  - Schistosomiasis
  - Strongyloidiasis
  - Amebiasis
  - Lassa fever
  - Hepatitis
- Imaging studies
  - Chest radiograph
  - Abdominal ultrasound

Definitive Diagnosis:

Fever in a returning traveler may be attributed to one or more of many infections; use ICD-9-CM code for specific diagnoses; for example:

Lassa fever	ICD-9-CM 078.89
African trypanosomiasis	ICD-9-CM 086.5
Chagas' disease	ICD-9-CM 086.2
Dengue fever	ICD-9-CM 061
Brucellosis	ICD-9-CM 023.9

Suggested Treatment:

- Specific treatment is tailored to definitive diagnosis
- Lassa fever:
  - Strict isolation procedures should be instituted
  - Ribavarin may be tried, but treatment is generally supportive
- African trypanosomiasis:

- No central nervous system (CNS)
  involvement:
  —Suramin 5 mg/kg intravenously (IV)
    on day 1, 10 mg/kg IV on day 3, and
    20 mg/kg IV every day on days 5, 11, 17,
    23, and 30
- CNS involvement present:
  —Suramin 5 mg/kg IV on day 1, 10 mg/kg
    IV on day 2, and 20 mg/kg IV on day
    3, and
      Melarsoprol 3.6 mg/kg/day by slow
        intravenous infusion for 4 days,
        rest 10 days, then repeat, rest
        another 10 days, then repeat, or
  —Elfornithine 100 mg IV every 6 hours for
    14 days, then 75 mg/kg orally every 6
    hours for 4 weeks
- New World or American Trypanosomiasis
  (Chagas' disease)
  - Nifurtimox 5 to 10 mg/kg/day orally 3
    times a day for 60 days, or
  - Beznidazole 100 mg orally 3 times a day
    after a meal for 60 days
- Dengue fever:
  - Uncomplicated disease:
    —Supportive therapy
    —Symptomatic relief with NSAIDs
    —Frequent monitoring for changes in
      neurologic and cardiac status,
      thrombocytopenia, and severe
      hypovolemia leading to
      hemoconcentration and shock
  - Hemorrhagic disease (dengue hemorrhagic
    fever; DHF):
    —Fluid resuscitation
      –Ringer's lactate or normal saline
        20 mg/kg intravenous bolus, and

–Plasma or dextran colloid fluids 10 to
  20 mg/kg IV as needed
—Close monitoring of volume status
—Close monitoring of hematocrit and
  platelet counts
—Transfusion as needed
—Heparin NOT indicated for disseminated
  intravascular coagulation (DIC)
- Brucellosis
  - Doxycycline 100 mg orally 2 times a day
    for 45 days, and
      Streptomycin 1 g intramuscularly once
        daily for first 14 days, or
  - Doxycycline 100 mg orally 2 times a day, and
      Rifampin 600 mg orally once daily for
        45 days
  - Chronic disease may be treated with one of
    the standard treatments above, then
      Doxycycline 100 mg orally 2 times a day
        for 3 months

Follow-Up:

- Outpatient care is generally sufficient except
  in life-threatening situations
- **Watch for:** signs and symptoms of
  - Volume depletion and shock
  - CNS deterioration
  - Ocular involvement
  - Hematologic collapse

References and Recommended Reading

GENERAL REFERENCES:

American College of Physicians. Clinical practice guidelines. Philadelphia: American College of Physicians, 1995.

American Medical Association. Directory of practice parameters. Chicago: AMA, 1996.

Bennett WM, Aronoff GR, Golper TA, et al. Drug prescribing in renal failure, 3rd ed. Philadelphia: American College of Physicians, 1994.

The choice of antibacterial drugs. Med Lett 1996;38:25–34.

Drug topics® red book. Montvale, NJ: Medical Economics, 1997.

Drugs for non-HIV viral infections. Med Lett 1997;39:69–76.

Facts and Comparisons. Drug facts and comparisons, 50th ed. St. Louis: Facts and Comparisons, 1996.

Fauci A, Braunwald E, Isselbacher KJ, et al, eds. Harrison's principles of internal medicine, 14th ed. New York: McGraw-Hill, 1997.

Hansten PD, Horn JR. Drug interactions analysis and management. Vancouver, WA: Applied Therapeutics, 1997.

International classification of diseases, 9th revision, Clinical modification, 4th ed. Los Angeles: PMIC, 1996.

Mandell GL, Bennett JE, Dolin R. Principles and practice of infectious diseases, 4th ed. New York Churchill Livingstone, 1995.

The Medical Letter. Handbook of antimicrobial therapy. New Rochelle, NY: The Medical Letter, 1996.

PDR Guide to drug interactions, side effects, indications, 50th ed. Montvale, NJ: Medical Economics, 1996.

Physicians' desk reference, 52nd ed. Montvale, NJ:
    Medical Economics, 1998.
Rakel RE. Conn's current therapy. Philadelphia: WB
    Saunders, 1997.
Systemic antifungal drugs. Med Lett 1997;39:86–88.
United States Pharmacopeial Convention. Advice for
    the patient. Drug information in lay language, vol. II,
    17th ed. Taunton, MA: Rand McNally, 1997.

CHAPTER 1—SKIN AND SOFT TISSUES:

Andreassi L, Flori L. Pharmacologic treatment of burns.
    Clin Dermatol 1992;9:453–458.
Baltimore RS. Treatment of impetigo: A review. Pediatr
    Inf Dis 1985;4:597–601.
Brook I. Microbiology of human and animal bite
    wounds in children. Pediatr Infect Dis 1987;6:29–32.
Chartier C, Grosshans E. Erysipelas. Int J Dermatol
    1990;29:459–467.
Elewski BE, ed. Cutaneous fungal infections. New York:
    Igaku-Shoin Med. Publ., 1992.
Elewski BE, Hazen PG. The superficial mycoses and the
    dermatophytes. J Am Acad Dermatol
    1989;21:655–673.
Elewski BE, Sullivan J. Dermatophytes as opportunistic
    pathogens. J Am Acad Dermatol 1994;30:1021–1022.
Esterly NB, Nelson DB, Dunn WM Jr. Impetigo. Am J
    Dis Child 1991;145:125–126.
George WL. Other infections of skin, soft tissue, and
    muscle. In: Finegold SM, George WL, eds. Anaerobic
    infections in humans. New York: Academic Press,
    1989;492–504.
Gill V, Cunha BA. Onychomycosis. Infect Dis Pract
    1997;21:5–8.
Giuliano A, Lewis F Jr, Hadley K, et al. Bacteriology of
    necrotizing fasciitis. Am J Surg 1977;134:52–57.
Goldstein EJC. Bite wounds and infection. Clin Infect
    Dis 1992;14:633–640.
Goldstein EJC, Citron DM. Comparative susceptibilities
    of 173 aerobic and anaerobic bite wound isolates to
    sparfloxacin, temafloxacin, clarithromycin and older
    agents. Antimicrob Agents Chemother
    1993;37:1150–1153.

Gupta AK, Sauder DN, Shear NH. Antifungal agents: An overview, part II. J Am Acad Dermatol 1994;30:911–933.

Gustafson TL, Band JD, Hutcheson RH Jr, Schaffner W. *Pseudomonas* folliculitis: An outbreak and review. Rev Infect Dis 1983;5:1–8.

Hay RJ. Onychomycosis. Agents of choice. Dermatol Clin 1993;11:161–169.

Hestrom SA. Treatment and prevention of recurrent staphylococcal furunculosis: Clinical and bacteriologic follow-up. Scand J Infect Dis 1985;17:55–58.

Hook EW, Hooton TM, Horton CA, et al. Microbiologic evaluation of cutaneous cellulitis in adults. Arch Int Med 1986;146:295–297.

Iorianni P, Oliver GC. Synergistic soft tissue infections of the perineum. Dis Colon Rectum 1992;35:640–644.

Karchmer AW, Gibbons GW. Foot infections in diabetes: Evaluation and management. In: Remington JS, Swartz MN, eds. Current clinical topics in infectious diseases. v. 14. Boston: Blackwell Scientific, 1994;7–10.

Kilborn JA, Manz LA, O'Brien M, et al. Necrotizing cellulitis caused by *Legionella micdadei*. Am J Med 1992;92:104–106.

Kost RG, Straus SE. Postherpetic neuralgia—pathogenesis, treatment, and prevention. N Engl J Med 1996;335:32–42.

Kremer M, Zuckerman R, Avraham Z, Raz R. Long-term antimicrobial therapy in the prevention of soft-tissue infections. J Infect 1991;22:37–40.

Melski JW, Arndt KA. Topical therapy for acne. N Engl J Med 1980;302:503–506.

Monafo WW, Freedman B. Topical therapy for burns. Surg Clin North Am 1987;67:133–145.

Moriarty RA, Margileth AM. Cat scratch disease. Infect Dis Clin North Am 1987;1:575–590.

Nickel JC, Morales A. Necrotizing fasciitis of the male genitalia (Fournier's gangrene). Can Med Assoc J 1983;129:445–448.

Parish LC, Witkowski JA. Cutaneous bacterial infections. Postgrad Med 1992;91:119–122, 125–126, 129–130.

Rea WJ, Wyrick WJ Jr. Necrotizing fasciitis. Ann Surg 1970;172:957–964.

Sachs MK. Cutaneous cellulitis. Arch Dermatol 1991;127:493–496.

Sachs MK. An optimum use of needle aspiration in the bacteriologic diagnosis of cellulitis in adults. Arch Int Med 1990;150:1907–1912.

Schwartz JJ, Myskowski PL. Molluscum contagiosum in patients with human immunodeficiency virus infection. A review of 27 patients. J Am Acad Dermatol 1992;27:583–588.

Shalita AR, Leyden JE Jr, Pochi PE, et al. Acne vulgaris. J Am Acad Dermatol 1987; 16:410–412.

Stevens DL, Musher DM, Watson DA, et al. Spontaneous nontraumatic gangrene due to *Clostridium septicum*. Rev Infect Dis 1990;12:286–296.

Webster GF. Inflammatory acne. Int J Dermatol 1990;29:313–317.

Whitley RJ, Weiss H, Gnann WJ Jr, et al. Acyclovir with and without prednisone for the treatment of Herpes zoster. Ann Intern Med 1996;125:376–383.

Zalar GL, Warmuth IP. Common cutaneous bacterial infections. Hosp Med 1996;41:31–39.

CHAPTER 2—CENTRAL NERVOUS SYSTEM AND EYE:

Aragones JV. The treatment of blepharitis; A controlled double blind study of combination therapy. Ann Ophthalmol 1973;5:49–52.

Baum JL. Initial therapy of suspected microbial corneal ulcers. I. Broad antibiotic therapy based on prevalence of organisms. Surv Ophthalmol 1979;24:97–105.

Baum JL, Barza M. Topical versus subconjunctival treatment of bacterial corneal ulcers. Ophthalmology 1983;90:162–168.

Bonadio WA. The cerebrospinal fluid: Physiologic aspects and alterations associated with bacterial meningitis. Pediatr Infect Dis J 1992;11:423–432.

Brewer NS, MacCarty CS, Wellamn WE. Brain abscess: A review of recent experience. Ann Intern Med 1975;82:571–576.

Connolly KJ, Hammer SM. The acute aseptic meningitis syndrome. Infect Dis Clin North Am 1990;4:599–622.

Darouiche RO, Hamill RJ. Bacterial spinal epidural abscess. Review of 43 cases and literature survey. Medicine 1992;71:369–385.

Feigin RD, McCracken GH Jr, Klein JO. Diagnosis and management of meningitis. Pediatr Infect Dis J 1992;11:785–814.

Greenlee JE. Approach to diagnosis of meningitis: Cerebrospinal fluid evaluation. Infect Dis Clin North Am 1990;4:583–598.

Harrison MJG. The clinical presentation of intracranial abscesses. Q J Med 1982;51:461–468.

Hsich G, Kenney K, Gibbs CJ Jr, et al. The 14-3-3 brain protein in cerebrospinal fluid as a marker for transmissible spongiform encephalopathies. N Engl J Med 1996;335:924–930.

Johnson JT, Yu VL, eds. Infectious diseases and antimicrobial therapy of the ears, nose, and throat. Philadelphia:WB Saunders, 1997.

Kricun R, Shoemaker EI, Chovanes GI, et al. Epidural abscess of the cervical spine: MR findings in five cases. Am J Roentgenol 1992;158:1145–1149.

Nussbaum ES, Rigamonti D, Standiford H, et al. Spinal epidural abscess: A report of 40 cases and review. Surg Neurol 1992;38:225–231.

Quagliarello VJ, Scheld WM. Treatment of bacterial meningitis. N Engl J Med 1997;336:708–716.

Rea GL, McGregor JM, Miller CA, et al. Surgical treatment of the spontaneous spinal epidural abscess. Surg Neurol 1992;37:274–279.

Scheld WM, Whitley RJ, Durack DT, eds. Infections of the central nervous system, 2nd ed. Philadelphia: Lippincott-Raven, 1996.

Silverberg AL, DiNubile MJ. Subdural empyema and cranial epidural abscess. Med Clin North Am 1985;69:361–374.

Sjoln J, Lilja A, Eriksson N, et al. Treatment of brain abscess with cefotaxime and metronidazole: Prospective study on 15 consecutive patients. Clin Infect Dis 1993;17:857–863.

Smolion G, Okumoto M. Staphylococcal blepharitis. Arch Ophthalmol 1977;95:812–816.

Stepanov S. Surgical treatment of brain abscess. Neurosurgery 1988;22:724–730.

Syed MA, Hyndiuk RA. Infectious conjunctivitis. Infect Dis Clin North Am 1992;6:789–805.

Tunkel AR, Scheld WM. Acute therapy of bacterial
meningitis. J Intensive Care Med 1991;6:229–237.
Tunkel AR, Scheld WM. Applications of therapy in
animal models to bacterial infection in human
disease. Infect Dis Clin North Am 1989;3:441–459.
Tunkel AR, Scheld WM. Therapy of bacterial
meningitis: Principles and practice. Infect Control
Hosp Epidemiol 1989;10:565–569.
Vaughan D, Asbury T, Riordan-Eva P. General
ophthalmology, 13th ed. Norwalk, CT: Appleton &
Lange, 1992.

CHAPTER 3—UPPER RESPIRATORY TRACT, TRACHEA, AND BRONCHI:

Bamberger DM. Antimicrobial treatment of sinusitis.
Semin Respir Infect 1991;6:77–84.
Barry W, Cockburn F, Cornall R, et al. Ribavirin aerosol
for acute bronchiolitis. Arch Dis Child
1986;61:593–594.
Bruce HM. Diagnosis of sinusitis in adults: History,
physical examination, nasal cytology, echo, and
rhinoscope. J Allergy Clin Immunol 1992;90:436–441.
Chow, AW. Life-threatening infections of the head and
neck. Clin Infect Dis 1992;14:991–1004.
Chow AW, Hall CB, Klein JO, et al. General guidelines
for the evaluation of new anti-infective drugs for the
treatment of respiratory tract infections. Clin Infect
Dis 1992;15:S62–S88.
Englund JA, Piedra PA, Jefferson LS, et al. High-dose,
short duration ribavirin aerosol therapy in children
with suspected respiratory syncytial virus infection.
J Pediatr 1990;117:313–320.
Greenspan D, Greenspan JS, Conant M, et al. Oral
''hairy'' leukoplakia in male homosexuals: Evidence
of association with both papillomavirus and a herpes-
group virus. Lancet 1984;2:831–834.
Gwaltney JM, Scheld WM, Sande MA, et al. The
microbial etiology and antimicrobial therapy of adults
with acute community-acquired sinusitis: A 15 year
experience at the University of Virginia and review of
other selected studies. J Allergy Clin Immunol
1992;90:457–462.
Influenza vaccine, 1996–1997. Med Lett 1996;38:86.

Johnston SL, Bloy H. Evaluation of rapid enzyme immunoassay for detection of influenza A virus. J Clin Microbiol 1993;31:142–143.

Ophir D, Bawnik J, Poria Y, et al. Peritonsillar abscess. A prospective evaluation of outpatient management by needle aspiration. Arch Otolaryngol Head Neck Surg 1988;114:661–663.

Pichichero ME. Assessing the treatment alternatives for acute otitis media. Pediatr Infect Dis J 1994;13:527–534.

Rivron RP, Murray JAM. Adult epiglottitis: Is there a consensus on diagnosis and treatment? Clin Otolaryngol 1991;16:338–344.

Schalen L, Ingvav E, Kamme C, et al. Erythromycin in acute laryngitis in adults. Ann Otol Rhino Laryngol 1993;102:209–214.

Schlossberg D, ed. Infections of the head and neck. New York: Springer Publishing, 1987.

Schuster GS, ed. Oral microbiology and infectious disease. Baltimore: Williams & Wilkins, 1983.

Sheikh KH, Mostow SR. Epiglottitis—an increasing problem for adults. West J Med 1989;151:520–524.

Stringer SP, Schaefer SD, Close LG. A randomized trial for outpatient management of peritonsillar abscess. Arch Otolaryngol Head Neck Surg 1988;114:296–298.

Todd JK. The sore throat: Pharyngitis and epiglottitis. Infect Dis Clin North Am 1988;2:149–162.

Topazian RG, Goldberg MH, eds. Oral and maxillofacial infections, 2nd ed. Philadelphia: WB Saunders, 1987.

Vukmir RB. Adult and pediatric pharyngitis: A review. J Emerg Med 1992;10:607–616.

Willis SE. Throat culture or rapid strep test? Postgrad Med 1990;88:111–114.

Wingfield WL, Pollack D, Grunert RR. Therapeutic efficacy of amantadine HCl and rimantadine HCl in naturally occurring influenza A2 respiratory illness in man. N Engl J Med 1989;281:579–584.

CHAPTER 4—LOWER RESPIRATORY TRACT AND MYCOBACTERIAL INFECTIONS:

Annas GJ. Control of tuberculosis—the law and the public's health. N Engl J Med 1993;328:585–588.

Bartlett JG, Gorbach SL, Tally FP, et al. Bacteriology and treatment of primary lung abscess. Am Rev Respir Dis 1974;109:510–518.

Bates JH, Campbell GD, Barron AL, et al. Microbial etiology of acute pneumonia in hospitalized patients. Chest 1992;101:1005–1012.

Brown RB. Community-acquired pneumonia: Diagnosis and therapy of older adults. Geriatrics 1993;48:43–50.

Centers for Disease Control and Prevention: CDC guidelines provide general recommendations to help prevent the emergence of MDR-TB. JAMA 1993; 11:270.

Davis SF, Sarosi GA. Pulmonary mycoses. In: Bone RC, Dantzker DR, George RB, et al., eds. Pulmonary and critical care medicine. Chicago: Mosby-Year Book, 1993:1–24.

Dismukes WE, Bradsher RW Jr, Cloud GC, et al. Itraconazole therapy for blastomycosis and histoplasmosis. Am J Med 1992;93:489–497.

Esposito AL. Current recommendations for community-acquired pneumonia. Contemp Intern Med 1995;7:47–60.

Fang GD, Fine M, Orloff J, et al. New and emerging etiologies for community-acquired pneumonia with implications for therapy. Medicine 1990;69:307–316.

Fine MJ, Auble TE, Yealy DM, et al. A prediction rule to identify low-risk patients with community-acquired pneumonia. N Engl J Med 1997;336:243–250.

Fine MJ, Smith DN, Singer DE. Hospitalization decision in patients with community-acquired pneumonia: A prospective cohort study. Am J Med 1990;89:713–721.

Flournoy DJ, Davidson LJ. Sputum quality: Can you tell by looking? Am J Infect Control 1993;21:64–69.

Frieden TR, Sterling T, Pablos-Mendez A, et al. The emergence of drug-resistant tuberculosis in New York City. N Engl J Med 1993;328:521–526.

Giron JM, Poey CG, Fajadet PP, et al. Inoperable pulmonary aspergilloma: Percutaneous CT-guided injection with glycerin and amphotericin B paste in 15 cases. Radiol 1993;188:825–827.

Goble M, Iseman MD, Madsen LA, et al. Treatment of 171 patients with pulmonary tuberculosis resistant to isoniazid and rifampin. N Engl J Med 1993;328:527–532.

Grayston JT, Diwan VK, Cooney M, et al. Community- and hospital-acquired pneumonia associated with *Chlamydia* TWAR infection demonstrated serologically. Arch Intern Med 1989;149:169–173.

Gudiol F, Manresa F, Pallares R, et al. Clindamycin vs penicillin for anaerobic lung infections. High rate of penicillin failures associated with penicillin-resistant *Bacteroides melaninogenicus.* Arch Intern Med 1990;150:2525–2529.

Jacoby GA. Prevalence and resistance mechanisms of common respiratory pathogens. Clin Infect Dis 1994;18:951–957.

Jackson M, Flower CDR, Shneerson JM. Aspergillomas with intracavitary instillation of amphotericin B through an indwelling catheter. Thorax 1993;48:928–930.

Lee KS, Kim HT, Kim YH, et al. Treatment of hemoptysis in patients with cavitary aspergilloma of the lung. Am J Radiol 1993;161:727–731.

Lemmer JH, Botham MJ, Orringer MD. Modern management of adult thoracic empyema. J Thorac Cardiovasc Surg 1985;90:849–855.

Levine DP, Lerner AM. The clinical spectrum of *Mycoplasma pneumoniae* infections. Med Clin North Am 1978;62:961–978.

Light RW. Management of empyema. Sem Respir Med 1992;13:167–176.

Mandell LA, ed. Toward 2001 in managing lower respiratory tract infection. Proceedings of a symposium. Am J Med 1995;99(Suppl 6B):1S–27S.

Mansel JK, Rosenow EC III, Smith TF, et al. *Mycoplasma pneumoniae* pneumonia. Chest 1989;95:639–646.

Marrie TJ, Durant H, Yates L. Community-acquired pneumonia requiring hospitalization: 5-year prospective study. Rev Infect Dis 1989;11:586–599.

Martin RE, Bates JH. Atypical pneumonia. Infect Dis Clin North Am 1991;5:585–601.

Massard G, Roeslin N, Wihlm J-M, et al. Pleuropulmonary aspergilloma. Clinical spectrum and results of surgical treatment. Ann Thorac Surg 1992;54:1159–1164.

Moreau P, Zahar J-R, Milpied N, et al. Localized invasive pulmonary aspergillosis in patients with neutropenia: Effectiveness of surgical resection. Cancer 1993;72:3223–3226.

Mroueh S, Spock A. Allergic broncholpulmonary
  aspergillosis in patients with cystic fibrosis. Chest
  1994;105:32–36.
Nguyen MH, Stout JE, Yu VL. Legionellosis. Infect Dis
  Clin North Am 1991;5:561–584.
Pappas PG, Pottage JC, Powderly WG, et al.
  Blastomycosis in patients with the acquired
  immunodeficiency syndrome. Ann Intern Med
  1992;116:847–853.
Ramsey BW. Management of pulmonary disease in
  patients with cystic fibrosis. N Engl J Med
  1996;335:179–188.
Rodnick JE, Gude JK. Diagnosis and antibiotic
  treatment of community-acquired pneumonia. West J
  Med 1991;154:405–409.

CHAPTER 5—CARDIAC INFECTIONS:

Aragam JR, Weyman AE. Echocardiographic findings in
  infective endocarditis. In: Weyman AE, ed. Principles
  and practice of echocardiography, 2nd ed.
  Philadelphia: Lea & Febiger, 1993;1178.
Bandyk DF, Esses GE. Prosthetic graft infection. Surg
  Clin North Am 1994;74:571–590.
Calderwood SB, Swinski LA, Karchmer AW, et al.
  Prosthetic valve endocarditis: Analysis of factors
  influencing outcome of therapy. J Thoracic
  Cardiovasc Surg 1986;92:776–778.
Daniel WG, Mugge A, Martin RP, et al. Improvement in
  the diagnosis of abscess associated with endocarditis
  by transesophageal echocardiography. N Engl J Med
  1991; 324:795–800.
Gaynes R, Marosok R, Mowry-Hanley J, et al.
  Mediastinitis following coronary artery bypass
  surgery: A 3 year review. J Infect Dis
  1991;163:117–121.
Hecht SR, Berger M. Right-sided endocarditis in
  intravenous drug users: Prognostic features in 102
  episodes. Ann Intern Med 1992;117:560–566.
Ilan Y, Oren R, Ben-Chetrit E. Acute pericarditis.
  Etiology, treatment and prognosis. Jpn Heart J
  1991;32:315–321.
Jaffe WM, Morgan DE, Pearlman AS, et al. Infective
  endocarditis, 1983–1988: Echocardiographic findings

and factors influencing morbidity and mortality. J Am Coll Cardiol 1990;15:1227–1233.

Johnson RA, Zajac RA, Evans ME. Suppurative thrombophlebitis: Correlation between pathogen and underlying disease. Infect Control 1986;7:582–585.

Kaye D. Treatment of infective endocarditis. Ann Intern Med 1996;124:606–608.

Maisch B, Herzum M, Schonian U. Immunomodulating factors and immunosuppressive drugs in the therapy of myocarditis. Scand J Infect Dis 1993;88:149–162.

Martin AB, Webber S, Fricker SJ, et al. Acute myocarditis: Rapid diagnosis by PCR in children. Circulation 1994; 90:330–339.

Park S, Bayer AS. Purulent pericarditis. Curr Clin Topics Infect Dis 1992;12:56–82.

Raoult D, Fournier PE, Drancourt M, et al. Diagnosis of 22 new cases of *Bartonella* endocarditis. Ann Intern Med 1996;125:646–652.

Saffle J, Gardner P, Schoenbaum SC, et al. Prosthetic valve endocarditis: The case for prompt valve replacement. J Thorac Cardiovasc Surg 1977;73:416–420.

Sagrista-Sauleda J, Barrabes JA, Permanyer-Miralda G, et al. Purulent pericarditis: Review of a 20 year experience in a general hospital. J Am Coll Cardiol 1993;22:1661–1665.

Sande MA, Kaye D, Root RK, eds. Endocarditis. London: Churchill Livingstone, 1984.

See DM, Tilles JG. Viral myocarditis. Rev Infect Dis 1991;13:951–956.

Sharp WJ, Hoballah JJ, Moran CR, et al. The management of the infected aortic prosthesis: A current decade of experience. J Vasc Surg 1994;19:844–850.

Stein JM, Pruitt BA. Suppurative thrombophlebitis: A lethal iatrogenic disease. N Engl J Med 1970;282:1452–1455.

Sterkelberg JM, Murphy JG, Ballard D, et al. Emboli in infective endocarditis: The prognostic value of echocardiography. Ann Intern Med 1991;114:635–640.

Durack DT, Lukes AS, Bright DK, et al. New criteria for diagnosis of infective endocarditis. Am J Med 1994; 96:200–209.

Vuille C, Nidorf M, Weyman AE, et al. Natural history of vegetations during successful medical management of endocarditis. Am Heart J 1994;128:1200–1209.

CHAPTER 6—GASTROINTESTINAL, INTRA-ABDOMINAL, AND PERITONEAL INFECTIONS:

Bai JC, Crosetti EE, Maurino EC, et al. Short-term antibiotic treatment in Whipple's disease. J Clin Gastroenterol 1991;13:303–307.

Banwell JG, Gorbach SL. Tropical sprue. Gut 1969;10:328–333.

Banwell JG, Kistler LA, Gianella RA, et al. Small intestinal bacterial overgrowth syndromes. Gastroenterology 1994;106:782–786.

Barkin RM. Ciguatera poisoning: A common source outbreak. South Med J 1974;67:13–16.

Bartlett JG. *Clostridium difficile:* Clinical considerations. Rev Infect Dis 1990;12:S243–S251.

Bean NH, Griffin PM. Foodborne disease outbreaks in the United States, 1973–1987: Pathogens, vehicles, and trends. J Food Protection 1990;53:804–817.

Blacklow N, Greenberg H. Viral gastroenteritis. N Engl J Med 1991;325:252–264.

Bohnen JMA, Solomkin JS, Dellinger EP, et al. Guidelines for clinical care: Anti-infective agents for intra-abdominal infections. Arch Surg 1992;127:83–89.

Centers for Disease Control and Prevention. Update: Multistate outbreak of *E. coli* O157:H7 infections from hamburgers—Western United States, 1992–1993. MMWR 1993;42:258–263.

Christie AB. Typhoid and paratyphoid fevers. In: Christie AB, ed. Infectious diseases: epidemiology and clinical practice, 2nd ed. New York: Churchill-Livingstone, 1974;55–130.

Do H, Lambiase RE, Deyoe L, et al. Percutaneous drainage hepatic abscesses: A multicenter study and review of the literature. Am J Surg 1987;157:1209–1212.

Drugs for treatment of peptic ulcers. Med Lett 1997;39:1–4.

Dupont HL. How safe is the food we eat? JAMA 1992;268:3240.

Fekety R, Shah AB. Diagnosis and treatment of *Clostridium difficile* colitis. JAMA 1993;269:71–75.

Fleming JL, Wiesner RH, Shorter RG. Whipple's disease: Clinical, biochemical, and histopathologic features and assessment of treatment in 29 patients. Mayo Clin Proc 1988;63:539–551.

Freed RC, Evenson ML, Reiser RF, et al. Enzyme-linked immunosorbent assay for detection of staphylococcal enterotoxins in foods. Appl Environ Microbiol 1982;44:1349–1355.

Glynn J. Tropical sprue—its aetiology and pathogenesis. J R Soc Med 1986;79:599.

Gorbach SL. Intra-abdominal infections. Clin Infect Dis 1993;17:961–967.

Griffin PM, Tauxe RV. The epidemiology of infections caused by *E. coli* O157:H7, other enterohemorrhagic *E. coli,* and the associated hemolytic uremic syndrome. Epidemiol Rev 1991;13:60–98.

Guerrant RL, Bobak DA. Bacterial and protozoal gastroenteritis. N Engl J Med 1991;325:327–340.

Hedberg CW, MacDonald KL, Osterholm MT. Changing epidemiology of food-borne disease. Clin Infect Dis 1994;18:671–682.

Hoofnagle JH, DiBisceglie AM. The treatment of chronic viral hepatitis. N Engl J Med 1997;336:347–356.

Hughes JM, Blumenthal JR, Merson MH, et al. Clinical features of types A and B food-borne botulism. Ann Intern Med 1981;95:442–445.

Hughes JM, Merson MH. Fish and shellfish poisoning. N Engl J Med 1976;295:1117–1120.

Kadakia SC. Biliary tract emergencies: Acute cholecystitis, acute cholangitis, and acute pancreatitis. Med Clin North Am 1993;77:1015–1036.

Kelly CP, Pothoulakis C, LaMont JT. Clostridium difficile colitis. N Engl J Med 1994;330:257–262.

Lederberg J, Shope RE, Oaks RC Jr, eds. Emerging infections: Microbial threats to health in the United States. Washington, DC: National Academy Press; 1992.

Lemon SM, Thomas DL. Vaccines to prevent viral hepatitis. N Engl J Med 1997;336:196–204.

Levinson MA. Percutaneous versus open drainage of intra-abdominal abscesses. Infect Dis Clin North Am 1992;6:525–544.

Lipsett PA, Pitt HA. Acute cholangitis. Surg Clin North Am 1990;70:1297–1312.

McCormick DJ, Avbel AJ, Gibbons RB. Nonlethal mushroom poisoning. Ann Intern Med 1979;90:332–335.

Mosdell DM, Morris DM, Voltura A, et al. Antibiotic treatment for surgical peritonitis. Ann Surg 1991;214:543–549.

Mueller PR, Simeone JF. Intra-abdominal abscess: Diagnosis by sonography and computed tomography. Rad Clin North Am 1983;21:425–443.

Nelken N, Isnatius J, Skinner M, et al. Changing clinical spectrum of splenic abscess: A multicenter study and review of the literature. Am J Surg 1987;154:27–34.

Niederau C, Heintges T, Lange S, et al. Long-term follow-up of HB$_e$Ag-positive patients treated with interferon alfa for chronic hepatitis B. N Engl J Med 1996;334:1422–1427.

Pavia AT. Approach to acute foodborne and waterborne disease. Semin Pediatr Infect Dis 1994;5:222–230.

Ranshoff DF, Gracie WA. Treatment of gallstones. Ann Intern Med 1993;119:606–619.

Rickles FR, Klipstein FA, Tomasini J, et al. Long-term follow-up of antibiotic-treated tropical sprue. Ann Intern Med 1972;76:203–210.

Rodriguez DC, Etzel RA, Hall S, et al. Lethal paralytic shellfish poisoning in Guatemala. Am J Trop Med Hyg 1990;42:267–271.

Sawyer MD, Dunn DL. Antimicrobial therapy of intra-abdominal sepsis. Infect Dis Clin North Am 1992;6:545–570.

Schlager SI, Hanauer SB. New therapeutic approaches to peptic ulcer disease: The role of *Helicobacter pylori*. Am J Therap 1996;3:586–596.

Shahara AI, Hunt CM, Hamilton JD. Hepatitis C. Ann Intern Med 1996;125:658–668.

Shandera WX, Tacket CO, Blake PA. Food poisoning due to *Clostridium perfringens* in the United States. J Infect Dis 1983;147:167–170.

Swift AEB, Swift TR. Ciguatera. Clin Toxicol 1993;31:1–29.

Tsutaoka B. Antibiotic-associated pseudomembranous enteritis due to *Clostridium difficile*. Clin Infect Dis 1994;18:982–984.

Waites WM, Arbuthnott JP. Foodborne illness: An overview. Lancet 1990;336:722–725.

Wilcox CM. Esophageal disease in the acquired immunodeficiency syndrome: Etiology, diagnosis, and management. Am J Med 1992;92:412–421.

CHAPTER 7—GENITOURINARY, GYNECOLOGIC, AND SEXUALLY TRANSMITTED DISEASES:

Abdullah AN, Drake SM, Wade AA, et al. Balanitis in patients attending a department of genitourinary medicine. Internat J STD AIDS 1992;3:128–129.

Ball TP Jr. Epididymitis and orchitis. In: Seidman PD, Hanno HA, ed. Current urologic therapy. Philadelphia: WB Saunders, 1994.

Centers for Disease Control and Prevention. 1993 sexually transmitted diseases treatment guidelines. MMWR 1993;42(RR-14):1–102.

Coultrip LL, Grossman JH. Evaluation of rapid diagnostic tests in the detection of microbial invasion of the amniotic cavity. Am J Obstet Gynecol 1992;167:1231–1242.

Gauthier DW, Meyer WJ. Comparison of gram stain, leukocyte esterase activity, and amniotic fluid glucose concentration in predicting amniotic fluid culture results in preterm premature rupture of membranes. Am J Obstet Gynecol 1992;167:1092–1095.

Genc M, Mardh P-A. A cost-effectiveness analysis of screening and treatment for *Chlamydia trachomatis* infection in asymptomatic women. Ann Intern Med 1996;124:1–7.

Holmes KK, Mardh P-A, Sparling PF, et al., eds. Sexually transmitted diseases, 2nd ed. New York: McGraw-Hill, 1990.

Hooton TM, Stamm WE. Management of acute uncomplicated urinary tract infection in adults. Med Clin North Am 1991;75:339–357.

Hutchinson CM, Hook EW III. Syphilis in adults. Med Clin North Am 1990;74:1389–1416.

Koutsky LA, Galloway DA, Holmes KK. Epidemiology of genital human papillomavirus infection. Epidemiol Rev 1988;10:122–163.

Kraus SJ, Stone KM. Management of genital infection caused by human papillomavirus. Rev Infect Dis 1990;12:S620–S632.

Kunin CM. Urinary tract infections in females. Clin Infect Dis 1994;18:1–12.

Landers DV, Sweet RL, eds. Pelvic inflammatory disease. New York: Springer-Verlag, 1997.

Ling MR. Therapy of genital human papillomavirus infection. Part II: Methods of treatment. Int J Dermatol 1992;31:769–776.

Lossick JG. Treatment of sexually transmitted vaginosis/vaginitis. Rev Infect Dis 1990;12:S665–S681.

Lugo-Miro VI, Green M, Mazur L. Comparison of different metronidazole therapeutic regimens for bacterial vaginosis. JAMA 1992;268:92–95.

Magid D, Douglas JM Jr, Schwartz JS. Doxycycline compared with azithromycin for treating women with genital *Chlamydia trachomatis* infections: An incremental cost-effectiveness analysis. Ann Intern Med 1996;124:389–399.

Martin DH, ed. Sexually transmitted diseases. Med Clin North Am 1990;74:1339–1697.

Millar LK, Wing DA, Paul RH. Outpatient treatment of pyelonephritis in pregnancy: A randomized controlled trial. Obstet Gynecol 1995;86:560–564.

Mroczkowski TF. Common nonvenereal genital lesions. Med Clin North Am 1990;74:1507–1528.

Norrby SR. Short-term treatment of uncomplicated lower urinary tract infections in women. Rev Infect Dis 1990;12:458–467.

Ronald AR, Nicolle LE, Harding GK. Standards of therapy for urinary tract infections in adults. Infection 1992;20:S164–S170.

Sacks SL, Aoli FY, Diaz-Mitoma F, et al. Patient-initiated, twice-daily oral famciclovir for early recurrent genital herpes. JAMA 1996;276:44–49.

Schmidt C, Sobel JD, Meriwether C. Bacterial vaginosis: Treatment with clindamycin cream versus oral metronidazole. Obstet Gynecol 1992;79:1020–1023.

Sobel JD. Bacterial vaginosis—an ecologic mystery. Ann Intern Med 1989;111:551–553.

Vuylsteke B, Laga M, Alary M, et al. Are clinical algorithms useful to screen women for the presence of gonococcal and chlamydial infection? Clin Infect Dis 1993;17:82–88.

CHAPTER 8—JOINTS AND OSTEOMYELITIS:

Gentry LO. Antibiotic therapy for osteomyelitis. Infect Dis Clin North Am 1990;4:485–499.

Gillespie WJ. Infection in total joint replacement. Infect Dis Clin North Am 1990;4:465–484.

Goldenberg DL. Bacterial arthritis. In: Kelly WN, Harris ED Jr, Ruddy S, et al., eds. Textbook of rheumatology, 4th ed. Philadelphia: WB Saunders, 1993;1449–1466.

Inman RD, Gallegos KV, Brause BD, et al. Clinical and microbial features of prosthetic joint infection. Am J Med 1984;77:47–53.

Lew DP, Waldvogel FA. Osteomyelitis. N Engl J Med 1997;336:999–1007.

Mader JT, Norden C, Nelson JD, et al. Evaluation of new anti-infective drugs for the treatment of osteomyelitis in adults. Clin Infect Dis 1992; 15:S155–S161.

Prober CD. Current antibiotic therapy of community-acquired bacterial infections in hospitalized children: Bone and joint infections. Pediatr Infect Dis 1992;11:156–159.

Sapico FL, Montgomerie JB. Vertebral osteomyelitis. Infect Dis Clin North Am 1990;4:539–550.

Schawecher DS, Braunstein EM, Wheat JC. Diagnostic imaging of osteomylelitis. Infect Dis Clin North Am 1990;4:441–463.

Smith JW. Infectious arthritis. Infect Dis Clin North Am 1990;4:523–538.

Smith JW, Piercy E. Infectious arthritis. Clin Infect Dis 1995;20:225–231.

Steckelberg JM, Osmon DR. Prosthetic joint infections. In: Bisno AL, Waldvogel FA, eds. Infections associated with indwelling medical devices, 2nd ed. Washington, DC: ASM Press, 1994;259–290.

Wilson MG, Kelley K, Thornhill TS. Infection as a complication of total knee-replacement arthroplasty: Risk factors and treatment in 67 cases. J Bone Joint Surg Am 1990;72:878–883.

CHAPTER 9—PARASITES, RICKETTSIAE, AND SPIROCHETES:

Cook GC, ed. Manson's tropical diseases, 7th edition. London: WB Saunders, 1995.

Davidson RA. Issues in clinical parasitology: The treatment of giardiasis. Am J Gastroenterol 1984;79:256–261.

Didier R, Drancourt M. Antimicrobial therapy of rickettsial diseases. Antimicrob Agents Chemother 1991;35:2457–2462.

Drugs for parasitic infections. Med Lett 1988; 30:15–24.

Drugs for parasitic infections. Med Lett 1998;40:1–12.

Gerber MA, Shapiro ED, Burke GS, et al. Lyme disease in children in southeastern Connecticut. N Engl J Med 1996;335:1270–1274.

Goodgame RW. Understanding intestinal spore-forming protozoa: Cryptosporidia, Microsporidia, *Isospora,* and *Cyclospora.* Ann Intern Med 1996;124:429–441.

Liu LX, Weller PF. Antiparasitic drugs. N Engl J Med 1996;334:1178–1184.

Luft BJ, Bosler EM, Dattwyler RJ. Diagnosis of Lyme borreliosis. In: Lyme disease: molecular and immunologic approaches. Cold Spring Harbor, NY: Cold Spring Harbor Laboratory Press, 1992;317–324.

Luft BJ, Dattwyler RJ, Johnson RC, et al. Azithromycin compared with amoxicillin in the treatment of erythema migrans. Ann Intern Med 1996;124:785–791.

Luft BJ, Steinman CR, Schubach WH, et al. Invasion of the central nervous system by *Borrelia burgdorferi* in acute disseminated infection. JAMA 1992;267:1364–1367.

Marmion BP, Ormsbee R, Kyrkou M, et al. Vaccine prophylaxis of abattoir-associated Q fever. Lancet 1984;2:1411–1414.

Mintz ED, Hudson-Wragg M, Mshar P, et al. Foodborne giardiasis in a corporate office setting. J Infect Dis 1993;167:250–253.

Pawlowski ZS. Efficacy of low doses of praziquantel in taeniasis. Acta Trop 1991;48:83–88.

Pawlowski ZS. Taeniasis and cysticercosis. In: Hui YH, Gorham JR, Murrell KD, et al., eds. Foodborne disease handbook, Vol. 2. New York: Marcel Dekker, 1994;199–254.

Petri WA Jr, Mann BJ. Molecular mechanisms of invasion by *Entamoeba histolytica.* Sem Cell Biol 1993;4:305–313.

Radvin JI, ed. Amebiasis: Human infection by *Entamoeba histolytica.* New York: Churchill Livingstone, 1988.

Radvin JI. *Entamoeba histolytica:* Pathogenic mechanisms, human immune response, and vaccine development. Clin Res 1990;38:215–225.

Raoult D, Drancourt M. Antimicrobial therapy of rickettsial diseases. Antimicrob Agents Chemother 1991;35:2457–2462.

Sawyer LA, Fishbein DB, McDade JE. Q fever: Current concepts. Rev Infect Dis 1987; 9:935–946.

Spach DH, Liles WC, Campbell GL, et al. Tick-borne diseases in the United States. N Engl J Med 1993;329:936–947.

Treatment of Lyme disease. Med Letter 1997;39:47–48.

Warren KS, Mahmoud AAF. Tropical and geographical medicine, 2nd ed. New York: McGraw-Hill, 1990.

White NJ. The treatment of malaria. N Engl J Med 1996;335:800–806.

Wolfe MS. Giardiasis. Clin Microbiol Rev 1992;5:93–100.

CHAPTER 10—IMMUNOCOMPROMISED HOSTS:

Armstrong D. Empiric therapy for the immunocompromised host. Rev Infect Dis 1991;13:S763–S769.

Bartlett JG. The Johns Hopkins Hospital 1996 guide to medical care of patients with HIV infection, 6th ed. Baltimore: Williams & Wilkins, 1996.

Bodey GP. Antibiotics in patients with neutropenia. Arch Intern Med 1984;144:1845–1851.

Bodey GP. Empirical antibiotic therapy for fever in neutropenic patients. Clin Infect Dis 1993;17:S378–S384.

Bodey GP, Faistein V, Elting LS, et al. Beta-lactam regimens for the febrile neutropenic patient. Cancer 1990;65:9–16.

Bow EJ, Mandell LA, Louie TJ, et al. Quinolone-based antibacterial chemoprophylaxis in neutropenic patients: Effect of augmented gram-positive activity on infectious morbidity. Ann Intern Med 1996;125:183–190.

Bozzette SA, Sattler FR, Chiu J, et al. A controlled trial of early adjunctive treatment corticosteroids for *Pneumocystis carinii* pneumonia in the acquired immunodeficiency syndrome. New Engl J Med 1990;323:1451–1457.

Carpenter CCJ, Fischl MA, Hammer SM, et al. Antiretroviral therapy for HIV infection in 1997. Updated recommendations of the International AIDS Society—USA panel. JAMA 1997;277:1962–1969.

Centers for Disease Control and Prevention. 1993 revised classification system for HIV infection and expanded surveillance case definition for AIDS among adolescents and adults. MMWR 1992;41:1–21.

Chaisson RE, Benson CA, Dube MP, et al. Clarithromycin therapy for bacteremic *Mycobacterium avium* complex disease. Ann Intern Med 1994;121:905–911.

Chambers HF, Morris DL, Tauber MG, et al. Cocaine use and the risk for endocarditis in intravenous drug users. Ann Intern Med 1987;104:833–836.

Cohen PT, Sande M, Volberding PA, eds. The AIDS knowledge base, 2nd ed. Boston: Little, Brown, 1995.

Cohn DL, Dobkin J. Treatment and prevention of tuberculosis in HIV infection. AIDS 1993;7:S195–S202.

Cotton D, Watts DH, eds. The medical management of AIDS in women. New York: John Wiley, 1996.

Dannemann B, McCutchan JA, Israelski D, et al. Treatment of toxoplasmic encephalitis in patients with AIDS. Ann Intern Med 1992;116:33–43.

Decker CF, Masur H. Current status of prophylaxis for opportunistic infections in HIV-infected patients. AIDS 1994;8:11–20.

Diagnostic tests for HIV. Med Lett 1997;39:81–83.

DiNubile MJ. Fever and neutropenia: Still a challenge. Contemp Intern Med 1995;7:35–45.

Drugs for HIV infection. Med Lett 1997;39:111–116.

Fischl MA, Richman DD, Grieco MH, et al. The efficacy of azidothymidine (AZT) in the treatment of patients with AIDS and AIDS-related complex. N Engl J Med 1987;317:185–191.

Fischl MA, Stanley K, Collier A, et al. Combination and monotherapy with zidovudine and zalcitabine in patients with advanced HIV disease. Ann Intern Med 1995;122:24–32.

Francis P, Walsh TJ. Current approaches to the management of fungal infections in cancer patients. Oncology 1992;6:81–91; 133–144.

Gallant JE, Moore RD, Chaisson RD. Prophylaxis for opportunistic infections in patients with HIV infection. Ann Intern Med 1994;120:932–944.

Gold J. HIV-1 infection, diagnosis, and management. Med Clin North Am 1992;76:1–18.

Holmberg SD, Moorman AC, Von Bargen JC, et al. Possible effectiveness of clarithromycin and Rifabutin for Cryptosporidiosis chemoprophylaxis in HIV disease. JAMA 1998;279:384–386.

Horsburgh CR Jr. *Mycobacterium avium* complex infection in the acquired immunodeficiency syndrome. N Engl J Med 1991;324:1332–1338.

Hughes WT, Armstrong D, Bodey GP, et al. Guidelines for the use of antimicrobial agents in neutropenic patients with unexplained fever: A statement by the Infectious Diseases Society of America. J Infect Dis 1990;161:381–396.

Jewett JF, Hecht FM. Preventive health care for adults with HIV infection. JAMA 1993;269:1144–1153.

Kahn JO, Lagakos SW, Richman DD, et al. A controlled trial comparing continued zidovudine with didanosine in human immunodeficiency virus infection. N Engl J Med 1992;327:582–587.

Karp JE, Merz WG, Charache P. Response to empiric amphotericin B during antileukemic therapy-induced granulocytopenia. Rev Infect Dis 1991;13:592–599.

Karp JE, Merz WG, Dick JD. Management of infections in neutropenic patients: New opportunities and emerging challenges. Curr Opin Infect Dis 1994;7:430–435.

Klastersky J. Empiric treatment of infection during granulocytopenia: A comprehensive approach. Infection 1989;17:59–64.

Kovacs JA, Masur H. Prophylaxis for *Pneumocystic carinii* pneumonia in patients infected with HIV. Clin Infect Dis 1992;14:1005–1009.

Lane HC, Laughon BE, Falloon J. Recent advances in the management of AIDS-related opportunistic infections. Ann Intern Med 1994;120:945–955.

Lee HH, Weiss SH, Brown LS, et al. Patterns of HIV-1 and HTLV I/II in intravenous drug abusers from the middle Atlantic and central regions of the USA. J Infect Dis 1990;162:347–352.

Levine DP, Sobel JD, eds. Infections in intravenous drug abusers. New York: Oxford University Press, 1991.

Luft BJ, Remington JS. Toxoplasmic encephalitis in AIDS. Clin Infect Dis 1992;15:211–222.

Masur H. Prevention and treatment of pneumocystis pneumonia. N Engl J Med 1992;327:1853–1860.

More new drugs for HIV and associated infections. Med Lett 1997;39:14–16.

New drugs for HIV infection. Med Lett 1996;38:35–38.

Nightingale SD, Byrd LT, Southern PM, et al. Incidence of *Mycobacterium avium-intracellulare* complex bacteremia in HIV-positive patients. J Infect Dis 1992;165:1082–1085.

Ong K, Iftikhar S, Glatt AE. Medical evaluation of the adult with HIV infection. Infect Dis Clin North Am 1994;8:289–301.

Pizzo PA. Management of fever in patients with cancer and treatment induced neutropenia. N Engl J Med 1993;328:1323–1332.

Roilides E, Pizzo PA. Perspectives on the use of cytokines in the management of infectious complications of cancer. Clin Infect Dis 1993;17:S385–S389.

Rolston KVI, Berkey P, Bodey GP, et al. A comparison of imipenem to ceftazidime with or without amikacin as empiric therapy in febrile neutropenic patients. Arch Intern Med 1992;152:283–291.

Rolston KVI, Bodey GP. Infections in patients with cancer. In: Holland JF, Frei E, Bast RC, et al., eds. Cancer medicine, 3rd ed. Philadelphia: Lea & Febiger, 1993;2416–2441.

Rubenstein EB, Rolston KVI, Benjamin RS, et al. Outpatient treatment of febrile episodes in low-risk neutropenic patients with cancer. Cancer 1993;71:3640–3646.

Rubin RH. Impact of cytomegalovirus infection on organ transplant recipients. Rev Infect Dis 1990;12:S754–S766.

Rubin RH. Infection in the organ transplant recipient. In: Rubin RH, Young LS, eds. Clinical approach to infection in the compromised host, 3rd ed. New York: Plenum, 1994;629–705.

Rubin RH. Nephrology forum: Infectious disease complications of renal transplantation. Kidney Int 1993;44:221–236.

Rubin RH, Tolkoff-Rubin NE. Antimicrobial strategies in the care of organ transplant recipients. Antimicrob Agents Chemother 1993;37:619–624.

Saag MS, Powderly WG, Cloud GA, et al. Comparison of amphotericin B with fluconazole in the treatment of acute AIDS-associated cryptococcal meningitis. N Engl J Med 1992;326:83–89.

Sable CA, Donowitz GR. Infections in bone marrow transplant recipients. Clin Infect Dis 1994;18:273–281.

Sande MA, Carpenter CCJ, Cobb CG, et al. Antiretroviral therapy for adult HIV-infected patients. JAMA 1993;270:2583–2589.

Sande MA, Volberding PA. The medical management of AIDS, 4th ed. Philadelphia: WB Saunders, 1995.

Sanford JP, Sande MA, Gilbert DN, et al. The Sanford guide to HIV/AIDS therapy. Dallas: Antimicrobial Therapy, 1994.

Schlager SI. Management of opportunistic infections in AIDS. I. Treatment. Amer J Therap 1998;5:45–49.

Selwyn PA, Hartel D, Lewis VA, et al. A prospective study of the risk of tuberculosis among intravenous drug users with HIV infection. N Engl J Med 1989;320:545–550.

Shearer WT, Paul ME, Smith CW, et al. Laboratory assessment of immune deficiency diseases. Immunol Allergy Clin North Am 1994;14:265–300.

Shlaes DM, Binczewski B, Rice LB. Emerging antimicrobial resistance and the immunocompromised host. Clin Infect Dis 1993;17:5527–5536.

Singh N, Carrigan DR. Human Herpesvirus-6 in transplantation: An emerging pathogen. Ann Intern Med 1996;124:1065–1071.

Smith P, Quinn T, Strober W, et al. Gastrointestinal infections in AIDS. Ann Intern Med 1992; 116:63–77.

Spach DH, Hooton TM, eds. The HIV manual: A guide to diagnosis and treatment. New York: Oxford University Press, 1996.

Studies of Ocular Complications of AIDS Research Group, ACTG. Mortality in patients with the acquired immunodeficiency syndrome treated with either foscarnet or ganciclovir for cytomegalovirus retinitis. N Engl J Med 1992;326:213–220.

Virella G, Patrick C, Goust JM. Diagnostic evaluation of lymphocyte functions and cell-mediated immunity. Immunol Ser 1993;58:291–310.

Wei X, Ghosh S, Taylor ME, et al. Viral dynamics in human immunodeficiency virus type 1 infection. Nature 1995;373:117–122.

Wheat LJ, Connolly-Stringfield PA, Baker RL, et al. Disseminated histoplasmosis in AIDS: Clinical findings, diagnosis, and treatment, and review of the literature. Medicine 1990;69:361–374.

Wilcox CM. Esophageal disease in AIDS: Etiology, diagnosis and management. Am J Med 1992;92:412–421.

CHAPTER 11—BACTEREMIA, SEPSIS, AND SHOCK:

Bone RC. Sepsis syndrome: New insights into its pathogenesis and treatment. Infect Dis Clin North Am 1991;5:793–805.

Bone RC. The pathogenesis of sepsis. Ann Intern Med 1991;115:457–469.

Bone RC. The systemic inflammatory response syndrome: Does the new name mean new therapies? Clin Immunother 1994;1:369–377.

Bone RC, Balk RA, Cerra FB, et al. Definitions for sepsis and organ failure and guidelines for the use of innovative therapies in sepsis. Chest 1992;101:1644–1655.

Bone RC, Fischer RJ, Clemmer TP, et al. A controlled clinical trial of high-dose methylprednisolone in the treatment of severe sepsis and septic shock. N Engl J Med 1989;317:653–658.

Corrigan JJ, Kiernat JF. Effect of heparin in experimental gram-negative septicemia. J Infect Dis 1975;131:138–143.

Demaria A, Hefferman JJ, Grindlinger GA, et al. Naloxone versus placebo in treatment of septic shock. Lancet 1985;1:1363–1365.

Jacobs R, Kaliner M, Shelhamer JH, et al. Blood histamine concentrations are not elevated in humans with septic shock. Crit Care Med 1989;17:30–35.

Harris RL, Musher DM, Bloom K, et al. Manifestations of sepsis. Arch Intern Med 1987;147:1895–1906.

Natanson C, Hoffman WD, Suffrendi AF, et al. Selected treatment strategies for septic shock based on proposed mechanisms of pathogenesis. Ann Intern Med 1994;120:771–783.

Ruokonen E, Takala J, Kari A, et al. Septic shock and multiple organ failure. Crit Care Med 1991;19:1146–1151.

Sheagren JN. Corticosteroids for the treatment of septic shock. Infect Dis Clin North Am 1991;5:875–882.

Sheagren JN. Mechanism-oriented therapy for multiple systems organ failure. Crit Care Clin 1989;5:393–409.

The Working Group on Severe Staphylococcal Infections. Defining the group A streptococcal toxic shock syndrome. JAMA 1993;269:390–391.

Todd JK. Therapy of toxic shock syndrome. Drugs 1990;39:856–861.

Young LS, Bone RC, Wenzel RP, Opal SM, eds. New immunotherapeutic strategies against gram-negative infections. Proceedings of the symposium on new immunotherapeutic strategies against gram-negative infections; 1992 Oct 14; Anaheim, CA. New York: Plenum, 1993.

CHAPTER 12—NOSOCOMIAL INFECTIONS AND FEVERS OF UNKNOWN ORIGIN:

Bach A, Boehrer H, Schmidt H, et al. Nosocomial sinusitis in ventilated patients. Nasotracheal versus orotracheal intubation. Anaesthesia 1992;47:335–339.

Bennett JV, Brachman PS, eds. Hospital infections, 3rd ed. Boston: Little, Brown, 1992.

Centers for Disease Control. Protection against viral hepatitis: Recommendations of the immunization practices advisory committee. MMWR 1990;39:17–22.

Cone JB, Bradsher R, Golladay S. Atypical surgical infections. Am J Surg 1988;156:522–523.

Dodd RY. Infectious complications of blood transfusion. Hematol Oncol Ann 1994;2:280–287.

Donowitz LG, Wenzel RP, Hoyt JW. High risk of hospital-acquired infection in the ICU. Crit Care Med 1982;10:355–357.

Dugdale DC, Ramsey PG. *Staphylococcus aureus* bacteremia in patients with Hickman catheters. Am J Med 1990;89:137–141.

Durack DT, Street AC. Fever of unknown origin—reexamined and redefined. Curr Clin Top Infect Dis 1991;11:35–51.

Fildes J, Bannon MP, Barret J. Soft-tissue infections after trauma. Surg Clin North Am 1991;71:371–384.

Gastinne H, Wolff M, Delatour F, et al. A controlled trial in intensive care units of selective decontamination of the digestive tract with nonabsorbable antibiotics. N Engl J Med 1992;326:594–599.

Geberding JL. Management of occupational exposures to blood-borne viruses. N Engl J Med 1995;332:444–451.

Goetz MB. Fever of unknown origin in the elderly. Infect Dis Clin Prac 1993;2:377–380.

Gold HS, Moellering RC Jr. Antimicrobial-drug resistance. N Engl J Med 1996;335:1445–1453.

Horan TC, Gaynes RP. CDC definitions of nosocomial surgical site infections, 1992. Am J Infect Control 1992;20:271–274.

Intravenous Immunoglobulin Collaborative Study Group. Prophylactic intravenous administration of standard immune globulin as compared with core lipopolysaccharide immune globulin in patients at high risk of postsurgical infection. N Engl J Med 1992;327:234–240.

Kazanjian PH. Fever of unknown origin: Review of 86 patients treated in community hospitals. Clin Infect Dis 1992;15:968–973.

Knockaert DC, Dujardin KS, Bobbaers HJ. Long-term follow-up of patients with undiagnosed fever of unknown origin. Arch Intern Med 1996;156:618–620.

Knockaert DC, Vanneste LJ, Vanneste SB, et al. Fever of unknown origin in the 1980s. Arch Intern Med 1992;152:51–55.

Larson EB, Featherstone HJ, Petersdorf RG. Fever of undetermined origin: Diagnosis and follow-up of 105 cases 1970—1980. Medicine 1982;61:269–292.

Mahul PH, Auboyer C, Jospe R, et al. Prevention of nosocomial pneumonia in intubated patients: Respective role of mechanical subglottic secretions drainage and stress ulcer prophylaxis. Intensive Care Med 1992;18:20–25.

Maki D, Jarrett F, Sarafin H. A semiquantitative method for identification of catheter-related infection in the burn patient. J Surg Res 1977;22:513–520.

Maki D, Weise C, Sarafin H. A semiquantitative method for identifying intravenous catheter-related infection. N Engl J Med 1977;296:1305–1309.

Maki DG, Alvarado CJ, Ringer MA. A prospective, randomized trial of povidone-iodine, alcohol, and chlorhexidine for prevention of infection with central venous and arterial catheters. Lancet 1991;338:339–343.

Maki DG, Ringer M. Risk factors for infusion-related phlebitis with small peripheral venous catheters. Ann Intern Med 1991;114:845–854.

Meakins JL, ed. Surgical infections: Diagnosis and treatment. New York: Scientific American, 1994.

Morrow JE, Braine HG, Kickler TS, et al. Septic reactions to platelet transfusions: A persistent problem. JAMA 1991;266:555–558.

Petersdorf RG. Fever of unknown origin: An old friend revisited. Arch Intern Med 1992;152:21–22.

Platt R, Polk BF, Murdock B, et al. Risk factors for nosocomial urinary tract infection. Am J Epidemiol 1986;124:977–985.

Raad I, Davis S, Becker M, et al. Low infection rate and long durability of nontunneled silastic catheters. Arch Intern Med 1993;153:1791–1796.

Raad I, Umphrey J, Khan A, et al. The duration of placement as a predictor of peripheral and pulmonary arterial catheter infections. J Hosp Infec 1993;23:17–26.

Rello J, Ausina V, Castella J, et al. Nosocomial respiratory tract infections in multiple trauma patients: Influence of level of consciousness with implications for therapy. Chest 1992;102:525–529.

Rodriguez JL, Gibbons KJ, Bitzer LG, et al. Pneumonia: Incidence, risk factors, and outcome in injured patients. J Trauma 1991;31:907–912.

Stamm WE. Catheter-associated urinary tract infections: Epidemiology, pathogenesis, and prevention. Am J Med 1991;91:65S–71S.

Stumacher RJ. Fever in the ICU (part I). Infect Dis Pract 1996;20:89–92.

Third international conference on hospital infections. J Hosp Infect 1995;30:1–253.

Wagner SJ, Friedman LI, Dodd RY. Transfusion-associated bacterial sepsis. Clin Microbiol Rev 1994;7:290–302.

Warren JW. The catheter and urinary tract infection. Med Clin North Am 1991;75:481–493.

Wenzel RP, ed. Prevention and control of nosocomial infections, 2nd ed. Baltimore: Williams & Wilkins, 1993.

Wong-Beringer A, Jacobs RA, Gugliemo BG. Treatment of funguria. JAMA 1992;267:2780–2785.

Yannelli B, Gurevich I, Schoch PE, et al. Yield of stool cultures, ova and parasite tests, and *Clostridium difficile* determinations in nosocomial diarrheas. Am J Infect Control 1988;16:246–249.

Zaza S, Tokars JI, Yomtovian R, et al. Bacterial contamination of platelets at a university hospital. Infect Control Hosp Epidemiol 1994;15:82–87.

CHAPTER 13—IMMUNIZATION:

ACP Taskforce on Adult Immunization and Infectious Diseases Society of America. Guide for adult immunization, 3rd ed. Philadelphia: American College of Physicians, 1994.

Averhoff FM, Williams WW, Hadler SC. Immunization of adolescents. Am Fam Phys 1997;55:159–167.

Centers for Disease Control and Prevention. Update on adult immunization. Recommendations of the immunization practices advisory committee (ACIP). MMWR 1991;40(RR-12):1–94.

Centers for Disease Control and Prevention. Recommendation of the ACIP: Diphtheria, tetanus, and pertussis: Guidelines for vaccine prophylaxis and other preventive measures. MMWR 1991;40(RR-10):1–28.

Centers for Disease Control and Prevention. Recommendations of the ACIP: Hepatitis B virus: A comprehensive strategy for eliminating transmission in the US through universal childhood vaccination. MMWR 1991;40(RR-13):1–25.

Centers for Disease Control and Prevention. Recommendations of the ACIP: Pneumococcal polysaccharide vaccine. MMWR 1989;64–68, 73–76.

Centers for Disease Control and Prevention. Recommendations of ACIP: Prevention and control of influenza. MMWR 1993;42(RR-6):1–14.

Centers for Disease Control and Prevention. Recommendations of the ACIP: Recommendations for use of *Haemophilus* b conjugate vaccines and a combined diphtheria tetanus pertussis and *Haemophilus* b vaccine. MMWR 1993;42(RR-13):1–31.

Centers for Disease Control and Prevention. Recommendations of the ACIP: Update on adult immunization. MMWR 1991;40(RR-12):1–94.

Centers for Disease Control and Prevention. Recommendations of the ACIP: Use of vaccines and immune globulins in persons with altered immunocompetence. MMWR 1993;42(RR-4):1–18.

Centers for Disease Control and Prevention. Standards for pediatric immunization practices recommended by the National Vaccine Advisory Committee, approved by the US Public Health Service. MMWR 1993;42(RR-5):1–13.

Committee on Infectious Diseases. American Academy of Pediatrics, report of the Committee on Infectious Diseases, 22nd ed. Elk Grove Village, IL:AAP, 1991.

Gardner P, Eickhoff T, Poland GA, et al. Adult immunizations. Ann Intern Med 1996;124:35–40.

Gardner P, Schaffner W. Immunization of adults. N Engl J Med 1993;328:1252–1258.

Immunization of adolescents [editorial]. JAMA 1997;277:202–207.

Influenza vaccine. Med Lett 1997;39:85–86.

Inni BL, Sritbhan R, Kunasol P, et al. Protection against hepatitis A by an inactivated vaccine. JAMA 1994;271:328–334.

Jong EC, McMullen R, eds. The travel and tropical medicine manual, 2nd ed. Philadelphia: WB Saunders, 1995.

Nichol KL, Lind A, Margolis KL, et al. The effectiveness of vaccination against influenza in healthy, working adults. N Engl J Med 1995;333:889–893.

Recommended childhood immunization schedule—United States, July–December 1996 [editorial]. JAMA 1996;276:775–776.

Recommended childhood immunization schedule—United States, 1997 [editorial]. JAMA 1997;277:371–372.

Recommended childhood immunization schedule—United States, 1998 [editorial]. JAMA 1998;279:495–496.

Waalen J. Vaccination rates for the elderly get a boost on several fronts. Ann Intern Med 1996;125:1–38.

Williams WW. CDC guideline for infection control in hospital personnel. Infect Control 1983;4:326–348.

Williamsen AR, Maish WA. It's here at last—the varicella vaccine. Clin Briefs Pharmacol 1996;5:23–25.

CHAPTER 14—PROPHYLAXIS:

American Thoracic Society. Control of tuberculosis in the United States. Am Rev Respir Dis 1992;146:1623–1633.

American Thoracic Society. Treatment of tuberculosis and tuberculosis infection I adults and children. Am J Respir Crit Care Med 1994;149:1359–1374.

Antimicrobial prophylaxis in surgery. Med Lett 1997;39:97–102.

Bayer AS, Nelson RJ, Slama TG. Current concepts in prevention of prosthetic valve endocarditis. Chest 1990;97:1203–1207.

Berrios X, del Campo E, Guzman B, et al. Discontinuing rheumatic fever prophylaxis in selected adolescents and young adults: A prospective study. Ann Intern Med 1993;118:401–406.

Brause BD. Prosthetic joint infections. Curr Opin Rheumatol 1989;1:194–198.

Centers for Disease Control. Antibiotic chemoprophylaxis for household or intimate contacts of serious meningococcal infection. MMWR 1976;25:56–74.

Classen DC, Evans RS, Pestonik SL, et al. The timing of prophylactic administration of antibiotics and the risk of surgical-wound infection. N Engl J Med 1992;32:281–286.

Committee on Isoniazid Preventive Treatment. Preventive treatment of tuberculosis. Chest 1985;875:1285–1325.

Dajani AS, Bisno AL, Chung KJ, et al. Prevention of bacterial endocarditis. Recommendations by the American Heart Association. JAMA 1990;264:2919–2922.

Dajani AS, Bisno AL, Chung KJ, et al. Prevention of rheumatic fever. A statement for health professionals by the Committee on Rheumatic Fever, Endocarditis, and Kawasaki Disease on the Council on Cardiovascular Diseases in the Young, AHA. Circulation 1988;78:1082–1086.

Dajani AS, Taubert KA, Wilson W, et al. Prevention of bacterial endocarditis. Recommendations by the American Heart Association. JAMA 1997;277:1794–1801.

Faro S, Martens MG, Hammill HA, et al. Antibiotic prophylaxis: Is there a difference? Am J Obstet Gynecol 1990;162:900–909.

Fong IW, Baker CB, McKee DC. The value of prophylactic antibiotics in aorta-coronary bypass operations: A double-blind randomized trial. J Thorac Cardiovasc Surg 1979;78:908–913.

Gantz NM. Applying the new guidelines for endocarditis prophylaxis. Contemp Intern Med 1991;11:14–20.

Horskotte D, Friedrichs W, Pippert H, et al. Benefits of endocarditis prevention in patients with prosthetic heart valves [German]. Z Kardiol 1986;75:8–11.

Kaiser AB. Drug therapy: Antimicrobial prophylaxis in surgery. N Engl J Med 1986;315:1129–1138.

Kaiser AB, Petracek MR, Lea JW IV, et al. Efficacy of cefazolin, cefamandole, and gentamicin as prophylactic agents in cardiac surgery. Ann Surg 1987;206:791–797.

Maderazo EG, Judson S, Pasternak H. Late infections of total joint prostheses: A review and recommendations for prevention. Clin Orthop 1988;229:131–142.

Nagachinta T, Stephens M, Reitz B. Risk factors for surgical-wound infection following cardiac surgery. J Infect Dis 1987;156:967–973.

Norden C. A critical review of antibiotic prophylaxis in orthopedic surgery. Rev Infect Dis 1983;5:928–932.

Page CP, Bohnen JMA, Fletcher JR, et al. Antimicrobial prophylaxis for surgical wounds: Guidelines for clinical care. Arch Surg 1993;128:79–88.

Penketh ARL, Wansbrough-Jones MH, Wright E, et al. Antibiotic prophylaxis for coronary artery bypass surgery. Lancet 1985;1:1500.

Platt R, Kaiser AB. International symposium on perioperative antibiotic prophylaxis. Rev Infect Dis 1991;13:S779–S894.

Simmons NA. Recommendations for endocarditis prophylaxis. J Antimicrob Chemother 1993;31:437–453.

CHAPTER 15—TRAVEL MEDICINE:

Advice for travelers. Med Lett 1996;38:17–20.

Centers for Disease Control and Prevention. Health information for international travel. Washington, DC: U.S. Government Printing Office, 1995.

DuPont HL, Ericsson CD. Prevention and treatment of traveler's diarrhea. N Engl J Med 1993;328:1821–1827.

Ericsson CD, DuPoint HL. Traveler's diarrhea: Approaches to prevention and treatment. Clin Infect Dis 1993;16:616–626.

Farthing MJG, Keusch GT, eds. Enteric infection: Mechanisms, manifestations, and management. New York: Raven Press, 1988.

Kelsall BL, Guerrant RL. Evaluation of diarrhea in the returning traveler. Infect Dis Clin North Am 1992;6:413–426.

Levine MM, Kaper JB. Live oral vaccines against cholera: An update. Vaccine 1993;11:207–212.

Lobel HO, Kozarsky PE. Update on prevention of malaria for travelers. JAMA 1997;278:1767–1771.

Lobel HO, Miani N, Eng T. Long-term malaria prophylaxis with weekly mefloquine. Lancet 1993;341:848–851.

MacLeod CI. The pregnant traveler. Med Clin North Am 1992;76:1313–1326.

Saxe SE, Gardner P. The returning traveler with fever. Infect Dis Clin North Am 1992;6:427–439.

Steffen R, Lobel HO, Haworth J, et al, eds. Travel medicine. Berlin: Springer-Verlag, 1989.

Sulaiman A, Ericsson CD. STDs: A travel risk. Contemp Intern Med 1995;7:49–50.

Swerdlow DL, Ries AA. Cholera in the Americas: Guidelines for the clinician. JAMA 1992;267:1495–1499.

Wolfe MS. Diseases of travelers. CIBA Clin Symp 1984;36(2):1–16.

Wood AJJ. Prevention and treatment of traveler's diarrhea. N Engl J Med 1993;328:1821–1827.

World Health Organization. International travel and health, vaccination requirements and health advice. Geneva: WHO, 1994.

Wyler DJ. Malaria chemoprophylaxis for the traveler. N Engl J Med 1993;329:31–37.

DRUG INDEX

1. Generic Drug Name [AWDP]

(Trade Names)   [AWDP]

I   II   III

Cat. D

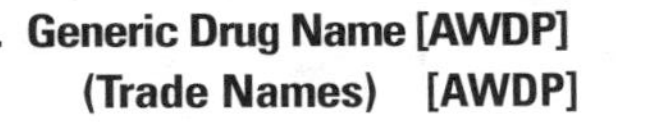

<u>Drug Interactions</u>

<u>Adverse Reactions</u>

VS:

LS: C:

FOOD: →   O:

ALCOHOL: →   R:

AWDP=average wholesale daily Rx price (based on 1997 Red Book prices); VS=very significant drug interaction, well documented for a potential for causing significant problems, including permanent damage to the patient or death; LS= less significant drug interaction which may occur but will likely not cause permanent harm to the patient; C=common reaction; O=reaction seen occasionally; R=rare reaction. [drug]=serum or plasma concentration of the drug.

PREGNANCY ICON indicates use in pregnancy ratings approved by FDA (X=contraindicated in pregnancy; D=positive evidence of risk in pregnancy; C=risk cannot be ruled out; B=no evidence of risk in humans; A=controlled studies showed no risk); and whether the drug is safe to use during breast feeding (1=safe to use; 2=not advisable to use during breast feeding, but must weigh the risk/benefit ratio, 3=contraindicated during breast feeding).

DOSAGE MODIFICATIONS ICONS indicate dosing changes for patients with renal or hepatic dysfunction. Renal dosing is based on GFR levels I (>50 ml/min), II (10–50 ml/min), or III (<10 ml/min).

Acyclovir [$5.10–7.73]
(Zovirax®) **[$5.43–8.20];**
(Zovirax® I.V.) **[$113.20]**

Dosage Modifications

	I	II	III
Cat. C ②	5 mg/kg q8h	5 mg/kg q12h	2.5 mg/kg q24h	None needed except in patients with cirrhosis

Drug Interactions

VS: Phenytoin →↓ [phenytoin]
Valproic acid →↓ [valproic acid]
LS: Probenecid →↑ [acyclovir]
Zidovudine → lethargy
FOOD: → NONE
ALCOHOL: → NONE

Adverse Reactions

C:
O: Abdominal pain
Anorexia
Headache
Injection site reaction
Nausea/vomiting
R: Encephalopathy
Reversible renal failure (IV only)

Albendazole [$1.40]
(Albenza®, Zentel®) [$3.50]

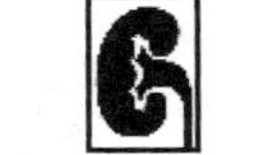 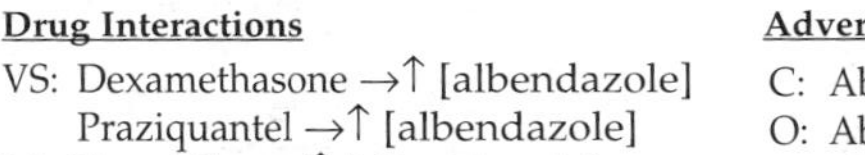

I II III

Drug Interactions

VS: Dexamethasone →↑ [albendazole]
    Praziquantel →↑ [albendazole]
LS: Cimetidine →↑ [albendazole]
FOOD: →↑ [albendazole]
ALCOHOL: → NONE

Adverse Reactions

C: Abnormal LFT's
O: Abdominal pain
   Nausea/vomiting
   Headache
R: Dizziness
   Meningeal signs
   Fever
   Rash
   Leukopenia

Cat. C
②

NONE

50% normal dose in patient with moderate to severe hepatic disease or extra-hepatic obstruction.

Amantadine HCl [$0.66]
(Symmetrel®) [$1.74]

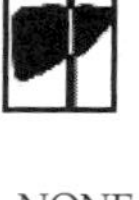 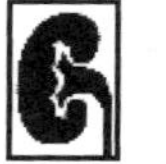 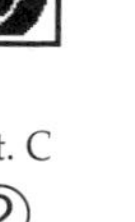 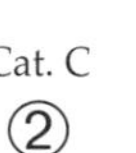

Dosage Modifications

Drug Interactions

VS: Trimethoprim →↑ [amantadine]
    Thiazides →↑ [amantadine]
    Anti-cholinergics → CNS effects
LS: Quinidine →↑ [amantadine]
FOOD: → NONE
ALCOHOL: → NONE

Adverse Reactions

C: Nausea
   Dizziness
   Insomnia
O: Anxiety
   Depression
   Hallucinations
   Irritability
   Confusion
   Anorexia
   Headache
   Abnl. dreams
   Dry nose/mouth
   Diarrhea
   Fatigue

R: CHF
   Psychosis
   Dyspnea
   Slurred speech
   ↑ BP
   ↓ Libido

Cat. C
②

I	200 mg × 1 on day 1, then 100 mg qd	
II	200 mg × 1 on day 1, then 100 mg qod	
III	200 mg q7d	

NONE

❶ **Not for use in children < 1 year of age!**

Amikacin sulfate
(Amikin®)   [$65.00]

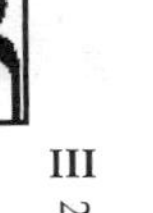

Dosage Modifications

Cat. D
①

I	II	III
60–90% of normal dose q12h	30–70% of normal dose q12–18h	20–30% of normal dose q24–48h

NONE

Drug Interactions

VS: Bumetanide → ototoxicity
Aminoglycosides → ototoxicity, nephrotoxicity
Furosemide → ototoxicity
NSAID's →↑ [amikacin]
Digoxin →↓ [digoxin]
Polypeptide → respiratory antibiotics depression
Cephalosporins → nephrotoxicity
Amphotericin B → nephrotoxicity
Penicillins →↓ amikacin activity

LS: Oral anticoagulants →↑ hypoprothrombinemia
Clindamycin → nephrotoxicity

FOOD: → NONE
ALCOHOL: → NONE

Adverse Reactions

C: Hearing loss
Loss of balance
↑ Serum creatinine (reversible)
O: Rash
R: Fever
Headache
Paresthesias
Tremor
Nausea
Arthralgia
Anemia
↓ BP
Muscle paralysis
Apnea

Amoxicillin [$0.24–0.92]
(Amoxil®, Polymox®, Wymox®, Trimox®)   [$0.63–1.68]

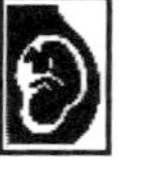

I — Normal dose q8h

II — Normal dose q8–12h

III — Normal dose q24h

Cat. B

① NONE

Drug Interactions

VS: Heparin →↑ risk of bleeding
Oral →↑ risk of bleeding anticoagulants
Methotrexate →↑ [methotrexate]
Chloramphenicol ⎫→ inhibit effect
Tetracyclines ⎭ of amoxicillin
LS: Atenolol →↓ effects of atenolol on BP and angina
Aminoglycosides →↓ [amoxicillin]
Oral contraceptives →↓ contraceptive effect
Allopurinol →↑ incidence of rash
FOOD: →↓ absorption
ALCOHOL: → NONE

Adverse Reactions

C: NONE
O: Nausea
Vomiting
Diarrhea
↑ SGOT (AST)
R: Rashes
Anemia
↓ Platelets
Agranulocytosis
Anxiety
Agitation
Confusion

❗ **Not for PCN-allergic patients!**

Amoxicillin + Clavulanic acid [$8.65]

(Augmentin®)   [$9.17];   (Pediatric)   [$4.51/10kg]

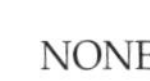 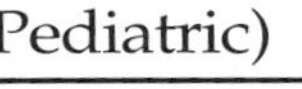

Drug Interactions

VS: Oral anticoagulants →↑ risk of
      bleeding
   Methotrexate →↑ [methotrexate]
   Tetracyclines   ⎫→↓ activity of
   Chloramphemicol   ⎭   amoxicillin
   Heparin →↑ risk of bleeding
   Atenolol →↓ atenol activity
         on BP + angina
LS: Erythromycin   ⎫→↓ activity of
   Aminoglycosides   ⎭   amoxicillin
   Oral contraceptives →↓ contraceptive
         effect
   Allopurinol →↑ incidence of rash
FOOD: ↓ absorption
ALCOHOL: → NONE

Adverse Reactions

C: Diarrhea
   Nausea
   Skin rash
   Urticaria
O: Vomiting
   Vaginitis
R: Abdominal pain
   Flatulence
   Headache
   Psuedomembranous colitis
   Stevens-Johnson syndrome
   ↑ LFT's
   Anemia

❶ **Not for PCN-allergic patients!**

Amphotericin B
(Fungizone®, ABLC®, Amphocin®, Abelcet®, AmBisome®)   [$16.60–38.50]

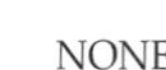

Dosage Modifications

| | Drug Interactions | Adverse Reactions | | | | | |

Drug Interactions

VS: Digoxin → digoxin toxicity
Corticosteroids →↓ K$^+$ and
    cardiotoxicity
Aminoglycosides → nephrotoxicity
Loop diuretics → nephrotoxicity
LS: Miconazole →↓ amphotericin
    activity
FOOD: → NONE
ALCOHOL: → NONE

Adverse Reactions

C: Fever, chills
↓ BP
Tachypnea
↓ Renal function
O: Flushing
Rash
Abnl LFT's
R: Shock
Cardiac failure
Pulmonary edema
Arrhythmias
Agranulocytosis
Tinnitus
Vertigo

Cat. B

②

I   II   III

Normal dose q24h

Normal dose q24h

Normal dose q24–36h

NONE

Ampicillin (oral) [$0.52]; (IV) [$7.96]

(Principen®, Marcillin®,
Omnipen®)   [$0.68–1.04];
(Totacillin®-N, Omnipen®-N)   [$15.52–17.11]

Drug Interactions

VS: Anticoagulants →↑ risk of bleeding
Cyclosporine →↑ [cyclosporine]
LS: Methotrexate →↑ [methotrexate]
Tetracyclines →↓ ampicillin effect
Chloramphenicol →↓ ampicillin effect
Atenolol →↓ [atenolol]
Erythromycin →↑ antibiotic effects
Aminoglycosides →↓ [ampicillin]
Oral contraceptives →↓ contraceptive effects
Allopurinol →↑ incidence of rash
FOOD: →↓ [ampicillin]
ALCOHOL: → NONE

Adverse Reactions

C: Nausea
Diarrhea
O: Dysgeusia
Vomiting
Glossitis
R: Skin rash
Urticaria
↑ SGOT (AST)
Anemia
Leukopenia
Fever

Dosage Modifications

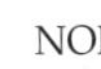

Cat. B ②

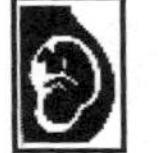

I Normal dose q8h
II Normal dose q12h
III Normal dose q24h

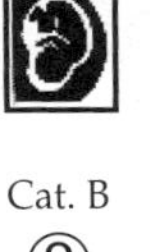

NONE

❶ Not for PCN-allergic patients!

Ampicillin + Sulbactam
(Unasyn®) [$29.98 – 54.92]

Drug Interactions

See Ampicillin

Adverse Reactions

C: Pain at injection site
O: Thrombophlebitis
   Diarrhea
   Rash
R: Nausea
   Pruritus
   Candidiasis
   Malaise
   Headache
   Abdominal discomfort
   Chills
   ↑ SGOT/SGPT (AST/ALT)
   Anemia
   Leukopenia

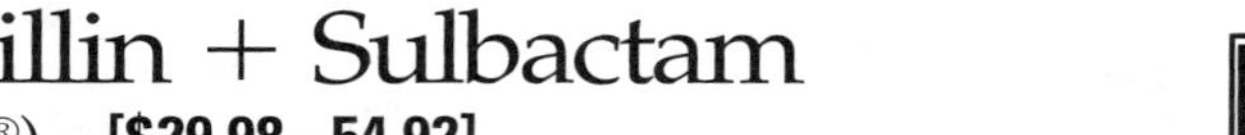

Cat. B
②

I   1.5–3.0 gm q6–8h

II   1.5–3.0 gm q12h

III   1.5–3.0 gm q24h

NONE

❶ **Not for PCN-allergic patients!**

Atovaquone
(Mepron®) **[$25.65]**

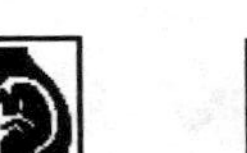

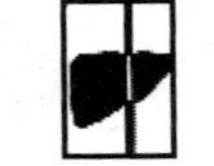

	I	II	III
Cat. C ②		NONE	NONE

Drug Interactions

VS: NONE
LS: Zidovudine→↑ [zidovudine]
    Rifampin → ↓ [atovaquone]
FOOD: →↑ atovaquone
      absorption 2X
      (*dose with food*)
ALCOHOL: → NONE

Adverse Reactions

C: Nausea
   Diarrhea
   Vomiting
O: Anorexia
   Dyspepsia
   Abdominal pain
   Constipation
   Oral monilial infections
R: Dizziness
   Anemia
   Neutropenia

Azithromycin
(Zithromax®) [$6.22]

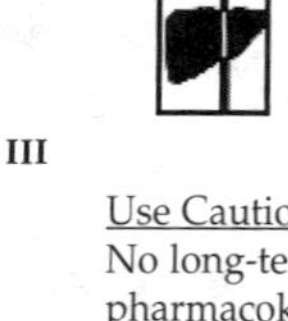

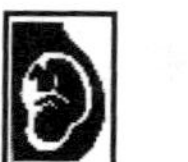

Dosage Modifications

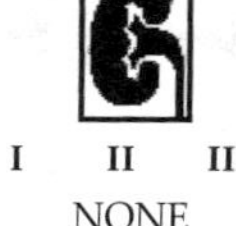

I	II	III

Drug Interactions

VS: None
LS: Tacrolimus →↑ risk of
         nephrotoxicity
FOOD: →↓ Azithromycin
         absorption
(Do not dose with food)
ALCOHOL: → NONE

Adverse Reactions

C: Diarrhea
   Nausea
   Abdominal pain
O: Dyspepsia
   Flatulence
R: Vaginitis
   Dizziness
   Headache
   Vertigo
   Fatigue
   Rash
   Angioedema

Cat. B
②

NONE

Use Caution
No long-term
pharmacoki-
netic data
available at
this time.

Aztreonam
(Azactam®)   [$36.22–108.65]

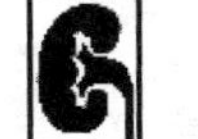

Drug Interactions

VS: NONE
LS: NONE
FOOD: → NONE
ALCOHOL: → NONE

Adverse Reactions

C: NONE
O: Abdominal cramps
R: Pseudomembranous
   colitis assoc/with
   C. difficile
   Rash
   Local phlebitis
     at injection site

Cat. B
①

I   II   III
     NONE   NONE
(But monitor renal and hepatic
function periodically while
drug is in use)

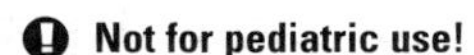 **Not for pediatric use!**

723

Bacitracin + neomycin + polymyxin solution
(Cortisporin® Ophthalmic/Otic)　[$25.59/15gm]

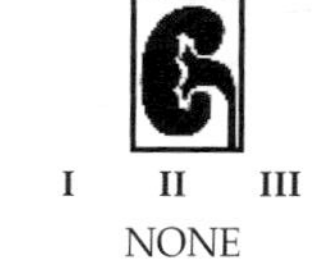

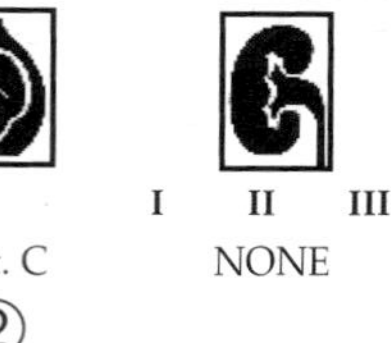

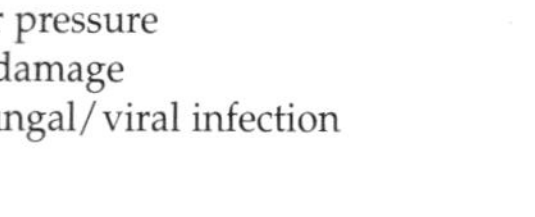

	I	II	III
Cat. C		NONE	NONE
②			

Drug Interactions
VS: NONE
LS: NONE
FOOD: → NONE
ALCOHOL: → NONE

Adverse Reactions
C: NONE
O: Conjunctival
　itching, swelling, erythema
R: Anaphylaxis
　↑ Intraocular pressure
　Optic nerve damage
　Secondary fungal/viral infection
　　of cornea

❶ **Not recommended for pediatric use!**

BCG vaccine
(Tice®)   **[$147.50]**

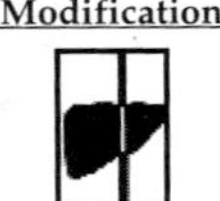

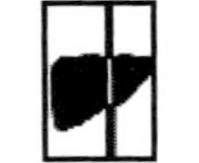

	Drug Interactions	Adverse Reactions		I	II	III

Drug Interactions

VS: Antibiotics →↓ immune response
to BCG
Immunosuppressive
agents →↓ immune response
to BCG
FOOD: → NONE
ALCOHOL: → NONE

Adverse Reactions

C: NONE
O: Regional lymphadenopathy
R: Osteomyelitis
Lupoid reaction
Disseminated BCG infection

Cat. C
②

I   II   III

NONE   NONE

Beznidazole
(Rochagan®)

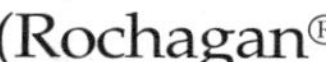

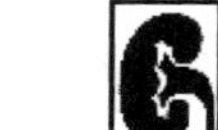
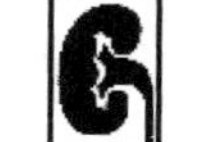

Drug Interactions

Adverse Reactions

Drug information is available from the Centers for Disease Control & Prevention, Center for Infectious Diseases, by calling (404) 639-3670 (8 AM–4:30 PM EST, M–F) or (404) 639-2888 (for emergencies).

Bismuth + metronidazole + tetracycline

(Helidac®)   [$5.55]

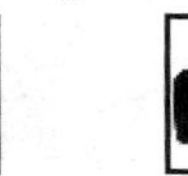 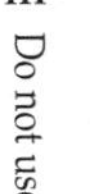 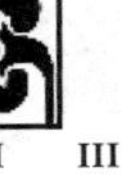 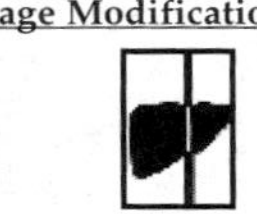

Drug Interactions	**Adverse Reactions**

VS: Methotrexate →↑ [methotrexate]
Corticosteroids →↑ risk of GI
    ulceration
Insulin → hypoglycemia
Oral antibiotics →↓ [antibiotic]
Anti-hypertensives →↓ effect on BP
Loop diuretics → salicylate toxicity
Anticoagulants →↑ risk of bleeding
Digitalis →↑ [digoxin]
LS: Cimetidine →↑ metronidazole
    toxicity
Carbamazepine →↑ [carbamazepine]
Phenytoin →↑ [phenytoin]
Iron →↓ [tetracycline]
FOOD: →↓ [tetracycline]
ALCOHOL: → disulfiram reaction

C: Nausea
   Diarrhea
   Abdominal pain
   Melena
O: Anal discomfort
   Anorexia
   Dizziness
   Paresthesia
   Vomiting
R: Asthenia
   Constipation
   Insomnia
   Pain
   URI
   Urticaria

Cat. D
③

I — Normal dose
II — Do not use
III — Do not use
Do not use

❶ **Not for pediatric use!**

(Burow's® solution) [$2.38/480 ml]

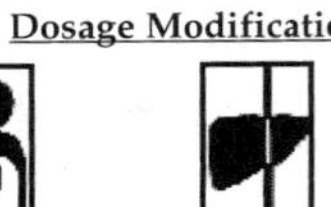 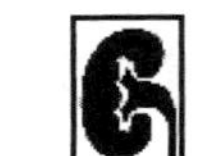 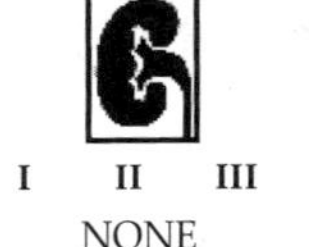 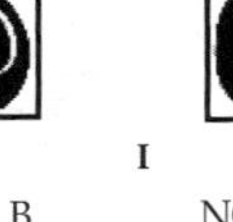 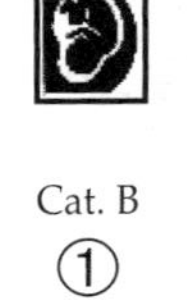

	I	II	III
Cat. B		NONE	NONE
①			

Drug Interactions

VS: NONE
LS: NONE
FOOD: → NONE
ALCOHOL: → NONE

Adverse Reactions

C: NONE
O: NONE
R: Local irritation

Capreomycin sulfate
(Capastat®)   [$22.53]

 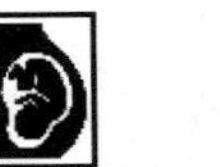

Drug Interactions

VS: Paromomycin → nephrotoxicity & respiratory depression
Cephalosporins → nephrotoxicity
Aminoglycosides → nephrotoxicity
LS: Methotrexate →↓ [methotrexate]
Phenothiazines → respiratory depression
Lidocaine → respiratory depression
FOOD: → NONE
ALCOHOL: → NONE

Adverse Reactions

C: Nephrotoxicity
Ototoxicity
Abnormal LFT's
O: Leukocytosis
Leukopenia
Injection site pain & induration
R: Bleeding at injection site
Sterile abcesses at injection site
Urticaria
Rash

Cat. C
②

	I	II	III
NONE	Not recom-mended	NONE

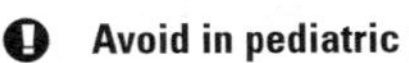 **Avoid in pediatric patients!**

Carbenicillin indanyl sodium
(Geocillin®)   [$7.68–15.36]

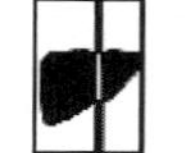
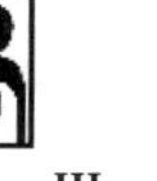
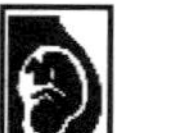

Drug Interactions

VS: Anticoagulants →↑ bleeding
    Cyclosporine →↕ [cyclosporine]
LS: Methotrexate →↑ [methotrexate]
    Tetracyclines →↓ carbenicillin
        effect
    Oral contraceptives →↓ contraceptive
        effect
    Chloramphenicol →↓ carbenicillin
        effect

FOOD: → NONE
ALCOHOL: → NONE

Adverse Reactions

C: Nausea
   Dysgeusia
   Diarrhea
   Flatulence
   Glossitis
O: Vomiting
   Abdominal cramps
   Dry mouth
R: Anemia
   Leukopenia
   Headache
   Itchy eyes
   Vaginitis
   ↑ SGOT (AST)

Cat. B
②

I   II   III

I   Normal dose q6h
II Normal dose q12h
III Normal dose q24h

NONE

❗ **Not for PCN-allergic patients!**
❗ **Avoid in pediatric patients!**

Cefaclor [$6.83]
(Ceclor®) [$9.83]; (PEDS) [$4.30/10kg]

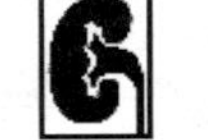

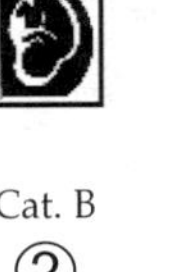

	I	II III
Cat. B	NONE	NONE
②		

Drug Interactions

VS: NONE

LS: Anticoagulants →↑ risk of
       bleeding

  Polypeptide
  antibiotics →↑ nephrotoxicity
  Aminoglycosides →↑ nephrotoxicity
  H2 blockers →↓ [cefaclor]
  Loop diuretics →↑ nephrotoxicity

FOOD: →↓ cefaclor absorption

ALCOHOL: → NONE

Adverse Reactions

C: Diarrhea

O: Eosinophilia
   Vaginitis

R: Serum sickness-like reaction
   Stevens-Johnson syndrome
   Hemolytic anemia
   Lymphocytosis
   Leukopenia
   Reversible hyperactivity
   Nausea
   Vomiting

❶ **Use with caution in PCN-allergic patients!**
❶ **Avoid in infants < 1 month old!**

Cefadroxil
(Duricef®) [$6.92–13.84]

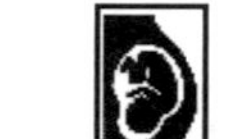
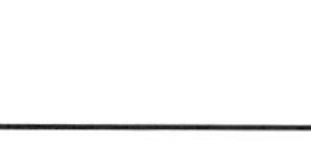
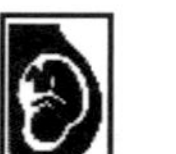 **Dosage Modifications**

Drug Interactions	Adverse Reactions				

Drug Interactions

VS: Oral anticoagulants →↑ risk of
      bleeding
    H2 antagonists →↓ [cefadroxil]
    Aminoglycosides →↑ nephrotoxicity
LS: Chloramphenicol →↓ cefadroxil
      activity
    Loop diuretics →↑ nephrotoxicity
FOOD: → NONE
ALCOHOL: → NONE

Adverse Reactions

C: Dyspepsia
   Nausea
O: Diarrhea
   Rash
   Urticaria
R: Vaginitis
   Neutropenia
   Stevens-Johnson syndrome
   Anaphylaxis

Cat. B
②

	I	II	III
	Normal dose q12h	Normal dose q24h	Normal dose q36h

NONE

❶ Use with caution in PCN-allergic patients!

Cefamandole
(Mandol®) [$36.26]

Dosage Modifications

	I	II	III	
Cat. B ②	1.2gm q4–6h	0.5–1.0 gm q8h	0.5gm q12h	NONE

Drug Interactions

VS: Aminoglycosides →↑ nephrotoxicity
FOOD: → NONE
ALCOHOL: → disulfiram-like
    reaction (nausea,
    vomiting, vasomotor
    instability)

Adverse Reactions

C: NONE
O: Pain at injection site
R: Nausea/vomiting
   Jaundice
   Rash
   Urticaria
   Anaphylaxis
   Thrombocytopenia
   Neutropenia
   ↑ SGOT/SGPT (AST/ALT)
   ↑ BUN

❗ **Use with caution in PCN-allergic patients!**

Cefazolin [$5.22]
(Ancef®, Kefzol®) [$11.19–14.52]

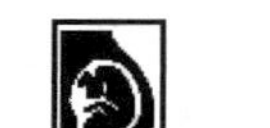 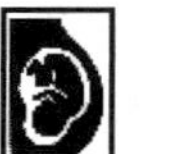 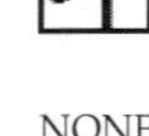

	I	II	III
Cat. B 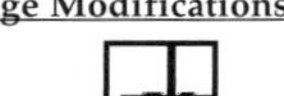	Normal dose q8h	Normal dose q12h	Normal dose q24–48h	NONE

Drug Interactions

VS: Oral antacids →↓ absorption
Oral anticoagulant →↑ risk of bleeding
Omeprazole
H-2 blockers } →↓ [cefazolin]
Aminoglycosides →↑ nephrotoxicity
LS: Chloramphenicol →↓ cefazolin activity
Loop diuretics →↑ nephrotoxicity
Probenecid →↑ [cefazolin]
FOOD: → NONE
ALCOHOL: → NONE

Adverse Reactions

C: Anaphylaxis in PCN-allergic patients
Diarrhea
O: Oral thrush
Nausea
Abdominal cramps
R: ↑ LFT's
Rash
Vomiting
Drug fever
Phlebitis at injection site

❶ **Use with caution in PCN-allergic patients!**

Cefixime

(Suprax®) [$7.21]

	I	II	III
Cat. B	400 mg qd	300 mg qd	200 mg qd	NONE
②			

Drug Interactions

VS: Antacids →↓ [cefixime]
Anticoagulant →↑ risk of bleeding
H2 antagonists →↓ [cefixime]
Aminoglycosides →↑ nephrotoxocity
LS: Chloramphenicol →↓ cefimine
activity
Loop diuretics →↑ nephrotoxicity
FOOD: → NONE
ALCOHOL: → NONE

Adverse Reactions

C: Diarrhea
Nausea
Dyspepsia
Flatulence
Abdominal pain
O: Vomiting
R: Skin rash
Urticaria
↑ SGPT/SGOT (ALT/AST)
↑ BUN/creatinine
Headache
Thrombocytopenia
Vaginitis
Anaphylaxis

❗ **Use with caution in PCN-allergic patients!**
❗ **Avoid in infants < 6 months old!**

Cefoperazone
(Cefobid®)   [$35.14 – 43.67]

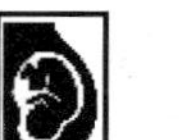 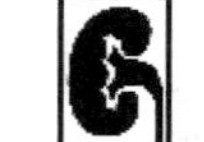 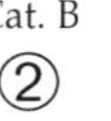

Drug Interactions

VS: Anticoagulants →↑ risk of bleeding
Aminoglycosides →↑ nephrotoxicity
LS: Loop diuretics →↑ nephrotoxicity
FOOD: → NONE
ALCOHOL: → disulfiram-like reactions
(nausea, vomiting,
vasomotor instability,
hypotension)

Adverse Reactions

C: Nausea
Dyspepsia
Diarrhea
O: Neutropenia
Anemia
R: ↑ SGOT/SGPT (AST/ALT)
↑ BUN/creatinine
Pain at injection site

Cat. B
②

	I	II	III
		NONE	NONE, but total daily dosage should not exceed 4gm

❶ Use with caution in PCN-allergic patients!
❶ Avoid in pediatric patients!

Cefotaxime
(Claforan®) [$45.08–84.64]

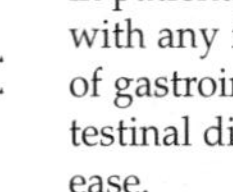 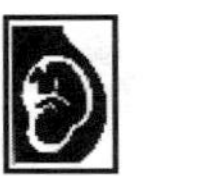 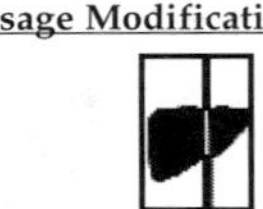

Drug Interactions

VS: Anticoagulants →↑ risk of bleeding
    Aminoglycosides →↑ nephrotoxicity
LS: Loop diuretics →↑ nephrotoxicity
FOOD: → NONE
ALCOHOL: → NONE

Adverse Reactions

C: Injection site pain & inflammation
O: Rash
   Pruritus
   Fever
   Diarrhea
   Nausea
   Vomiting
R: Arrhythmias
   Neutropenia
   Thrombocytopenia
   Vaginitis
   Headache
   ↑ SGOT/SGPT (AST/ALT)
   ↑ BUN/creatinine
   Pseudomembranous colitis

Cat. B
②

I — Normal dose

II — 50% normal dose

III — 50% normal dose

NONE, but use with caution in patients with any form of gastrointestinal disease.

❶ Use with caution in PCN-allergic patients!

Cefotetan
(Cefotan®)   **[$23.16–46.32]**

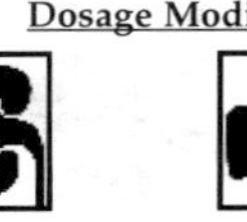

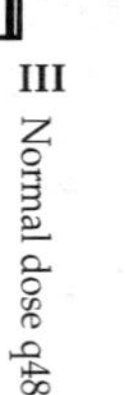

Drug Interactions

VS: Anticoagulants →↑ risk of bleeding
Aminoglycosides →↑ nephrotoxicity
LS: Loop diuretics →↑ nephrotoxicity
FOOD: → NONE
ALCOHOL: → disulfiram-like reaction
(nausea, vomiting,
vasomotor instability,
hypotension,
flushing, headache)

Adverse Reactions

C: Diarrhea
Nausea
O: Eosinophilia
Thrombocytosis
⊕ Coombs test
↑ SGOT/SGPT (AST/ALT)
↑ BUN/creatinine
R: Agranulocytosis
Hemolytic anemia
↑ Prothrombin time
Nephrotoxicity
Fever
Pseudomembranous colitis

Cat. B
②

I   II   III

Normal dose q12h
Normal dose q24h
Normal dose q48h

NONE, but use
with caution
in patients
with any form
of gastroin-
testinal dis-
ease.

❶ **Use with caution in PCN-allergic patients!**
❶ **Avoid use in pediatric patients!**

Cefoxitin
(Mefoxin®)   **[$41.28–78.84]**

Drug Interactions

VS: Anticoagulants →↑ risk of bleeding
Aminoglycosides →↑ nephrotoxicity
LS: Loop diuretics →↑ nephrotoxicity
FOOD: → NONE
ALCOHOL: → NONE

Adverse Reactions

C: Pain and tenderness at injection
site
Diarrhea
O: Thrombophlebitis
R: Rash
Nausea/vomiting
Exacerbation of myasthenia gravis
Eosinophilia
Leukopenia
Anemia
↑ SGOT/SGPT (AST/ALT)
↑ BUN/creatinine

Cat. B
②

	I	II	III
	1–2 gm q8–12h	1–2 gm q12–24h	0.5–1 gm q24–48h
			NONE

❗ **Use with caution in PCN-allergic patients!**
❗ **Avoid in infants < 3 months old!**

Ceftazidime

(Fortaz®, Ceptaz®, Tazicef®, Tazidime®)   **[$42.68–82.80]**

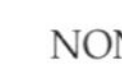

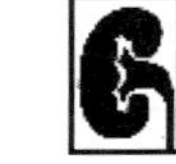

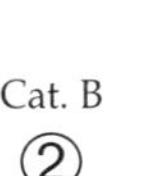

Drug Interactions

VS: Anticoagulants → ↑ risk of bleeding
    Aminoglycosides → ↑ nephrotoxicity
LS: Loop diuretics → ↑ nephrotoxicity
FOOD: → NONE
ALCOHOL: → NONE

Adverse Reactions

C: Local pain and inflammation at
    injection site
O: Diarrhea
    Nausea/vomiting
    Abdominal pain
    Rash
    Pruritus
    Fever
    Eosinophilia
R: Headache
    Dizziness
    Pseudomembranous colitis
    Vaginitis
    Hemolytic anemia
    ↑ SGOT/SGPT (AST/ALT)
    Renal dysfunction

Cat. B
②

	I	II	III
	1 gm q12h	1 gm q24h	500 mg q24–48h
			NONE

❗ **Use with caution in PCN-allergic patients!**

Ceftizoxime

(Cefizox®)   [$23.05–69.15]

Drug Interactions

VS: Anticoagulants →↑ risk of bleeding
Aminoglycosides →↑ nephrotoxicity
LS: Loop diuretics →↑ nephrotoxicity
FOOD: → NONE
ALCOHOL: → NONE

Adverse Reactions

C: NONE
O: Rash
Fever
↑ SGOT/SGPT (AST/ALT)
Eosinophilia
Thrombocytosis
⊕ Coombs test
Injection site burning
Diarrhea
R: Numbness
Anaphylaxis
↑ BUN/creatinine
Anemia
Vaginitis
Pseudomembranous colitis

Cat. B
②

I   II   III

500 mg q8h   250–500 mg q12h   500 mg q48h   NONE

❶ **Use with caution in PCN-allergic patients!**
❶ **Avoid in infants < 6 months old!**

Ceftriaxone
(Rocephin®) [$70.57–141.14]

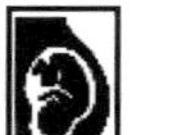

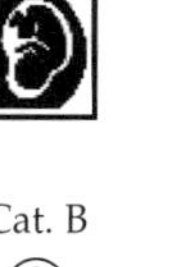

I   II   III

Drug Interactions	**Adverse Reactions**

VS: Anticoagulants →↑ risk of bleeding
    Aminoglycosides →↑ nephrotoxicity
LS: Loop diuretics →↑ nephrotoxicity
FOOD: → NONE
ALCOHOL: → NONE

C: Injection site reactions
   Rash
   Diarrhea
   Eosinophilia
   ↑SGOT/SGPT (AST/ALT)
   Thrombocytosis
O: Leukopenia
   ↑ BUN
R: Pruritus
   Fever
   Anemia
   Nausea
   ↑ Creatinine
   Vaginitis
   Diaphoresis
   Jaundice

Cat. B
②

NONE needed with dosages up
to 2 gm/day

❶ **Use with caution in PCN-allergic patients!**

Cefuroxime axetil (oral) [$6.55–13.10]
(Ceftin®) [$6.64–13.28]

Drug Interactions

VS: Loop diuretics →↑ nephrotoxicity
Antacids →↓ absorption of
cefuroxime
FOOD: →↑ absorption of cefuroxime
(37–52%)
ALCOHOL: → NONE

Adverse Reactions

C: Diarrhea
Nausea
↑ SGOT/SGPT (AST/ALT)
Eosinophilia
O: ↑ LDH
R: Abdominal pain
Flatulence
Headache
Vaginitis
Rash
Dysuria
Chest pain
Shortness of breath
Mouth ulcers
⊕ Coombs test
Tachycardia

I II III

Cat. B
②

Avoid in
patients with
renal dysfunc-
tion.

NONE

❶ **Use with caution in PCN-allergic patients!**

Cefuroxime sodium (IV) [$37.26]
(Kefurox®, Zinacef®) **[$40.38–41.82]**

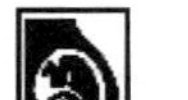

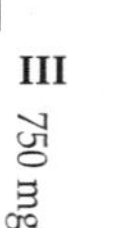

Drug Interactions

VS: Anticoagulants →↑ risk of bleeding
Aminoglycosides →↑ nephrotoxicity
LS: Loop diuretics →↑ nephrotoxicity
FOOD: → NONE
ALCOHOL: → NONE

Adverse Reactions

C: Local injection site reactions
Thrombophlebitis
O: Diarrhea
Nausea
Rash
Pruritus
Anemia
Eosinophilia
↑ SGOT/SGPT (AST/ALT)
↑ LDH
R: Neutropenia
Colitis
↑ Prothrombin time

Cat. B
②

I   II   III

I   750 mg–1.5 gm q8h
II 750 mg q12h
III 750 mg q24h
NONE

 Use with caution in PCN-allergic patients!
Avoid in patients < 3 months old!

Cephalexin [$2.56–5.04]
(Keflex®, Bio-Cef®)   **[$5.96–11.48]**;
PED-(Ed-A-Ceph®)   **[$3.58–6.89]**

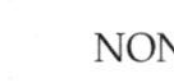 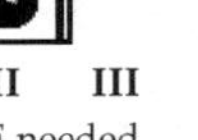 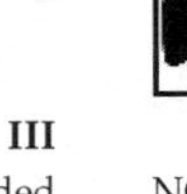

Drug Interactions

VS: Anticoagulants →↑ risk of bleeding
    Aminoglycosides →↑ nephrotoxicity
LS: Loop diuretics →↑ nephrotoxicity
    H2 antagonists →↓ absorption
FOOD: →↓ cephalexin absorption
ALCOHOL: → NONE

Adverse Reactions

C: Diarrhea
   Dyspepsia
   Gastritis
O: Rash
   Urticaria
R: Vaginitis
   Jaundice
   ↑ SGPT/SGOT (AST/ALT)
   Headache
   Confusion
   Eosinophilia
   Neutropenia
   Thrombocytopenia

Cat. B⊕
③

I   II   III

NONE needed   NONE
with dosages
up to 2gm/day

❶ †But safety for use during pregnancy has *not* been established!
❶ Use with caution in PCN-allergic patients!

Cephalothin
(Keflin®)   [$64.80]

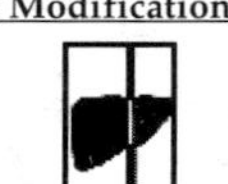

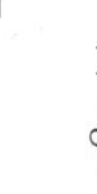
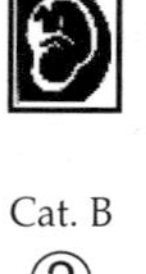

	I	II	III
Cat. B 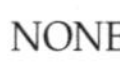	2 gm q6h	1–1.5 gm q6h	0.5 gm q6–8h	NONE

Drug Interactions

VS: Anticoagulants →↑ risk of bleeding
    Aminoglycosides →↑ nephrotoxicity
LS: Loop diuretics →↑ nephrotoxicity
FOOD: → NONE
ALCOHOL: → NONE

Adverse Reactions

C: Local injection site irritation
   Nausea
   Dyspepsia
O: Diarrhea
   ↑ SGOT/SGPT (AST/ALT)
   Anemia
   Eosinophilia
   Rash
   Thrombocytosis
R: ⊕ Coomb's test
   ↑ Creatinine
   Colitis
   Vaginitis

❶ Use with caution in PCN-allergic patients!

Cephradine (oral) [$1.24]
(Velosef®) **[$3.24]**

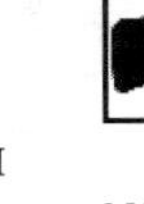

	I	II	III
Cat. B 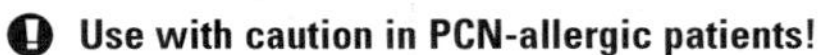	500 mg q6h	250 mg q6h	250 mg q12h	NONE

Drug Interactions

VS: Antacids →↓ absorption
Anticoagulants →↑ risk of
bleeding
H2 antagonists →↓ absorption
Aminoglycosides →↑ nephrotoxicity
LS: Loop diuretics →↑ nephrotoxicity
FOOD: →↓ absorption
ALCOHOL: → NONE

Adverse Reactions

C: Nausea
Dyspepsia
O: Diarrhea
Rash
↑ SGOT/SGPT (AST/ALT)
Anemia
Eosinophilia
Thrombocytosis
R: ⊕ Coomb's test
↑ Creatinine
Colitis
Vaginitis

❶ **Use with caution in PCN-allergic patients!**

Chloramphenicol succinate [$12.45]
(Chloromycetin®); (Chloromycetin® Kapseals)

Drug Interactions

VS: Phenytoin →↑ [phenytoin]
Anticoagulants →↑ risk of
    bleeding
Oral hypoglycemics →↑ hypoglycemic
    effects
Barbiturates →↑ [barbiturate]
LS: Rifampin →↓ [chloramphenicol]
PCN →↓ PCN activity
Iron →↑ [iron]
Vitamin B_{12} →↓ B_{12} effects
FOOD: → NONE
ALCOHOL: → NONE

Adverse Reactions

C: *Bone marrow depression →*
   aplastic anemia
   Pancytopenia
O: Nausea/vomiting
   Glossitis
   Stomatitis
   Colitis
   Headache
   Confusion
   Delirium
   "Gray syndrome" in children
R: Leukemia

I	II	III
Cat. D	NONE	Monitor chloramphenicol serum levels q2–4 days, and adjust dosage to achieve peak levels of 10–20 µg/ml and trough levels of 5–10 µg/ml
③		

❶ **Do not give intramuscularly! Change to oral therapy promptly!**
❶ **Use only in *serious* infections in hospital!**

Chloroquine phosphate [$3.77]
(Aralen®) [$3.89]

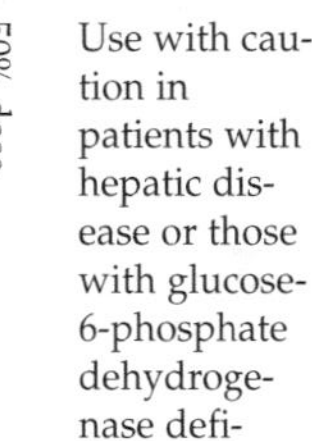

	I	II	III
Cat. C ②	Normal dose	Normal dose	50% dose	Use with caution in patients with hepatic disease or those with glucose-6-phosphate dehydrogenase deficiency.

Drug Interactions

VS: Digoxin →↑ [digoxin] → toxicity
Cyclosporine → nephrotoxicity
Praziquantel →↓ [praziquantel]

LS: Antacids →↓ chloroquine absorption
Methotrexate →↓ methotrexate effect on rheumatic disease
Cimetidine →↑ chloroquine effect

FOOD: → NONE
ALCOHOL: → NONE

Adverse Reactions

C: Nausea
Abdominal cramps
Anorexia

O: Diarrhea
Vomiting

R: Retinal damage
Seizures
Pleomorphic skin eruptions
Muscular weakness

❶ **Avoid in patients with psoriasis!**

Cholera vaccine [$9.69]

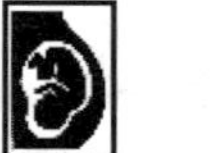 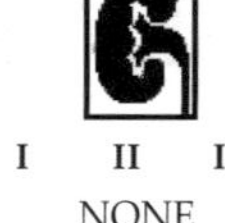

	I	II	III
Cat. C 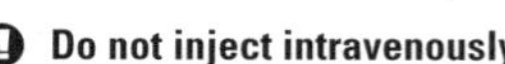	NONE		NONE

Drug Interactions

VS: Concomitant yellow fever vaccine →↓ levels of antibody response to both vaccines (should be given at least 3 weeks apart)

FOOD: → NONE

ALCOHOL: → NONE

Adverse Reactions

C: Local injection reaction (pain, redness)
Malaise
Headache
Fever for 48 to 72 hr

❶ Do not inject intravenously!

Ciclopirox topical cream 1%
(Loprox®)   [$11.58/15 gm]

Drug Interactions
NONE
FOOD: → NONE
ALCOHOL: → NONE

Adverse Reactions
C: None
O: Application site reactions
   Pruritus
   Burning
R: None

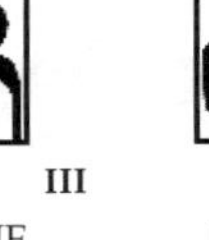

I   II   III

Cat. B   NONE   NONE
②

❗ **Avoid use in children < 10 years old!**

Cidofovir
(Vistide®)   [$706.80]

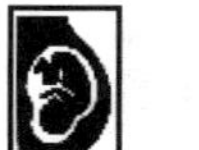

Dosage Modifications

Drug Interactions	Adverse Reactions		I	II	III
VS: Probenecid → ↑ [cidofovir] FOOD: → NONE ALCOHOL: → NONE	C: *Nephrotoxicity* *Neutropenia* Proteinuria O: Fanconi's syndrome ↑ Creatinine Fever Dyspnea Nausea/vomiting Diarrhea Asthenia/anorexia R: Ocular hypotony Allergic reaction Oral candidiasis	Cat. C ③	Do not use in patients with creatinine clearance rate < 55 ml/min. Monitor renal function prior to each dose		NONE

- Avoid use in pediatric patients!
- Administer with Probenecid!
- Administer only after IV prehydration!

Ciprofloxacin

(Cipro® oral)   [$6.84];   (Cipro® IV)
[$30.01–60.02]

Drug Interactions

VS: Iron →↓ [ciprofloxacin] (oral)
Antacid →↓ [ciprofloxacin] (oral)
Theophylline →↑ [theophylline]
Anticoagulant →↑ risk of bleeding
H2 blocker→↓ [ciprofloxacin] (oral)
LS: Mitoxanthone →↓ [ciprofloxacin]
(oral)
Caffeine →↑ caffeine effects
Valium →↑ [valium]
Mexiletene →↑ [mexiletene]
Procainamide →↑ [procamamide]
FOOD (dairy): →↓ ciprofloxacin
oral absorption
ALCOHOL: → NONE

Adverse Reactions

C: Nausea
Diarrhea
Vomiting
Dyspepsia
O: Headache
Restlessness
Rash
↑ SGPT/SGOT (ALT/AST)
R: Eosinophilia
Leukopenia
Thrombocytosis
Vaginitis
↑ Creatinine

Cat. C
③

I II III

Normal dose
50% normal dose q12–18h
25–50% normal dose q18–24h
NONE

❗ **Do not use in patients < 18 years old!**

Ciprofloxacin ophthalmic solution 0.3%

(Ciloxan®)   [$11.88/2.5 ml]

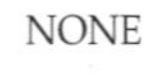

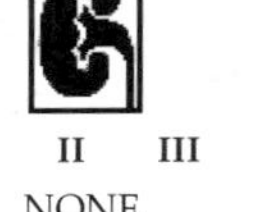 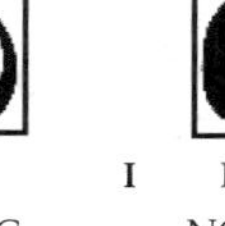 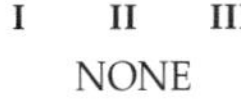

	I	II	III
Cat. C ②		NONE	NONE

Drug Interactions

NONE
FOOD: → NONE
ALCOHOL: → NONE

Adverse Reactions

C: Local burning and discomfort
O: Lid margin crusting
   Conjunctival hyperemia and itching
R: Corneal staining
   Keratopathy
   Allergic reactions
   Lid edema
   Tearing
   Photophobia
   Nausea
   ↓ Vision

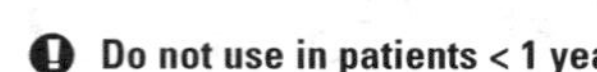 **Do not use in patients < 1 year old!**

Clarithromycin
(Biaxin®) [$6.90–11.35]

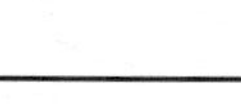
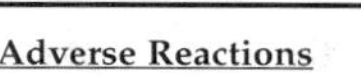

Drug Interactions

VS: *Terfenadine* → *cardiac arrhythmias*
Anticoagulants →↑ risk of bleeding
Digoxin →↑ [digoxin]
Cisapride → cardiotoxicity
Cyclosporine → nephrotoxicity & neurotoxicity
Ergot alkaloids →↑ ergot toxicity
Theophylline →↑ [theophylline]

LS: Zidovudine →↓ [zidovudine]
Carbamazepine →↑ [carbamazepine]

FOOD: → NONE
ALCOHOL: → NONE

Adverse Reactions

C: Diarrhea
Nausea
Dysgeusia
Dyspepsia
Headache

O: Personality changes
Urticaria

R: ↑ SGOT/SGPT (AST/ALT)
Leukopenia
↑ Prothrombin time
↑ BUN/creatinine

Cat. C⊕
②

I   500 mg q8h–q12h
II   250 mg q12h
III 250 mg q24h

NONE

❶ †Use in pregnant women should be avoided!
❶ Do not use in patients < 6 months old!
❶ Do not use with Terfenadine!

Clindamycin (oral) [$2.97–5.95]; (IV) [$12.33]
(Cleocin®) **[$3.81–7.59]**; (Cleocin® I.V.) **[$33.95]**

	I	II	III
		NONE	NONE

Drug Interactions

VS: Antacids →↓ clindamycin oral
absorption
Muscle relaxants and
neuromuscular blocking
agents →↑ neuromuscular
blockade and
respiratory depression

LS: Aminoglycosides →↑ nephrotoxicity
Erythromycin →↓ antibiotic
effectiveness of
both drugs

FOOD: → NONE
ALCOHOL: → NONE

Adverse Reactions

C: Nausea
Vomiting
Abdominal pain

O: Dysgensia
Rash
Severe colitis
↑ SGOT/SGPT (AST/ALT)
Jaundice
Neutropenia

R: Hypotension
Polyarthritis
Renal dysfunction

Safety for
use during
pregnancy
has not
been
estab-
lished

③

Clindamycin 1% solution/gel

[$9.75/30 ml]

(Cleocin® T)   [$12.80/30 ml]

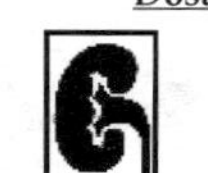

	I	II	III
Cat. B ②		NONE	NONE

Drug Interactions

VS: Erythromycin topical
gel → antagonism
with Cleocin T
FOOD: → NONE
ALCOHOL: → NONE

Adverse Reactions

C: Burning
Itching
Dryness
Erythema
Peeling
O: Abdominal pain
R: Severe colitis

❗ Use with caution in atopic patients!
❗ Do not use in patients < 12 years old!

Clindamycin vaginal cream 2%
(Cleocin® vaginal) [$30.23/40 gm]

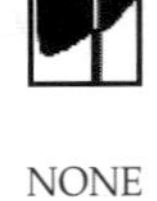 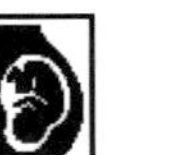 

	I	II	III
	Cat. B	NONE	NONE
	②		

Drug Interactions

See clindamycin
(oral/IV)—up to
11% of vaginally
administered dose
is absorbed systemically
after 7 days of dosing

Adverse Reactions

C: Cervicitis
   Vaginitis
   Amnionitis
   Endometritis
   UTI
O: Labor disorders
   Preeclampsia
   Labor induction
   Abruptio placenta
   Hypertention
   Gestational diseases
   Headache
R: Dyspepsia
   Constipation

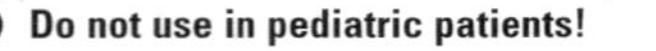 **Do not use in pediatric patients!**

Clofazimine
(Lamprene®)   **[$0.28]**

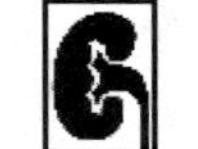

I   II   III

Cat. C   NONE   NONE

③

Drug Interactions

VS: NONE
LS: Dapsone →↓ activity of
        clofazimine
FOOD: → NONE
ALCOHOL: → NONE

Adverse Reactions

C: Discoloration of skin to
      brownish-black
   Ichthyosis
   Abdominal pain
   Diarrhea/vomiting
O: Rash
   Pruritus
   Conjunctional discoloration
R: Phototoxicity
   GI bleeding
   Hepatitis
   Depression

❶ **Avoid use in pediatric patients!**

Clotrimazole cream/lotion, 1%

[$9.44/15 gm cream; $15.52/30 ml lotion]
(Lotrimin®)   [$12.86/15 gm cream;
$24.66/30 ml lotion]

Dosage Modifications

I   II   III

Cat. B   NONE   NONE

②

Drug Interactions

NONE
FOOD: → NONE
ALCOHOL: → NONE

Adverse Reactions

C: Skin irritation
   Erythema
   Stinging
O: Peeling
   Pruritus
   Urticaria
R: Burning
   Blistering
   Edema

Clotrimazole oral solution/ troche, 10 mg [$3.94]
(Mycelex®) [$4.10]

Dosage Modifications

	I	II	III
Cat. C		NONE	NONE
②			

Drug Interactions

NONE
FOOD: → NONE
ALCOHOL: → NONE

Adverse Reactions

C: ↑ SGOT (AST)
O: Nausea
   Vomiting
   Dysgeusia
   Pruritus
R: NONE

❗ **Do not use in patients < 3 years old!**

Clotrimazole vaginal cream 1%
(Gyne Lotrimin®, Mycelex® G)   [$27.63/90 gm]

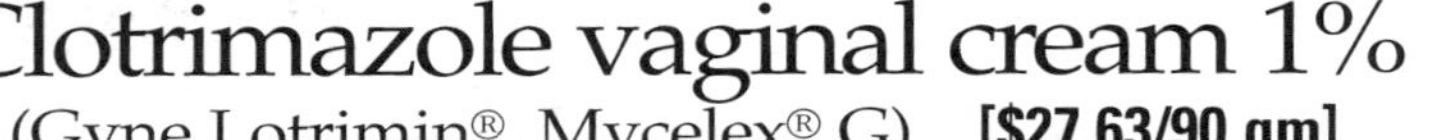 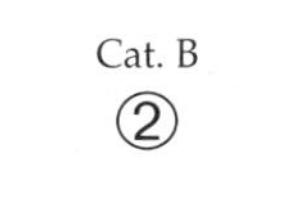 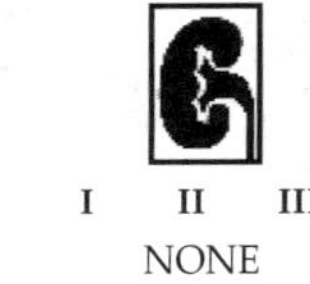

	I	II	III

Drug Interactions

NONE
FOOD: → NONE
ALCOHOL: → NONE

Adverse Reactions

C: NONE
O: Vulvar irritation
   Pruritus
   Abdominal discomfort
R: Dyspareunia
   Irritation in sexual partner

Cat. B
②

NONE   NONE

Clotrimazole + betamethasone topical cream
(Lotrisone®)   [$20.03/15 gm]

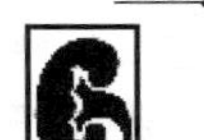

Dosage Modifications

	I	II	III
Cat. B ②		NONE	NONE

Drug Interactions

Dependent on degree of systemic absorption

↑Absorption augmented by
— Prolonged use
— Use over large surface areas
— Use under occlusive dressings

⊕ AVOID ALL OF THE ABOVE.

Adverse Reactions

C: Erythema
Stinging
Blistering
Peeling of skin
Pruritus

O: Paresthesia
Rash

R: Contact dermatitis
Secondary infection
Skin atrophy
Miliaria
Suppression of HPA axis

❗ **Do not use in patients < 12 years old!**

CMV Immune Globulin
(CytoGam®) [$290.61/20 ml]

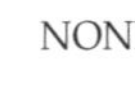

	I	II	III
Cat. C ③		NONE	NONE

Drug Interactions

VS: Live virus vaccines
(M-M-R) →↓ response
to live virus vaccines
(should be deferred for
3 months afer CMV-IG)
FOOD: → NONE
ALCOHOL: → NONE

Adverse Reactions

C: Flushing
Chills
Muscle cramps
Back pain
Fever
Nausea
Arthralgia
O: None
R: Anaphylaxis
Hepatitis
HIV infection

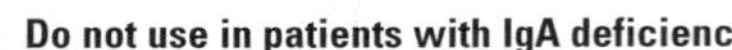 **Do not use in patients with IgA deficiency!**

Colistin sulfate
(Coly-mycin S®)   [$2.68 – 8.03]

Drug Interactions

VS: Aminoglycosides → ↑ risk of respiratory depression & nephrotoxicity

Muscle relaxants → respiratory depression

Cephalosporins → ↑ nephrotoxicity

LS: Phenothiazines → ↑ respiratory depression

FOOD: → NONE
ALCOHOL: → NONE

Adverse Reactions

C: Nausea
Diarrhea
Abdominal discomfort

O: Bacterial/fungal superinfection

R: Neurotoxicity
Nephrotoxicity
$\downarrow K^+/Ca^{++}/Mg^{++}$

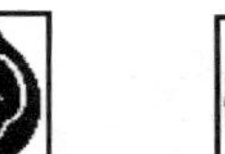

Dosage Modifications

Cat. C
②

I	II	III
NONE, but renal function must be assessed prior to and during therapy. *Use with extreme caution* in patients with renal insufficiency.		NONE

Cycloserine
(Seromycin®) **[$7.09–14.18]**

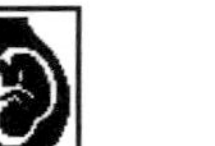 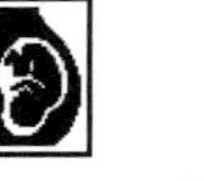 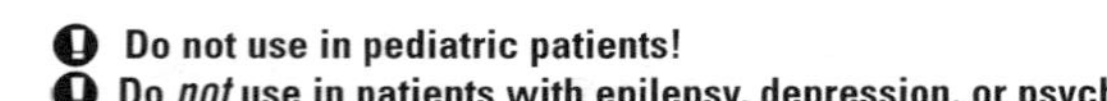

	I	II	III
Cat. C	Do not use in patients with renal impairment		NONE
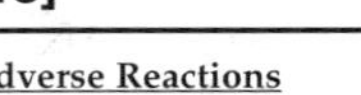			

Drug Interactions

VS: Ethionamide → ↑ neurotoxicity
    Isoniazid → dizziness or drowsiness
FOOD. → NONE
ALCOHOL: → SEIZURES

Adverse Reactions

C: Seizures
   Drowsiness
   Headache
   Tremor
   Confusion
   Personality changes
   Irritability
O: Rash
   ↑ SGOT/SGPT (AST/ALT)
R: Congestive heart failure

❶ **Do not use in pediatric patients!**
❶ **Do *not* use in patients with epilepsy, depression, or psychosis!**

Dapsone [$0.18]

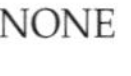 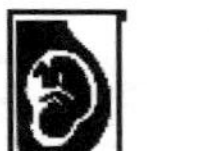 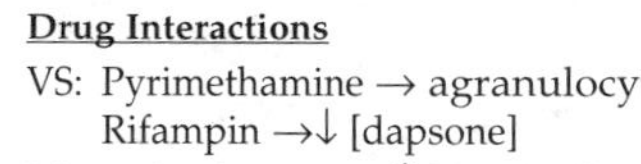

	I	II	III
Cat. C ③		NONE	NONE

Drug Interactions

VS: Pyrimethamine → agranulocytosis
    Rifampin →↓ [dapsone]
LS: Trimethoprim →↑ [dapsone] +
      ↑ [trimethoprim]
FOOD: → NONE
ALCOHOL: → NONE

Adverse Reactions

C: Hemolysis
   Anemia
O: Nausea
   Vomiting
   Hyperexcitability
   Abdominal pain
R: Peripheral neuropathy
   Pancreatitis
   Bullous dermatitis
   Toxic erythema multiforme
   Toxic epidermal necrolysis
   Lupus erythematosus

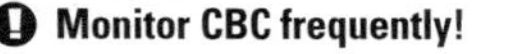 **Monitor CBC frequently!**

Dehydroemetine
(Mebadin®)

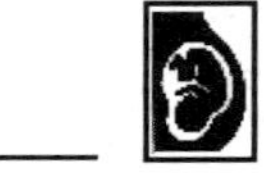

Drug Interactions

Adverse Reactions

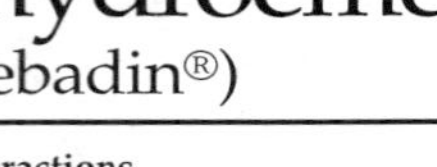

- Drug information available only from Centers for Disease Control & Prevention, Center for Infectious Disease, by calling (404) 639–3670 (8 A.M.–4:30 P.M. EST, M–F) or (404) 639–2888 (for emergencies).

Delavirdine mesylate
(Rescriptor®) **[$7.40]**

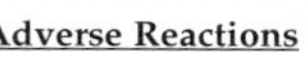

I II III

Drug Interactions

VS: Astemizole
Benzodiazepines ↑ toxicity
Cisapride and
Clarithromycin *cardiac arrhythmias!*
Terfenadine
Didanosine →↓ [didanosine] &
 ↓ [delavirdine]
Indinavir → toxicity } *Requires*
Nelfinavir → toxicity } *monitoring*
Rifabutin
Rifampin → toxicity—*Do not use!*
Saquinavir →↑ [saquinavir]
LS: Antacids →↓ [delavirdine]
Ketoconazole →↑ [delavirdine]
FOOD: → NONE
ALCOHOL: → NONE

Adverse Reactions

C: Nausea
Skin rash
Headache
Fatigue
Neutropenia
↑ SGOT/SGPT (AST/ALT)
O: Diarrhea
Vomiting
Pruritus
Maculopapular rash
R: Anemia
↑ Bilirubin
Angioedema

Cat. C
③

NONE

Use with caution and monitor clinical and laboratory parameters of liver function frequently

❶ **Do not use in patients < 16 years old!**
❶ **Consult PDR for list of important drugs which should *not* be co-administered with Delavirdine!**

Dicloxacillin [$2.84]
(Dycill®) [$3.04];
PEDS — (Dynapen®) [$1.86/10kg]

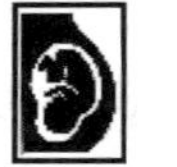

Drug Interactions

VS: Anticoagulants →↑ risk of bleeding
FOOD: →↓ dicloxacillin absorption rate
ALCOHOL: → NONE

Adverse Reactions

C: Nausea
Vomiting
Epigastric discomfort
Flatulence
Loose stools
O: Skin rash
Urticaria
Pruritus
Eosinophilia
R: ↑ SGOT (AST)
⊕ Coomb's test

Safety for use during pregnancy has not been established ②

I   II   III

NONE—But monitor renal function periodically   NONE

❶ **Do not use in PCN allergic patients!**

Didanosine (ddI)
(Videx®) [$6.20]

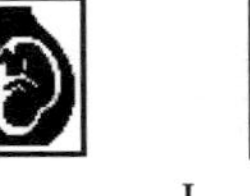 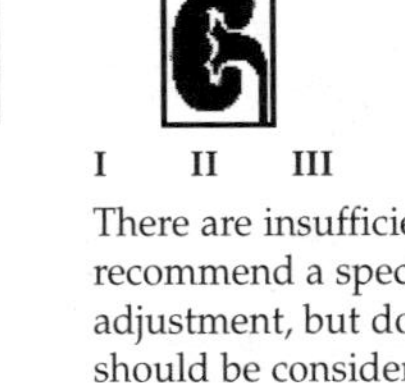 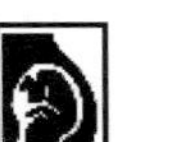

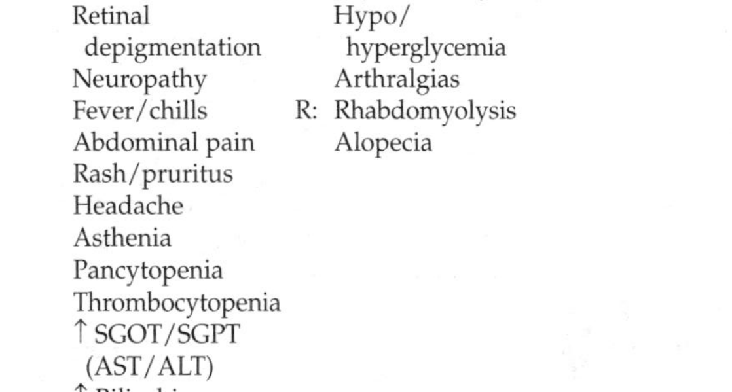

I II III

Drug Interactions

VS: Pentamidine IV →↑ pancreatic toxicity
LS: Tetracycline →↓ [tetracycline]
    Quinolones →↓ [quinolone]
FOOD: →↓ absorption by up to 50%
ALCOHOL: →↑ risk of pancreatitis

Adverse Reactions

C: *Pancreatitis*
    Hepatitis
    Hyperuricemia
    Diarrhea
    Retinal
      depigmentation
    Neuropathy
    Fever/chills
    Abdominal pain
    Rash/pruritus
    Headache
    Asthenia
    Pancytopenia
    Thrombocytopenia
    ↑ SGOT/SGPT
      (AST/ALT)
    ↑ Bilirubin

O: Anorexia
    Dyspepsia
    Flatulence
    Dry mouth/eyes
    Hypo/
      hyperglycemia
    Arthralgias

R: Rhabdomyolysis
    Alopecia

Cat. B
③

There are insufficient data to recommend a specific dose adjustment, but dose reduction should be considered

Diethylcarbamazine
(Benocide®)

 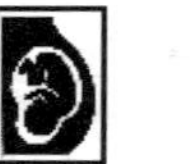 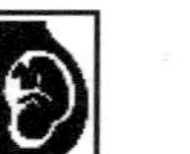

I   II   III

Drug Interactions

- Requests for drug & drug information should be directed to:
  Drug Service
  Centers for Disease Control
   & Prevention
  (404) 639-3670
  (404) 639-2888 (in emergencies)

Adverse Reactions

C: Headache
   Malaise
   Weakness
   Arthralgia
   Anorexia
   Nausea
   Vomiting
O: Severe pruritus
   Edema of the skin
   Fever
   Eosinophilia
   Lymphadenopathy
   Splenomegaly
   Proteinuria
R: Psychotic reactions

Diloxanide furoate
(Furamide®)

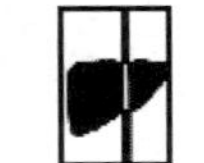 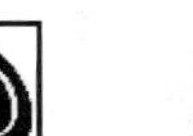 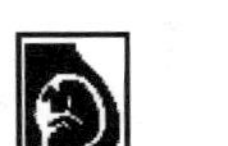

Dosage Modifications

I   II   III

Drug Interactions

Adverse Reactions

Drug information is available only from the Centers for Disease Control & Prevention, Center for Infectious Diseases, by calling (404) 639–3670 (8 A.M.–4:30 P.M. EST, M–F) or (404) 639–2888 (for emergencies).

Diphtheria-Tetanus-Acellular Pertussis (DTaP) vaccine
(Tripedia®)   [$25.45]

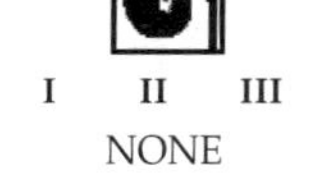
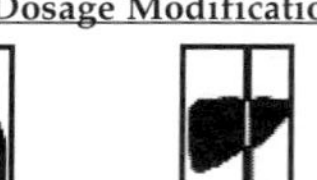
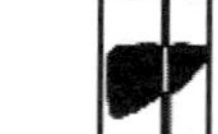

	I	II	III
Cat. C		NONE	NONE

Drug Interactions

- Do not give DTaP in patients who demonstrated the following after a previous immunization:
  - –Anaphylactic reaction
  - –Encephalopathy within 7 days following DTP
- Give DTaP *cautiously* where
  - –Temp >40.5°C within 48h of DTP
  - –Shock-like state within 48h of DTP
  - –Persistent crying for >3h within 48h of DTP
  - –Convulsions within 72h of DTP

Adverse Reactions

C: Injection site inflammation
   Fever
   Drowsiness
   Irritability
   Anorexia
O: Diarrhea
   Vomiting
   Crying
R: Arthus reaction
   Neuropathy

❗ Do not use in patients 7 years old and older!
❗ Do not use in patients < 15 months old!

❗ Do not use during course of any febrile illness/infection!
❗ Do not use for primary immunization—Use only as 4th or 5th dose in immunization schedule!

Diphtheria+tetanus toxoids+pertussis vaccine adsorbed and Haemophilus B conjugate vaccine
(Tetramune®)   **[$34.59/dose]**

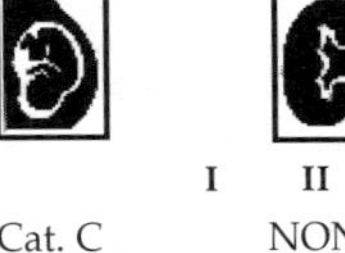 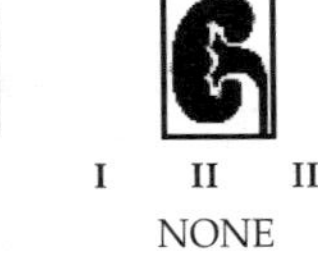 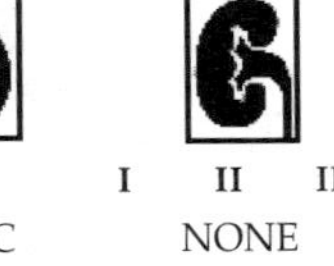

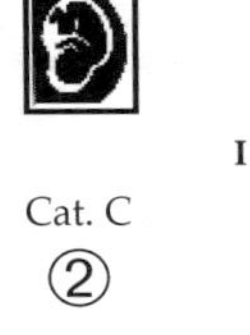

Drug Interactions

VS: Immunosuppressive agents
   →↓ antibody response
Influenza virus vaccine
   →↓ response to both vaccines
     if given within 3 days of
     each other
FOOD: → NONE
ALCOHOL: → NONE

Adverse Reactions

C: Local inflammation at injection site
Fever
Irritability
Drowsiness
Restless sleep
O: Loss of appetite
Vomiting
Diarrhea
Rash
R: Inconsolable, persistent crying
Fever >40.5°C
Shock-like episode
Convulsions

Cat. C
②

NONE NONE

❶ **Not recommended for patients >7 years old or < 6 weeks old!**

Domeboro solution [$2.04]

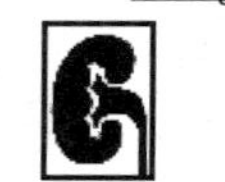

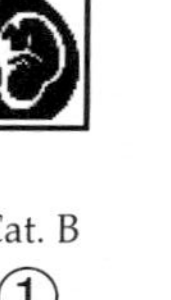 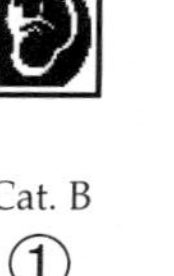

	I	II	III
Cat. B		NONE	NONE
①			

Drug Interactions

VS: NONE
LS: NONE
FOOD: → NONE
ALCOHOL: → NONE

Adverse Reactions

C: NONE
O: NONE
R: Local irritation

Doxycycline (oral) [$0.90];

(Doxy-D®, Doryx®, Vibramycin®,
Vibra-tabs®) **[$2.68–7.53]**
(Vibramycin® IV) **[$21.07– 42.14]**

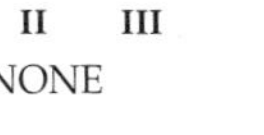 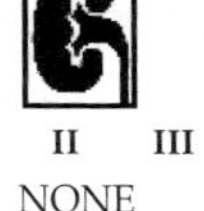 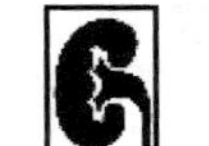

	I	II	III
Cat. D		NONE	NONE
③			

Drug Interactions

VS: Anticoagulants →↑ risk of bleeding
Penicillin →↓ penicillin activity
Antacids →↓ absorption of oral
    doxycycline
Bismuth →↓ absorption of oral
    doxycycline

LS: Barbiturates
Phenytoin →↑ [doxycycline]
Carbamazepine
Methoxyflurane → nephrotoxicity
Oral contraceptives
  →↓ contraceptive effect
FOOD: →↓ oral absorption
ALCOHOL: →↑ doxycycline clearance

Adverse Reactions

C: Nausea
Diarrhea
Anorexia
Glossitis
Tooth discoloration (children
  < 8-years old)
O: Esophagitis
Photosensitivity
Rash
↑ BUN
↓ Prothrombin time
R: Hemolytic anemia
Thrombocytopenia
Eosinophilia
Urticaria

❶ **Do not use in patients < 8 years old!**

Dronabinol
(Marinol®) [$2.99–5.87]

I   II   III

Cat. C   NONE   NONE

③

Drug Interactions

VS: Amphetamines ⟩ → hypertension, possible cardiotoxicity
    Cocaine

Anticholinergic →↑ tachycardia, drowsiness
    agents

Tricyclic →↑ tachycardia, hypertension, drowsiness
    antidepressants

CNS depressants →↑ CNS depression

LS: Theophylline →↑ [theophylline]

FOOD: → NONE

ALCOHOL: → NONE

Adverse Reactions

C: Anxiety
   Nervousness
   Confusion
   Nausea
   Abdominal pain

O: Dizziness
   Paranoid reaction
   Somnolence

R: Hypotension
   Diarrhea
   Flushing

❶ Avoid in pediatric patients!
❶ Note potential for drug abuse and dependence!

Econazole topical cream 1%
(Spectazole®)   [$12.60/15gm]

Drug Interactions	Adverse Reactions
NONE	C: Local skin irritation
FOOD: → NONE	O: NONE
ALCOHOL: → NONE	R: Pruritic rash

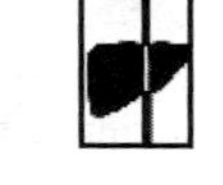

Dosage Modifications

Cat. C
②

I II III
NONE NONE

Erythromycin (oral) [$1.08–2.16]

(Ery-tab®) [$0.96–1.64]; (EES®–400) [$0.92];

(PCE® 333–500) [$4.98–6.56];

(EryC®) [$1.76–3.52];

PEDS(Eryped®) [$0.92/10kg]

Dosage Modifications

Cat. B ②

I II III

NONE

Avoid use in patients with hepatic dysfunction. Pharmacokinetics of drug excretion into bile has not been well characterized in these patients.

<u>Drug Interactions</u>

VS: Colchicine →↑ [colchicine]
Digoxin →↑ [digoxin]
Terfenadine ⎱
Astemizole ⎰ → cardiac arrhythmias
Cyclosporine →↑ [cyclosporine]
Ergot alkaloids →↑ ergot toxicity
Carbamazepine →↑ [carbamazepine]
Warfarin →↑ risk of bleeding
LS: Methylprednisolone →↑ steroid effects
Quinidine →↑ [quinidine]
Theophylline →↑ [theophylline]
Calcium channel blockers →↑ [CCB]
Chlorpropamide → hepatic toxicity
Penicillins →↓ PCN effect
FOOD: →↓ erythromycin absorption
ALCOHOL: → NONE

<u>Adverse Reactions</u>

C: Nausea
Vomiting
Abdominal pain
Diarrhea
O: ↑ SGOT/SGPT (AST/ALT)
Confusion
Vertigo
R: Colitis
Cardiac arrhythmias
Palpitations
Chest pain
Hearing loss

Erythromycin IV [$44.17]
(Ilotycin®) [$100.28]

Drug Interactions

See Erythromycin (oral)
FOOD: → NONE
ALCOHOL: → NONE

Adverse Reactions

C: ↑ SGPT/SGOT (AST/ALT)
O: Urticaria
R: Hearing loss
Ventricular arrhythmias
Torsades de pointes

Cat. B
②

See Erythromycin (oral)

Erythromycin ophthalmic
ointment, 0.5% [$3.60/3.5 gm]
(Ilotycin® ophthalmic ointment) [$5.58/3.5 gm]

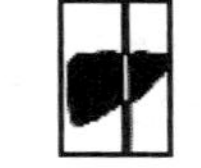

Drug Interactions

NONE
FOOD: → NONE
ALCOHOL: → NONE

Adverse Reactions

C: Ocular irritation & redness
O: Hypersensitivity reactions
R: NONE

Cat. B
②

NONE   NONE

✸ **May be used in neonates.**

Erythromycin 2% gel [$15.74/30 gm]

(A/T/S® 2%, Emgel® 2%,
T-stat® 2%, Erygel®)   **[$18.97/30 gm]**

Dosage Modifications

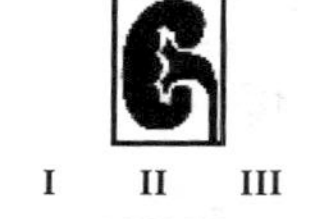

I   II   III

Cat. B	NONE	NONE
②		

Drug Interactions

VS: Topical acne →↑ irritatancy
    medications   effect
    (peeling,
    desquamating,
    abrasive agents)
FOOD: → NONE
ALCOHOL: → NONE

Adverse Reactions

C: Local burning
O: Peeling
    Dryness
    Itching
    Erythema
    Oiliness
R: Urticaria

❶ **Avoid use in pediatric patients!**

Ethambutol HCl
(Myambutol®) [$5.16]

Drug Interactions

VS: Kaolin-pectin→↓ [ethambutol]
Antacids →↓ [ethambutol]
FOOD: → NONE
ALCOHOL: → NONE

Adverse Reactions

C: ↓ Visual acuity due to optic neu-
ritis.
↑ SGOT/SGPT (AST/ALT)
O: Dermatitis
Joint pain
Anorexia
Nausea
Dyspepsia
Fever
Malaise
Headache
Disorientation
R: Peripheral neuritis
Hyperuricemia/gout

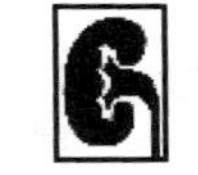

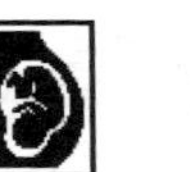

Cat. C
③

I	II	III
Follow serum levels of ethambutol & be prepared to ↓ dose if [drug] begins to increase		NONE

❶ **Avoid in patients with optic neuritis!**
❶ **Avoid in patients < 13 years old!**

Ethionamide
(Trecator®-SC) [$3.84–7.68]

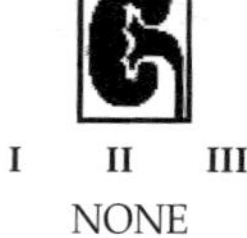

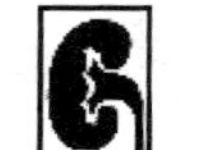

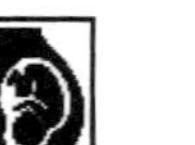

	I	II	III

Drug Interactions

VS: Other antituberculous drugs
→↑ incidence/severity of adverse
events
Cycloserine → seizures
FOOD: → NONE
ALCOHOL: → NONE

Adverse Reactions

C: Anorexia
Nausea
Vomiting
Diarrhea
Dysgeusia
O: Hepatitis
Jaundice
Stomatitis
Optic neuritis
R: Mental depression
Postural hypotension
Rash
Thrombocytopenia
Worsening diabetes mellitus
Impotence

Cat. D
③

NONE

NONE, although few patients can tolerate dosages >500 mg/day without some hepatic impairment

Famciclovir
(Famvir®)   [$18.45]

Drug Interactions

NONE
FOOD: → NONE
ALCOHOL: → NONE

Adverse Reactions

C: Nausea
Diarrhea
Vomiting
Constipation
Anorexia
Headache
O: Paresthesia
Fatigue
R: Pruritus

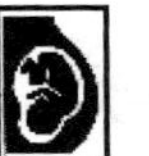

Cat. B
②

I   500 mg q8h

II   500 mg q12–24h

III 250 mg q48h

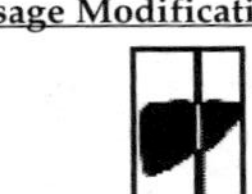

NONE

❶ **Do not use in patients < 18 years old!**

785

Fluconazole (oral)
(Diflucan®)   [$11.25]

	I	II	III
Cat. C ③	Normal dose	50% dose	50% dose

NONE, but LFTs should be monitored periodically

Drug Interactions

VS: Anticoagulants →↑ risk of bleeding
Terfenadine ⎫
Astemizole ⎭ → cardiac arrhythmias
Cisapride → cardiotoxicity
Cimetidine →↓ [fluconazole]
HCTZ →↑ [fluconazole]
Rifampin →↓ [fluconazole]
Phenytoin →↑ [phenytoin]
Cyclosporine →↑ [cyclosporine]
Zidovudine →↑ [zidovudine]
Theophylline →↑ [theophylline]
Oral hypoglycemics → hypoglycemia
FOOD: → NONE
ALCOHOL: → NONE

Adverse Reactions

C: Nausea
Headache
Rash
Vomiting
Abdominal pain
Diarrhea
O: ↑ SGOT/SGPT (AST/ALT)
R: Hepatic failure

Flucytosine
(Ancobon®) **[$14.21 – 42.63]**

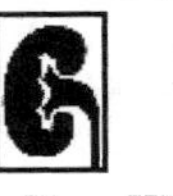
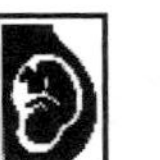
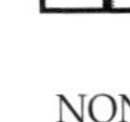

Drug Interactions

NONE
FOOD: → NONE
ALCOHOL: → NONE

Adverse Reactions

C: Nausea
   Dry mouth
O: Bone marrow depression
   Hepatotoxicity
   Colitis
   Rash
   Pruritus
R: Dyspnea
   Chest pain
   GI hemorrhage
   Renal failure
   Neuropathy
   Confusion

Cat. C
②

I — Normal dose q12h
II — Normal dose q16h
III — Normal dose q24h
NONE

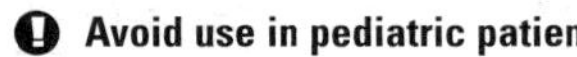 **Avoid use in pediatric patients!**

Fluorouracil topical cream/solution

(Efudex®, Fluoroplex®) [$36.90/25 gm 5% cream]; [$22.97/10 ml 2% solution]

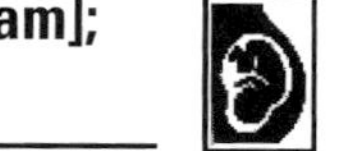

<u>Dosage Modifications</u>

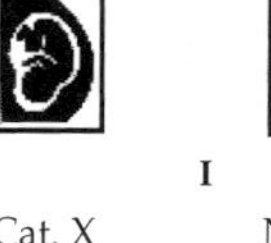

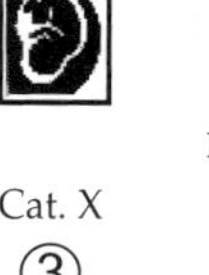

I II III

Drug Interactions

(Approx 6% of topical dose is absorbed systemically)
VS: Anticoagulants →↑ risk of bleeding
Cimetidine →↑ [fluorouracil]
Metronidazole →↑ fluorouracil toxicity

FOOD: → NONE
ALCOHOL: → NONE

Adverse Reactions

C: Local skin irritation
O: Hyperpigmentation
Leukocytosis
R: Ulceration
Eosinophilia
Thrombocytopenia
Alopecia
Blistering

Cat. X
③

NONE

NONE

❶ **Do not use in pediatric patients!**

Foscarnet

(Foscavir®)   **[$73.28–145.93]**

Drug Interactions	**Adverse Reactions**

VS: Cyclosporine → ↑ nephrotoxicity
LS: Quinolones → seizures
FOOD: → NONE
ALCOHOL: → NONE

C: Fever
Headache
Paresthesias
Neuropathy
Seizures
Anorexia
Nausea
Diarrhea
Abdominal pain
Anemia
Granulocytopenia
↓ K^+, Ca^{++}, Mg^{++}, PO_4
Renal failure
Vision abnormalities
O: Chest pain
Fungal infections
Hypertension

Palpitations
EKG abnormalities
Tremor
Ataxia
Dysphagia
Melena
Pancreatitis
↑ SGPT/SGOT
(AST/ALT)
↓ Weight
↑ BUN
Acidosis
Eye pain
Urinary retention
R: Cardiac failure
Encephalopathy
Glomerulonephritis

Cat. C
②

I — Normal dose
II — Normal dose q24h
III — Not recommended

NONE

(See PDR for full dosing nomogram)

❶ **Avoid use in pediatric patients!**

Furazolidone
(Furoxone®)   [$9.28]

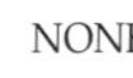

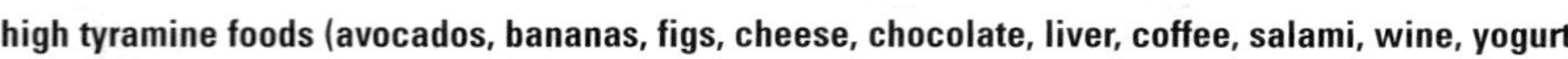

	I	II	III
Cat. C ③	NONE		NONE

Drug Interactions

VS: Sympathomimetics
Dopamine
Ephedrine
Phenylephrine
Epinephrine
Amphetamines
⟩ severe hypertensive crisis with possible intracranial hemorrhage

Levodopa → hypertension
MAO Inhibitors
(Antidepressants) ⟩ hypertension, seizures, delirium

FOOD (High Tyramine): → hypertensive crisis

ALCOHOL: → disulfiram-like reactions

Adverse Reactions

C: Urticaria
Fever
Arthralgia
Rash
O: Nausea
Vomiting
Headache
Malaise
Hemolysis

❶ **Avoid high tyramine foods (avocados, bananas, figs, cheese, chocolate, liver, coffee, salami, wine, yogurt)!**

Ganciclovir (oral)
(Cytovene®) [$23.40– 46.80]

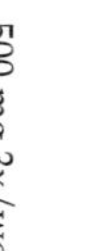

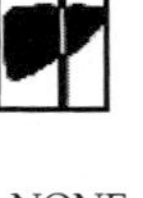

Drug Interactions

VS: Zidovudine → hematologic toxicity
Didanosine →↑ [didanosine]
Imipenem-cilastatin → seizures
FOOD: → NONE
ALCOHOL: → NONE

Adverse Reactions

C: Fever
Abdominal pain
Chills
Vomiting
Leukopenia
Anemia
Thrombocytopenia
Granulocytopenia
O: Asthenia
Malaise
↑ SGOT/SGPT
(AST/ALT)
Dry mouth
Insomnia
Weight loss

R: Allergic reaction
Cardiac
conduction
abnormalitites
SIADH
Memory loss

Cat. C
③

I 1500–3000 mg/day

II 500–1000 mg/day

III 500 mg 3x/week

NONE

❶ **Carcinogenic/caused aspermatogenesis in animal studies!**
❶ **Do not use in pediatric patients unless absolutely necessary!**

Garamycin ophthalmic ointment, 3%
[$17.33/3.5 gm]

Dosage Modifications

	I	II	III
Cat. C		NONE	NONE
②			

Drug Interactions

NONE
FOOD: → NONE
ALCOHOL: → NONE

Adverse Reactions

C: Irritation
O: Conjunctivitis
R: Allergic reactions

Gentamicin [$6.75–9.84]
(Garamycin®, G-mycin®)   [$7.88–21.02]

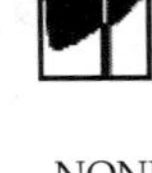
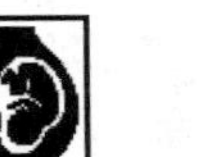
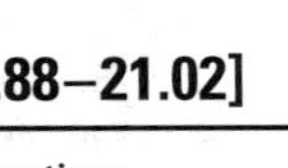

Drug Interactions

VS: Bumetanide → ototoxicity
Methoxyflurane → nephrotoxicity
Muscle relaxants → respiratory
depression
Furosemide→ ototoxicity/
nephrotoxicity
NSAIDs→↑ [gentamicin]
LS: Digoxin →↑ [digoxin]
Cephalosporins→↑ nephrotoxicity
Amphotericin B→↑ nephrotoxicity
Cyclosporine→↑ nephrotoxicity
Anticoagulants→↑ risk of bleeding
FOOD: → NONE
ALCOHOL: → NONE

Adverse Reactions

C: *Nephrotoxicity*
Neurotoxicity
O: Muscle weakness
R: Respiratory depression
Nausea
Vomiting
Stomatitis
↑ Salivation
Anorexia
↑ SGOT/SGPT (AST/ALT)

Cat. C
③

I Normal dose

II 25–50% normal dose

III 10–20% normal dose

NONE

See PDR for exact dosing
nomogram. In patients with
impaired renal function, serum
concentrations of gentamicin
should be monitored when
feasible (peak ≤ 12 µg/ml,
trough ≤ 2 µg/ml)

Granulocyte colony stimulating factor (G–, CSF; Filgrastim)
(Neupogen®)   [$156.10]

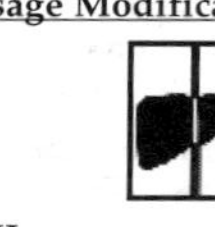

Drug Interactions

VS: Cytotoxic chemotherapy (24h before or after) →↑ risk of carcinogenesis to myeloid cells
Radiation therapy (24h before or after) →↑ risk of carcinogenesis to myeloid cells

FOOD: → NONE

ALCOHOL: → NONE

Adverse Reactions

C: Nausea
Vomiting
Diarrhea
Anorexia

O: Stomatitis
Constipation
Skeletal pain
↑ Uric acid
↑ LDH
↑ Alkaline phosphatase

R: Hypotension
Cardiac events
Anaphylaxis

Granulocyte-macrophage colony stimulating factor (GM–CSF; Sargramostim)
(Leukine®)   [$221.71]

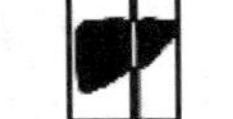

Dosage Modifications

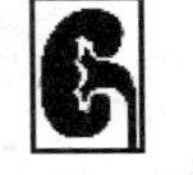

I   II   III

Drug Interactions

VS: Cytotoxic chemotherapy (24h before or after) →3 risk of carcinogenesis
Radiation therapy (24h before or after) →↑ risk of carcinogenesis

FOOD: → NONE

ALCOHOL: → NONE

Adverse Reactions

C: Peripheral edema
Pericardial effusion

O: Nausea
Diarrhea
Vomiting
Anorexia
Dyspepsia
Stomatitis
↑ SGOT/SGPT (AST/ALT)

R: Pleural effusion
Arrhythmias
↑ Creatinine
Anaphylaxis

Cat. C
②

NONE, but monitoring renal and hepatic function weekly during therapy is recommended

Griseofulvin (microcrystalline)

[$1.77]

(Fulvicin® P/G, Grifulvin® V)   [$1.61–1.95]

(Gris-PEG® ultramicrocrystalline)   [$0.97–1.54]

<u>Dosage Modifications</u>

I   II   III

Cat. X   NONE   NONE

③

Drug Interactions

VS: Salicylates →↓ [salicylate]
  Anticoagulants →↓ anticoagulant
      effect
LS: Barbiturates →↓ griseofulvin
      absorption
  Oral contraceptives →↓ contraceptive
      effect
  Cyclosporine →↓ [cyclosporine]
FOOD: →↑ griseofulvin absorption
ALCOHOL: → disulfiram-like reaction
      (tachycardia, flush)

Adverse Reactions

C: Skin rash
  Urticaria
O: Oral thrush
  Nausea
  Vomiting
  Epigastric pain
  Diarrhea
  Headache
  Fatigue
  Dizziness
  Insomnia

R: Proteinuria
  Leukopenia
  ↑ SGOT/SGPT
    (AST/ALT)
  GI bleeding
  Menstrual
    irregularities

❶ Do not use in patients with porphyria or hepatic failure!

Haemophilus influenzae type b vaccine
(ActHIB®[1], HibTITER®[2], PedvaxHIB®[3])   [$18.13–23.35]

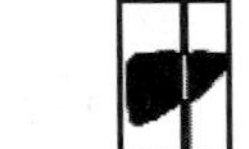

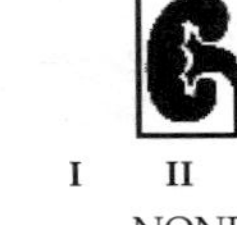

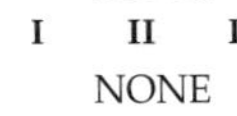

Drug Interactions

VS: Immunosuppressives
→↓ vaccine effect
FOOD: → NONE
ALCOHOL: → NONE

Adverse Reactions

C: NONE
O: Local injection site reaction
Fever
Irritability
Lethargy
Anorexia
Cough
R: Vomiting
Seizures
Urticaria
Renal failure
Guillain-Barré syndrome
Anaphylactic reactions

Cat. C
③

NONE

NONE

[1] ActHIB® is also conjugated with tetanus toxoid
[2] HibTITER® is also conjugated with diphtheria protein
[3] PedvaxHIB® is also conjugated with meningococcal protein.

Hepatitis A vaccine
(Havrix®, Vaqta®)   **[$20.40–28.58]**

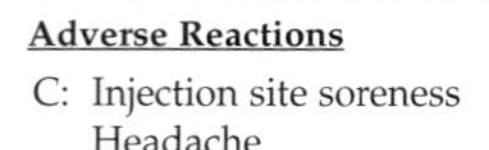

Dosage Modifications

	I	II	III
Cat. C ②	NONE		NONE

Drug Interactions

NONE
FOOD: → NONE
ALCOHOL: → NONE

Adverse Reactions

C: Injection site soreness
   Headache
O: Fatigue
   Fever
   Malaise
   Anorexia
   Nausea
R: Rash
   Anaphylaxis
   Urticaria
   Diarrhea
   Vomiting
   Dysgeusia
   Arthralgia
   Lymphadenopathy

❶ **Not for use in patients < 2 years old!**

Hepatitis B immune globulin
(Hyperhep®, Hep-B-Gammagee®, H-BIG®)   [$80.00–167.50]

Dosage Modifications

	I	II	III
Cat. C ②		NONE	NONE

Drug Interactions

VS: Live virus vaccines
→↓ immune response to
vaccination (defer vaccines ≥ 3
months after use of Hepatitis B I.G.)
FOOD: → NONE
ALCOHOL: → NONE

Adverse Reactions

C: Local rejection reaction
   Urticaria
O: Angioedema
R: Anaphylaxis

Hepatitis B vaccine
(Engerix®-B, Recombivax® HB)   [$54.35-Adults; $23.45-Pediatric]

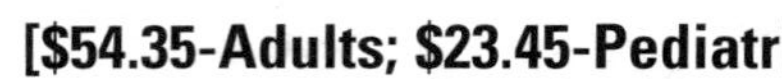

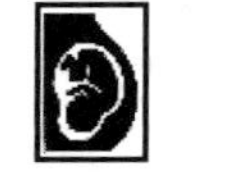 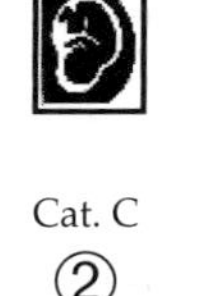

	I	II	III

Drug Interactions

NONE
FOOD: → NONE
ALCOHOL: → NONE

Adverse Reactions

C: Injection site soreness
    Fatigue
O: Fever
    Headache
    Dizziness
R: Pain
    Pruritus
    Chills
    Weakness
    Flushing
    Hypotension
    Dysuria

Cat. C
②

I II III
NONE NONE

Idoxuridine ophthalmic solution, 0.1%

(Herplex®)   [$12.75/15 ml]

Drug Interactions

VS: Boric acid solution → ocular irritation
FOOD: → NONE
ALCOHOL: → NONE

Adverse Reactions

C: Local irritation
O: Pain
   Pruritus
   Inflamation/edema of eyelids
   Photophobia
   Allergic reaction
R: Corneal clouding
   Corneal stippling

Dosage Modifications

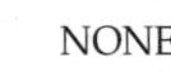

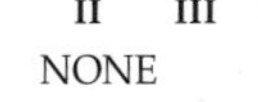

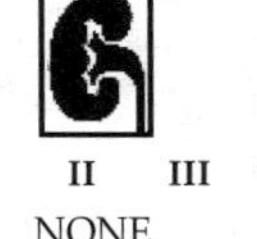

	I	II	III
Cat. C ②		NONE	NONE

❶ Do not use in pediatric patients!

Imipenem + cilastatin
(Primaxin®)   [$52.92–211.68]

Drug Interactions

VS: Cyclosporine → ↑ CNS toxicity
LS: Theophylline → seizures
FOOD: → NONE
ALCOHOL: → NONE

Adverse Reactions

C: Injection site inflammation
   Nausea
   Diarrhea
   Vomiting
O: Rash
   Fever
R: Hypotension
   Seizures
   Anaphylaxis
   Colitis
   Hepatitis
   Glossitis
   Pancytopenia
   ↑ BUN/Creatinine

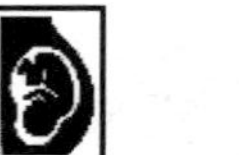

Cat. C
②

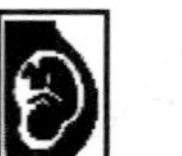

I   1–2 gm/day

II   500–750 mg/day given q8–12h

III   250–500 mg/day given q12h

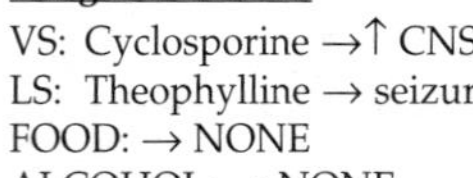

NONE

(See PDR for complete dosing nonograms)

❶ **Use with caution in PCN-allergic patients!**
❶ **Do not use in patients < 12 years old!**

Indinavir sulfate
(Crixivan®)   **[$15.00]**

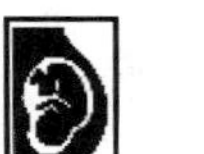  

				I	II	III

Drug Interactions

VS: Astemizole \
Terfenadine ⟩ → *cardiotoxicity* \
Cisapride /

Benzodiazepines →↑ *sedation* \
& respiratory \
depression

Rifampin →↓ [indinavir] \
Didanosine→↓ indinavir effect \
Ketoconazole→↑ [indinavir]

FOOD: →↓ absorption \
ALCOHOL: → NONE

Adverse Reactions

C: Nephrolithiasis \
Nausea \
Diarrhea \
Vomiting \
↑ Bilirubin

O: Anorexia \
Dry mouth \
Palpitations \
↑ SGOT/SGPT (AST/ALT)

R: Cardiac arrythmias \
GERD \
Peripheral neuropathy \
Anemia \
Thrombocytopenia \
Neutropenia

Cat. C \
③

NONE

600 mg q8h (normal dose is 800 mg q8h)

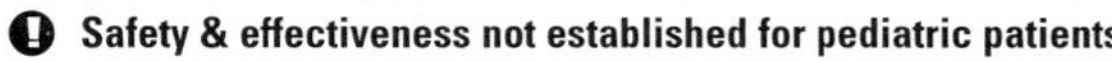 **Safety & effectiveness not established for pediatric patients!**

Influenza virus vaccine
(Fluvirin®, Fluzone®)   [$42.50–47.10]

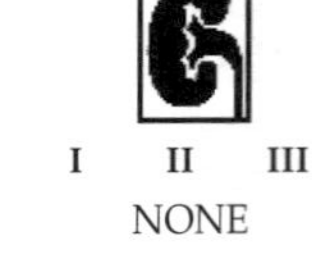
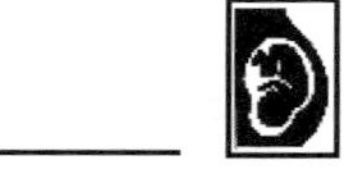
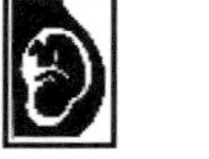

I   II   III

Cat. C	NONE	NONE
②		

Drug Interactions

LS: Anticoagulant →↑ risk of bleeding
Phenytoin → variations in [phenytoin]
Theophylline →↑ [theophylline]
FOOD: → NONE
ALCOHOL: → NONE

Adverse Reactions

C: Local injection site inflammation
O: Fever
Malaise
Myalgia
R: Hives
Angioedema
Allergic asthma
Anaphylaxis

❶ Do not use in patients < 6 months old!
❶ Do not use in patients with an acute febrile illness!
❶ Do not use in patients with allergy to eggs, chicken, or thimerosal!
❶ Do not use in patients with an active neurological disorder!

Interferon Alfa-n3 / Alfa-2b

(Alferon®-N) **[$15.91]** (Intron®-A) **[$11.30]**
(Roferon®-A) **[$32.94]**

I II III

Cat. C   NONE   NONE
②

Drug Interactions

VS: NONE
LS: NONE
FOOD: → NONE
ALCOHOL: → NONE

Adverse Reactions

C: Fever
   Chills
   Flu-like symptoms
   Fatigue
   Malaise
O: Dizziness
   Headache
   Myalgias
R: Pruritus
   Dyspepsia
   Nausea

❗ **Avoid use in patients < 18 years old!**

Iodoquinol
(Diquinol®, Yodoxin®)   [$3.69]

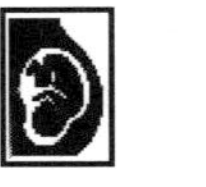
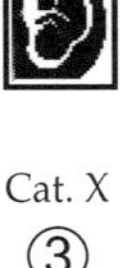

	I	II	III

Drug Interactions

VS: Thyroid function tests
  → iodoquinol interferes with
    these tests
FOOD: → NONE
ALCOHOL: → NONE

Adverse Reactions

C: Pustular or bullous skin eruptions
   Nausea
   Vomiting
   Dyspepsia
   Diarrhea
   Pruritus ani
O: Fever
   Chills
   Headache
   Thyroid enlargement
R: Optic neuritis
   Optic atrophy
   Peripheral neuropathy

Cat. X
③

NONE

Do not use
in patients
with hepatic
damage

❗ **Do not use long-term—May lead to optic neuritis, peripheral neuropathy!**

Isoniazid (INH) [$0.53]

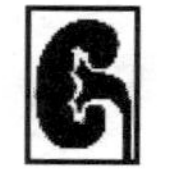

I   II   III

Drug Interactions

VS: Phenytoin →↑ [phenytoin]
    Carbamazepine→↑ [carbamazepine]
    Meperidine → hypotension &
        CNS depression
    Rifampin →↑ hepatotoxicity
    Ketoconazole →↓ [ketoconazole]
LS: Acetaminophen → hepatotoxicity
    Antacids →↓ INH absorption
    Anticoagulants →↑ risk of bleeding
    Corticosteroids →↓ INH effectiveness
    Enflurane → nephrotoxicity
    Cycloserine → CNS toxicity
    Theophylline →↑↓ [theophylline]
FOOD: →↓ absorption of INH
ALCOHOL: →↑ hepatotoxicity

Adverse Reactions

C: Peripheral neuropathy
   ↑ SGOT/SGPT (AST/ALT)
   ↑ Bilirubin
   Jaundice
O: Nausea
   Vomiting
   Dyspepsia
   Fever
R: Fatal hepatitis
   Skin eruptions
   Vasculitis
   Agranulocytosis
   SLE-like syndrome

Cat. C
②

Monitor patients with hepatic
or renal dysfunction frequently.
If evidence of worsening
hepatic/renal function occur,
discontinue drug. Reinstitute in
very small doses after symptoms and/or lab abnormalities
have normalized.

Isoniazid + rifampin
(Rifamate®)   [$4.86]

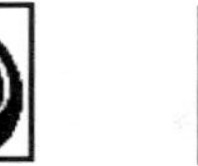

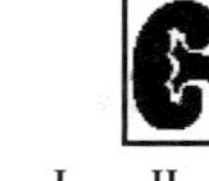

I   II   III

Drug Interactions   **Adverse Reactions**

See listings for Isoniazid and Rifampin. Rifamate is simply a combination capsule of the two drugs.

Isoniazid + Rifampin + Pyrazinamide
(Rifater®)   [$10.80]

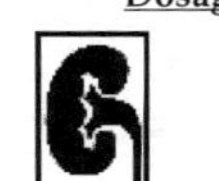

Dosage Modifications

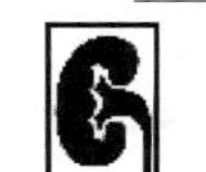

I   II   III

Drug Interactions

Adverse Reactions

See listings for Isoniazid, Rifampin, & Pyrazinamide. Rifater is simply a combination tablet containing the three drugs.

❶ **Avoid this combination in patients < 15 years old!**

Itraconazole
(Sporanox®)   [$11.64]

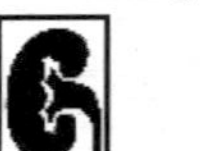 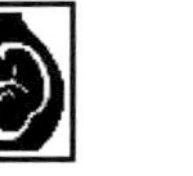 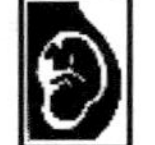

Drug Interactions

VS: Oral anticoagulants →↑ risk of
bleeding

Phenytoin →↓ [itraconazole]

Terfenadine ⎫
Astemizole ⎭ → *cardiac arrhythmias!*

Felodipine →↑ [felodipine]

Digoxin →↑ [digoxin]

Benzodiazepines →↑ *sedative effect!*

Rifabutin ⎫
Rifampin ⎭ →↓ [itraconazole]

Didanosine →↓ itraconazole effect

Cyclosporine →↑ [cyclosporine]

Cisapride → *ventricular arrhythmias!*

FOOD: →↑ absorption → dose with meals

ALCOHOL: → NONE

Adverse Reactions

C: Nausea
Vomiting
Diarrhea
Edema
Rash
Headache
Hypertension
↑ SGOT/SGPT
(AST/ALT)

O: Anorexia
Fever
Malaise
Pruritus

Dizziness
↓ Libido
Somnolence
↓ K+
Impotence

R: Allergic reactions
Hepatitis
Neuropathy
↑ Triglycerides

I II III

Cat. C
③

NONE

NONE, but monitor LFT's and plasma concentrations of Itraconazole carefully in patients with hepatic impairment.

❶ **Avoid in pediatric patients!**

Ivermectin

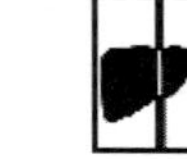

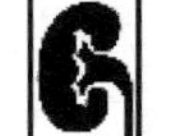 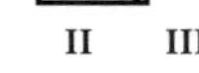

I II III

Drug Interactions　　　　　**Adverse Reactions**

Available in the U.S. only from:
Drug Service
Centers for Disease Control & Prevention
(404) 639-3670
(404) 639-2888 (in emergencies)

Japanese encephalitis B vaccine
(JE-VAX®)   [$57.33]

Drug Interactions

NONE
FOOD: → NONE
ALCOHOL: → NONE

Adverse Reactions

C: Local injection inflammation
   Fever/chills
   Headache
   Malaise
   Rash
   Dizziness
   Myalgia
   Nausea/vomiting
   Abdominal pain
O: Flu-like symptoms
R: Hives
   Facial edema

I   II   III

Cat. C
②

NONE   NONE

❶ Do not use in patients < 1-year old!
❶ Do not use in patients allergic to Thimerosal!

Kanamycin Sulfate
(Kantrex®) [$6.65]

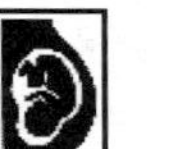

I II III

Drug Interactions

VS: Bumetanide → ototoxicity
Methoxyflurane → nephrotoxicity
Muscle relaxants → respiratory
depression
Loop diuretics → ototoxicity
Torsemide → ototoxicity
Succinylocholine → apnea
LS: NSAIDs →↑ nephrotoxicity
Digoxin →↓ [digoxin]
Cephalosporin →↑ nephrotoxicity
Amphotericin B →↑ nephrotoxicity
Penicillin →↓ kanamycin effect
Cyclosporine →↑ nephrotoxicity
Methotrexate →↓ methotrexate
effect
Cisplatin→↑ nephrotoxicity
FOOD: → NONE
ALCOHOL: → NONE

Adverse Reactions

C: *Nephrotoxicity!*
Neurotoxicity!
O: Nausea
Vomiting
R: Anorexia
↑ SGOT/SGPT (AST/ALT)
Respiratory
depression

Cat. D

③

NONE

→ Dosing interval by the following: Serum creatinine × 9 = dosage interval (h)

NONE

Follow renal function in all patients

Ketoconazole (oral);
(topical cream, 2%)
(Nizoral®)   [$2.92]; [$14.53/15 gm]

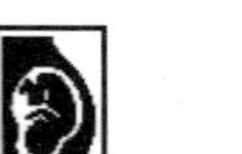

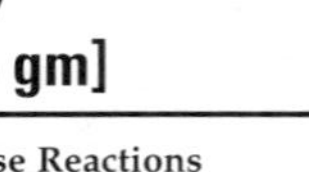

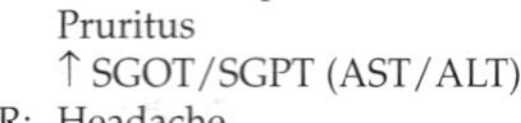

Drug Interactions (oral)

VS: Anticoagulants →↑ risk of bleeding
Terfenadine ⎫
Astemizole ⎬ → *cardiac arrhythmias!*
Cisapride → cardiac toxicity!

LS: Antacids →↓ [ketoconazole]
Oral hypoglycemics → hypoglycemia
Corticosteroids →↑ steroid effects & toxicity
Isoniazid →↓ ketoconazole effect
Benzodiazepines →↑ sedation
Rifabutin →↓ effect of both drugs
Didanosine →↓ ketoconazole effect
Theophylline →↓ [theophylline]
H2 blockers →↓ ketoconazole effect
Cyclosporine →↑ [cyclosporine]
Indinavir →↑ [indinavir]

FOOD: →↓ Absorption
ALCOHOL: → Disulfiram-like reaction

Adverse Reactions

C: Nausea
Vomiting
O: Abdominal pain
Pruritus
↑ SGOT/SGPT (AST/ALT)
R: Headache
Dizziness
Somnolence
Fever/chills
Thrombocytopenia
Leukopenia
Hemolytic anemia
Impotence
Hepatitis
Neuropsychiatric disturbances

Cat. C
③

NONE

NONE, but frequent monitoring of liver function is needed. Drug should be discontinued if there is clinical or laboratory evidence of worsening hepatic status

❶ **Avoid use in pediatric patients!**

Lactulose syrup

(Heptalac®, Duphalac®, Constilac®, Constulose®, Enulose®)

[$23.95–34.40/approx. 500 ml]

<u>Dosage Modifications</u>

	I	II	III
Cat. B		NONE	NONE
②			

Drug Interactions

VS: Antacids →↓ lactulose effect
FOOD: → NONE
ALCOHOL: → NONE

Adverse Reactions

C: Flatulence
   Abdominal cramps
O: Nausea
   Vomiting
   Diarrhea
R: $\downarrow K^+$
   $\downarrow Na^+$

❶ **Avoid use in pediatric patients!**

Lamivudine (3TC)
(Epivir®) [$7.68]

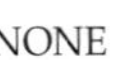 Cat. C ③

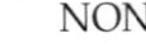 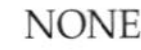

I	II	III
150 mg BID	150 mg × 1, then 100 mg qd	50–150 mg × 1, then 25–50 mg qd
		NONE

Drug Interactions

LS: Zidovudine →↑ [zidovudine]
    TMP-SMX →↑ [lamivudine]
FOOD: → NONE
ALCOHOL: → NONE

Adverse Reactions

C: Nausea
   Diarrhea
   Vomiting
   Anorexia
   Abdominal pain
   Dyspepsia
   Headache
   Neutropenia
   Anemia
O: Neuropathy
   Insomnia
   Depression
   Dizziness
   Cough
   Nasal congestion

R: Rash
   Arthralgia
   Pancreatitis
   Thrombocyto-
    penia

❶ **Avoid use in pediatric patients!**

Leucovorin (oral)
(Wellcovorin®)   [$21.02]

I   II   III

Cat. C   NONE   NONE

②

Drug Interactions

VS: Phenobarbital ⎫ →↑ seizure activity
    Phenytoin ⎬ in susceptible
    Primidone ⎭ children

LS: Intrathecal →↓ methotrexate
    Methotrexate effect on CNS
    Fluorouracil →↑ toxicity

FOOD: → NONE

ALCOHOL: → NONE

Adverse Reactions

C: Allergic sensitization

❶ **Use with caution in pediatric patients on anti-epileptic therapy!**

Lomefloxacin HCl
(Maxaquin®) [$6.60]

<u>Dosage Modifications</u>

Cat. C ③

	I	II	III
	400 mg qD	400 mg × 1, then 200 mg qD	400 mg × 1, then 200 mg qD	NONE

Drug Interactions

VS: Iron ⟩ →↓ [lomefloxacin]
    Zinc
    Antacids →↓ [lomefloxacin]
    Warfarin →↑ risk of bleeding
    H2 blockers →↓ [lomefloxacin]
    Theophylline →↑ [theophylline]
    Vincristine ⟩ →↓ [lomefloxacin]
    Cytarabine
    Cyclosporine →↑ nephrotoxicity
    Beta blockers →↑ beta blocker effect
LS: Loop diuretic →↑ [lomefloxacin]
FOOD: →↓ Absorption (especially with
       dairy products)
ALCOHOL: → NONE

Adverse Reactions

C: Phototoxicity/photosensitivity
   Nausea
   Diarrhea
   Vomiting
   Headache
   Dizziness
O: Dry mouth
   Dyspepsia
   Thrombocytopenia
R: ↑ SGOT/SGPT (AST/ALT)
   ↑ BUN
   ↓ K^+
   ↑ Bilirubin
   Vaginitis

❗ **Do not use in patients < 18 years old!**

Mafenid acetate cream
(Sulfamylon®) [$18.50/60 gm]

Dosage Modifications

Drug Interactions

NONE
FOOD: → NONE
ALCOHOL: → NONE

Adverse Reactions

C: Local burning
    Rash
O: Itching
R: Hyperventilation
    $\downarrow$pCO$_2$
    Metabolic acidosis
    Hemolytic anemia
    DIC
    Porphyria
    Bone marrow depression
    Respiratory alkalosis

Cat. C
②

I   II   III

NONE, but
follow renal
function and
acid-base bal-
ance closely
in patients
with more
than local
minor burns

NONE

Measles-rubella vaccine
(M-R-VAX® II) **[$27.41]**

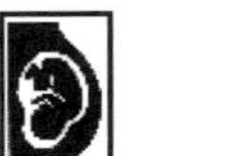 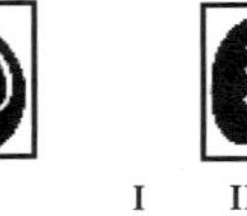 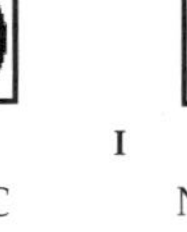 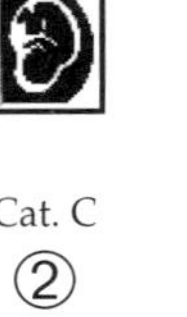 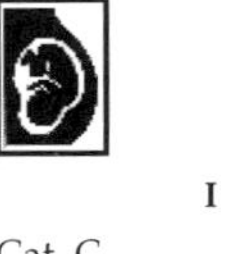

	I	II	III
Cat. C ②	NONE		NONE

Drug Interactions

VS: Immunosuppressive
   agents → *do not use*
FOOD: → NONE
ALCOHOL: → NONE

Adverse Reactions

C: Irritation at injection site
   URI symptoms
O: Fever
   Rash
   Nausea
   Diarrhea
   Local lymphadenopathy
R: Vasculitis
   Anaphylaxis
   Seizures
   Syncope
   Erythema multiforme

❶ Do *not* give to immunocompromised patients!
❶ Do *not* give vaccine to pregnant women!
❶ Do *not* give to patients with allergy to eggs!

Measles-mumps-rubella vaccine
(M-M-R® II)   [$37.64]

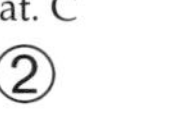

Drug Interactions

VS: Immunosuppressive
   agents → *do not use*
FOOD: → NONE
ALCOHOL: → NONE

Adverse Reactions

C: Irritation at injection site
   URI symptoms
O: Fever
   Rash
   Nausea
   Diarrhea
   Local lymphadenopathy
R: Vasculitis
   Anaphylaxis
   Seizures
   Syncope
   Erythema multiforme

Cat. C
②

I	II	III
	NONE	NONE

❶ Do *not* give to immunocompromised patients!
❶ Do *not* give vaccine to pregnant women!
❶ Do *not* give to patients with allergy to eggs!

Mebendazole
(Vermox®) [$10.44]

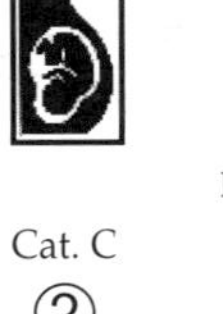

Dosage Modifications

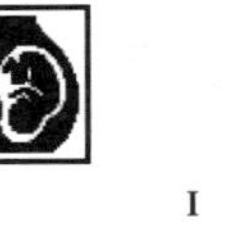 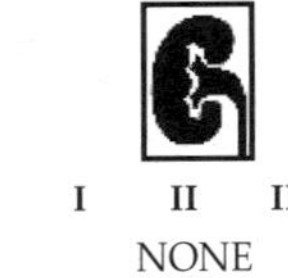 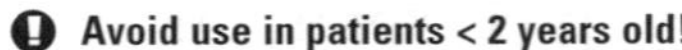

	I	II	III
Cat. C ②		NONE	NONE

Drug Interactions

VS: Phenytoin →↓ mebendazole effect

Carbamazepine →↓ mebendazole effect

Cimetidine →↑ [mebendazole]

FOOD: →↑ absorption

ALCOHOL: → NONE

Adverse Reactions

C: Abdominal pain
   Diarrhea
O: NONE
R: Rash
   Urticaria
   Angioedema

❶ **Avoid use in patients < 2 years old!**

Mefloquine HCl
(Lariam®)   [$35.23]

Dosage Modifications

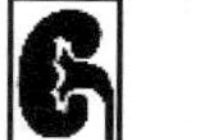

I	II	III
Cat. C ②	NONE	NONE

Drug Interactions

VS: Halofantrine → *Fatal prolongation of QT_c interval!*

Quinine ⎫
Quinidine ⎬ → *Do not use!*

Valproic acid → Loss of seizure control

LS: Metoclopramide →
↑ [mefloquine]
Propranolol → cardiotoxicity

FOOD: → NONE
ALCOHOL: → NONE

Adverse Reactions

C: Vomiting
O: Dizziness
Syncope
Extrasystoles
Myalgia
Fever/chills
Diarrhea
Rash
Fatigue
Anorexia
R: Bradycardia
Hair loss
Emotional disturbances
Seizures

❶ **Avoid use in pediatric patients!**

Megestrol acetate
(Megace®)   **[$5.40]**

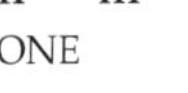 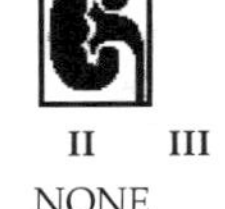 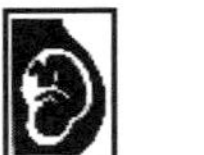

	I	II	III
Cat. D ③		NONE	NONE

Drug Interactions

VS: Phenytoin →↓ megestrol
        effect
    Rifampin →↓ [megestrol]
LS: Aminoglutethimide →
        ↓ [megestrol]
FOOD: → NONE
ALCOHOL: → NONE

Adverse Reactions

C: Weight gain
O: Nausea
    Vomiting
    Edema
    Alopecia
R: Pituitary-adrenal axis abnormality
    Thromboembolic phenomena
    Hypertension
    Rash

❶ Do *not* use during first 4 months of pregnancy!
❶ Do *not* use in pediatric patients!

Melarsoprol
(Arsobal®)

Dosage Modifications

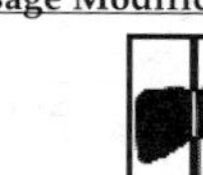 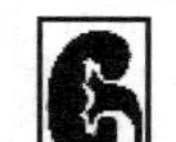 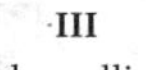

I II III

Drug Interactions

Adverse Reactions

Drug information is available from the Centers for Disease Control & Prevention, Center for Infectious Diseases, by calling (404) 639-3670 (8 AM–4:30 PM EST, M–F) or (404) 639-2888 (for emergencies).

Meningococcal vaccine
(Menomune®-A/C/Y/W-135)   [$57.63]

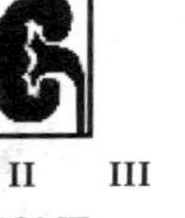

Dosage Modifications

Drug Interactions

VS: Immunosuppressive
    agents →↓ vaccine effect
FOOD: → NONE
ALCOHOL: → NONE

Adverse Reactions

C: Local injection reactions
O: Fever
R: Hypersensitivity reaction

Cat. C
③

	I	II	III
Cat. C		NONE	NONE

❶ Do not use in pregnant women!
❶ Do not use in patients with allergy to thimerosal!
❶ Do not use in patients < 2 years old!

Meropenem
(Merrem®) [$155.43]

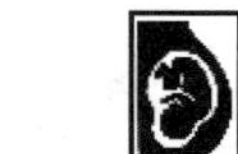 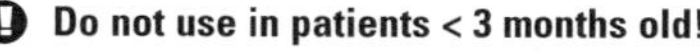

	I	II	III	
Cat. B ②	1.0 gm IV q8–12h	0.5 gm IV q12h	0.5 gm IV q24h	NONE

Drug Interactions

VS: Probenecid →↑ [meropenem]
FOOD: → NONE
ALCOHOL: → NONE

Adverse Reactions

C: Injection site inflammation
   Diarrhea
   Nausea
   Vomiting
   Headache
O: Phlebitis
   Rash
   Pruritus
   Apnea
   Constipation
R: Pain at injection site
   Bleeding events (systemic)
   ↑ SGPT/SGOT (AST/ALT)
   ↑ LDH
   ↑ BUN/Creatinine
   Hypersensitivity reactions

❶ **Do not use in patients < 3 months old!**

Metrifonate

Dosage Modifications

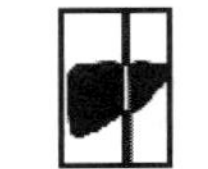 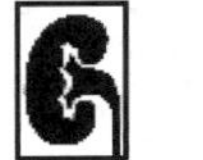 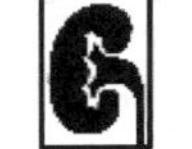

I II III

Drug Interactions

Adverse Reactions

Drug and dose information is available from Bayer Pharmaceuticals by calling (800) 468-0894 or (203) 812-2000.

Metronidazole (oral) [$3.90–11.70]; (IV) [$36.76]

(Flagyl®) **[$4.23–12.69]**;   (Flagyl® IV) **[$75.52]**

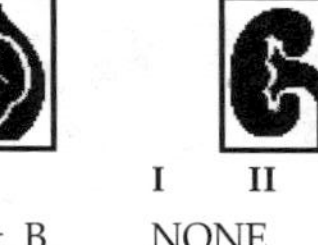 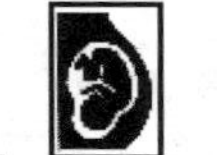 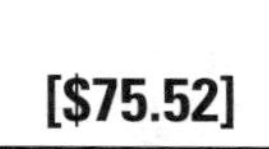

Drug Interactions

VS: Anticoagulants →↑ risk of
                bleeding
    Barbiturates →↓ [metronidazole]
    Fluorouracil →↑ FU toxicity
Cyclosporine →↑ [cyclosporine]
    Lithium →↑ lithium toxicity
LS: Antacid →↓ [metronidazole] (oral)
    Phenytoin →↑ phenytoin effect
    H2 blockers →↑ [metronidazole]
    Carbamazepine →↑ [carbamazepine]
    Cholestyramine →↓ oral absorption
                of metronidazole
FOOD: → NONE
ALCOHOL: → Disulfiram-like reaction

Adverse Reactions

C: Nausea
   Vomiting
   Diarrhea
   Constipation
   Epigastric pain
   Dysgeusia
   Anorexia
O: Glossitis
   Vaginitis
R: Seizures
   Peripheral neuropathy
   Pancreatitis
   Neutropenia
   Thrombocytopenia
   Urticaria

Cat. B
③

NONE   NONE
(In elderly patients, may need
to monitor serum levels of
metronidazole to adjust dosing)

❶ Do not use in pediatric patients except to treat amebiasis!

Metronidazole gel 0.75%
(Metrogel®)   [$25.00/30 gm]

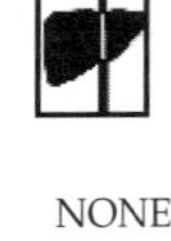

	I	II	III
Cat. B ②		NONE	NONE

Drug Interactions

NONE
FOOD: → NONE
ALCOHOL: → NONE

Adverse Reactions

C: Burning at local site
   Skin irritation
   Dryness
   Erythema
O: Dysgeusia
R: Peripheral neuropathy
   Nausea

❶ **Do not use in pediatric patients!**

Mezlocillin
(Mezlin®)   [$26.70–53.40]

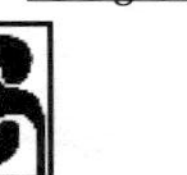

Drug Interactions

VS: Oral anticoagulants →↑ risk of
                bleeding
    Cyclosporine →↑ [cyclosporine]
    Methotrexate →↑ [methotrexate]
    Tetracyclines →↓ mezlocillin
           effect
    Aminoglycosides →↓ aminoglycoside
           effect
    Oral contraceptives →↓ contraceptive
           effect
LS: Chloramphenicol →↓ mezlocillin
           effect

FOOD: → NONE
ALCOHOL: → NONE

Adverse Reactions

C: Nausea
   Vomiting
   Diarrhea
   Dysgeusia
O: Leukopenia
   Thrombocytopenia
   Eosinophilia
   ⊕Coombs' test
   Anemia
   ↑ SGOT/SGPT (AST/ALT)
   ↑ BUN/Creatinine
R: Anaphylaxis
   Seizures
   Thrombophlebitis

Cat. B
②

I   Normal dose

II   1.5–3.0 gm q8h

III   1.5 gm q8h

NONE

❶ **Not for PCN-allergic patients!**

Miconazole cream, vaginal suppositories/cream

(Monistat®-Derm   [$13.50/15 gm]; Monistat® 3 [$8.70]; Monistat® Dual-Pak)   [$28.44]

Dosage Modifications

	I	II	III
Cat. C ②		NONE	NONE

Drug Interactions

NONE
FOOD: → NONE
ALCOHOL: → NONE

Adverse Reactions

C: Irritation
   Burning
O: Maceration
R: Contact dermatitis
   Headaches

❗ **Do not use vaginal preparation in the first trimester of pregnancy unless essential to the welfare of the patient!**

Minocycline HCl
(Minocin®, Dynacin®)   **[$2.96]**

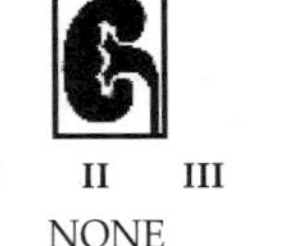 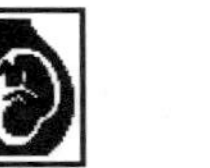 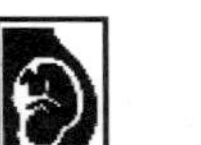

I   II   III

Drug Interactions

VS: Antacids →↓ minocycline
    absorption
Digoxin →↑ [digoxin]
Methoxyflurane → nephrotoxicity
Anticoagulants →↑ risk of
    bleeding
Penicillin →↓ effect of PCN
Insulin →↑ hypoglycemic
    effect
Colestipol →↓ [minocycline]
Bismuth →↓ [minocycline]

LS: Diuretics→↑ BUN/uremia
Oral contraceptives→↓
    contraceptive effect
Theophylline→↑ theophylline
    toxicity
Lithium→↑ lithium toxicity
FOOD: → NONE
ALCOHOL: →↓ [minocycline]

Adverse Reactions

C: Nausea
Vomiting
Diarrhea
Glossitis
Stomatitis
Photosensitivity
↑ BUN

O: Anemia
Thrombocytopenia
Neutropenia
Eosinophilia
Headache

R: Hepatitis
Dermatitis
Colitis
Acute renal failure
Anaphylaxis
Vertigo
Dizziness

Cat. D
③

NONE   NONE

❶ Do not use in patients < 8 years old!

Mupirocin ointment 2%
(Bactroban®)   [$16.50/15 gm]

Drug Interactions

NONE
FOOD: → NONE
ALCOHOL: → NONE

Adverse Reactions

C: Burning
  Stinging
  Local pain
O: Itching
R: Rash
  Nausea
  Erythema
  Dry skin
  Contact dermatitis
  Increased exudate

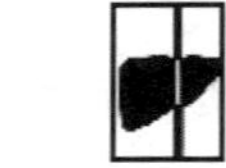

Cat. B
③

Dosage Modifications

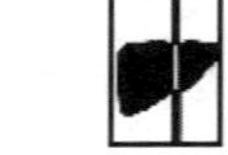

I   II   III

NONE   NONE

Nafcillin oral [$5.06];
Nafcillin IV [$10.72]
(Unipen®) **[$9.68]**;
(Unipen® IV, Nallpen®) **[$13.72–24.40]**

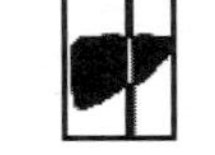

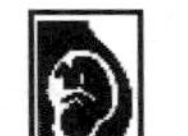

	I	II	III
Cat. B ②	250–1000 mg q4–6h	250–500 mg q6–8h	250–500 mg q12–24h	NONE

Drug Interactions

VS: Oral anticoagulant →↑ risk
    of bleeding
    (IV only)
Cyclosporine →↑ [cyclosporine]
Methotrexate →↑ [methotrexate]
Tetracyclines
Chloramphenicol ⟩ →↓ nafcillin effect
Atenolol →↓ [atenolol]

LS: Erthromycin →↓ nafcillin effect
Aminoglycosides →↓ [nafcillin]
Oral contraceptives →↓ contraceptive effect

FOOD: →↓ absorption of nafcillin
ALCOHOL: → NONE

Adverse Reactions

C: Nausea
Vomiting
Diarrhea
Dysgeusia

O: Leukopenia
Thrombocytopenia
Eosinophilia
⊕ Coombs' Test
↑ SGOT/SGPT (AST/ALT)
↑ BUN/↓K$^+$

R: Anaphylaxis
Thrombophlebitis (IV form)

❶ **Not for PCN-allergic patients!**
❶ **Avoid use of Nafcillin given orally; it is erratically absorbed!**

Natamycin ophthalmic solution, 5%

(Natacyn®)   **[$100/15 ml]**

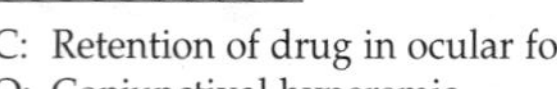

Dosage Modifications

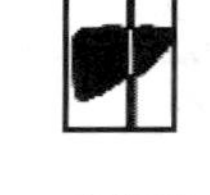 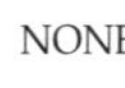 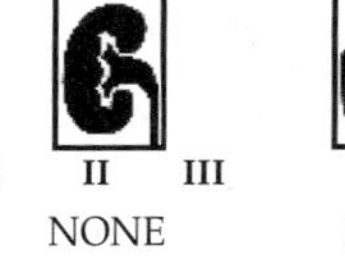

I   II   III

Drug Interactions	**Adverse Reactions**			
NONE	C: Retention of drug in ocular fornices	Cat. C	NONE	NONE
FOOD: → NONE	O: Conjunctival hyperemia	②		
ALCOHOL: → NONE	R: Chemosis			
	Allergic reactions			

❶ **Do not use in pediatric patients!**

Nelfinavir
(Viracept®) [$18.58]

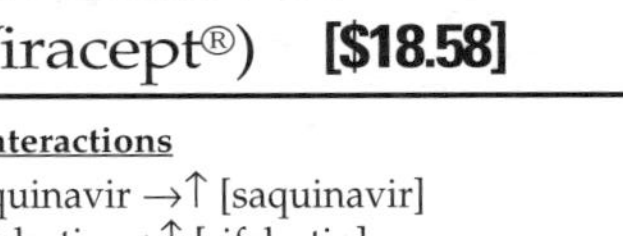  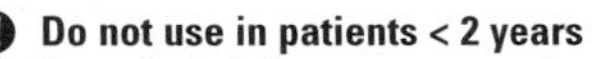

I   II   III

Drug Interactions

VS: Saquinavir →↑ [saquinavir]
   Rifabutin →↑ [rifabutin]
   Rifampin →↓ [nelfinavir]
   Ritonavir →↑ [nelfinavir]
LS: Lamivudine →↑ [lamivudine]
   Zidovudine →↓ [zidovudine]
   Oral contraceptives →↓ contraceptive
                effect
   Indinavir →↑ [indinavir]
   Ketoconazole →↑ [ketoconazole]
   Anticonvulsants→↓ [nelfinavir]
FOOD: →↑ nelfinavir
        absorption
ALCOHOL: → NONE

Adverse Reactions

C: Diarrhea
   Nausea
   Flatulence
   Rash
O: Neutropenia
   ↑ SGOT/SGPT (AST/ALT)
   ↑ CPK
R: ↑ Bleeding in hemophilia
   Hyperglycemia

Cat. B
③

NONE

Monitor LFTs frequently during use. Discontinue drug if clinical or laboratory evidence of hepatic injury occurs.

❶ Do not use in patients < 2 years old!
❶ Do *not* administer concurrently with Terfenadine, Astemizole, Cisapride, Triazolam, Midazolam, Ergots, Amiodarone, or Quinidine!

Neomycin + dexamethasone ophthalmic ointment/solution
(NeoDecadron®)   [$6.34/3.5 gm]

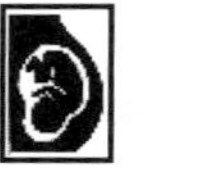

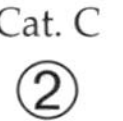

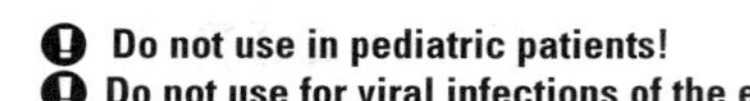

	I	II	III
Cat. C		NONE	NONE
②			

Drug Interactions

NONE
FOOD: → NONE
ALCOHOL: → NONE

Adverse Reactions

C: Allergic reactions
　 ↑ Intraocular pressure
O: Glaucoma
　 Secondary infections (viral/fungal)
R: Subcapsular cataract formation
　 Optic nerve damage

❶ **Do not use in pediatric patients!**
❶ **Do not use for viral infections of the eye!**

Neomycin sulfate oral solution
(Mycifradin®, Neofradin®)   [$31.34/500 ml]

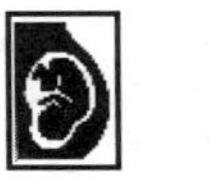 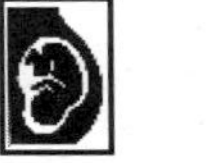 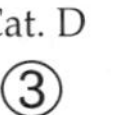

I	II	III
Cat. D	NONE	NONE
③		

Drug Interactions

VS: Bumetanide → ototoxicity
Muscle relaxants → respiratory depression & apnea

Diuretics → ototoxicity
Torsemide → ototoxicity
NSAIDs → ↑ [neomycin] & ↓ GFR
Digoxin → ↑↓ [digoxin]
Cephalosporins → nephrotoxicity
Amphotericin B → ↑ nephrotoxicity
Penicillins → ↓ neomycin effect
Cyclosporine → ↑ nephrotoxicity

LS: Oral anticoagulants → ↑ risk of bleeding
Methotrexate → ↓ MTX effect
Cisplatin → ↑ nephrotoxicity

FOOD: → NONE
ALCOHOL: → NONE

Adverse Reactions

C: Nausea
Vomiting
Diarrhea

O: ↑ BUN/creatinine
↓ K^+/Mg^{++}
↑ LDH
↑ Bilirubin
↓ Na^+

R: Respiratory depression
Anorexia
↑ SGOT/SGPT (AST/ALT)

Nevirapine
(Viramune®)   [$4.13–8.26]

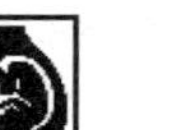 

Dosage Modifications

	I	II	III
Cat. C ③	No data available		NONE, but drug should be discontinued in patients experiencing moderate or severe LFT abnormalities, then restarted at 50% of the previous dosage level after LFT's have returned to baseline

Drug Interactions

VS: HIV protease inhibitors → ↓ [protease inhibitor]
Oral contraceptives →↓ contraceptive effect

LS: Rifampin / Rifabutin →↓↑ [Rifampin or Rifabutin]

FOOD: → NONE
ALCOHOL: → NONE

Adverse Reactions

C: Rash
Fever
Nausea
Headache
Diarrhea
Abdominal pain
Stomatitis
Hepatitis

O: *Life-threatening rash*
↑ SGOT/SGPT (AST/ALT)
Neutropenia

R: Myalgia
Paresthesia

❶ Do not use in pediatric patients!

Nifurtimox
(Lampit®)

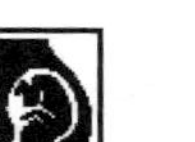

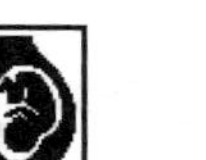

I II III

Drug Interactions

- Requests for drug & drug information
  should be directed to:
    Division of Host Factors Drug Service
    Centers for Disease Control
     & Prevention
    (404) 639-3670
    (404) 639-2888 (in emergencies)

Adverse Reactions

C: Nausea
   Vomiting
   Diarrhea
   Abdominal discomfort
   Peripheral neuropathy
   Anorexia
   Restlessness
   Disorientation
   Insomnia
O: Twitching
   Paresthesias
   Polyneuritis
   Weakness
   Stiffness
R: Convulsions
   Rash
   Neutropenia
   Decreased sperm count

Nitrofurantoin [$2.40–4.04]
(Macrodantin®) [$3.08–5.24]

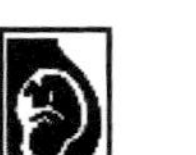

	I	II	III
Cat. B		NONE	NONE
②			

Drug Interactions

VS: Antacids →↓ [nitrofurantoin]
Probenecid
Sulfinpyrazone ⟩ →↑ [nitrofurantoin]
FOOD: →↑ nitrofurantoin absorption
ALCOHOL: → NONE

Adverse Reactions

C: Pulmonary hypersensitivity
reactions!
Nausea
Vomiting
Anorexia
O: ↑ SGOT/SGPT (AST/ALT)
Anemia
Eosinophilia
Thrombocytopenia
R: Hepatitis
Hepatic necrosis
Cholestatic jaundice
Peripheral neuropathy
Asthenia
Vertigo
Nystagmus
Transient alopecia
Stevens-Johnson syndrome
Diarrhea
Pseudomembranous colitis

❶ **Do not use in patients < 1 month old!**

Norfloxacin
(Noroxin®)   [$5.58]

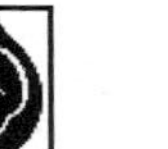 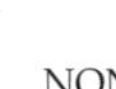

Cat. C
②

	I	II	III
	400 mg q12h	400 mg qd	400 mg qd

NONE

Drug Interactions

VS: Theophylline →↑ [theophylline]
Cyclosporine →↑ [cyclosporine]
Oral anticoagulants →↑ risk of
bleeding
Nitrofurantoin →↓ norfloxacin
effect

Multivitamins
Sucralfate   →↓ absorption of
Antacids   norfloxacin

LS: Caffeine →↑ caffeine effects
FOOD: →↓ Absorption of
norfloxacin
ALCOHOL: → NONE

Adverse Reactions

C: Dizziness
Nausea
Headache
Abdominal cramps
O: Anorexia
Diarrhea
Constipation
Dyspepsia
Flatulence
Vomiting
↑ SGOT (AST)
Leukopenia
R: Thrombocytopenia
Anemia

❶ **Do not use in patients < 18 years old!**

Norfloxacin ophthalmic solution, 0.3%
(Chibroxin®)　[$18.70/5 ml]

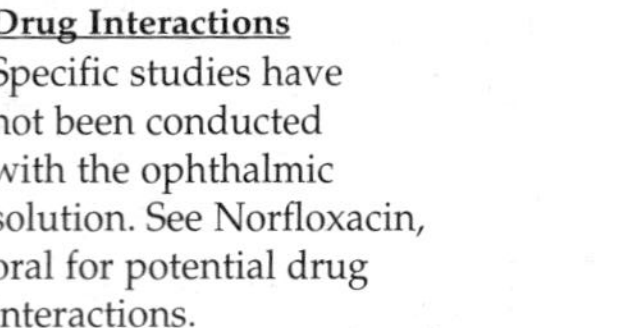

Dosage Modifications

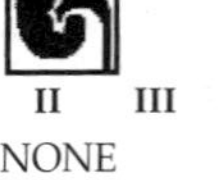

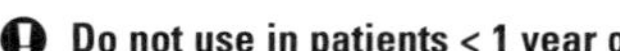

	I	II	III
Cat. C		NONE	NONE
②			

Drug Interactions

Specific studies have not been conducted with the ophthalmic solution. See Norfloxacin, oral for potential drug interactions.

Adverse Reactions

C: Local burning
O: Conjunctival hyperemia
　　Chemosis
　　Photophobia
R: Bitter taste after instillation

❶ Do not use in patients < 1 year old!

Nystatin oral suspension/pastilles

(Mycostatin pastilles®) **[$1.05/pastille]**
(Nystatin suspension®) **[$20.96/60 ml]**

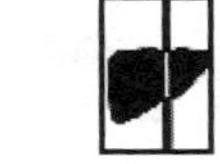

Dosage Modifications

	I	II	III
Cat. C		NONE	NONE
②			

<u>Drug Interactions</u>

NONE
FOOD: → NONE
ALCOHOL: → NONE

<u>Adverse Reactions</u>

C: NONE
O: Nausea
   Diarrhea
   Abdominal distress
   Vomiting
R: Oral irritation
   Rash
   Urticaria
   Stevens-Johnson syndrome

Nystatin topical ointment
(+ triamcinolone)
(Mycostatin®)   **[$22.68/30 gm];**
(Mytrex®, Myco-Triacet® II)   **[$20.30/30 gm]**

<u>Dosage Modifications</u>

	I	II	III
Cat. C		NONE	NONE
①			

Drug Interactions

NONE
FOOD: → NONE
ALCOHOL: → NONE

Adverse Reactions

C: NONE
O: Local irritation
R: NONE

Ofloxacin (oral); (IV)

(Floxin®) [$8.34];   (Floxin® IV)   [$26.40–52.80]

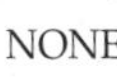 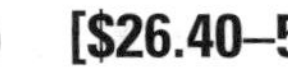 

Drug Interactions

VS: Vitamins ⎱
   Sucralfate ⎭ →↓ absorption of
   Antacids ⎰   oral ofloxacin
   Oral anticoagulants →↑ *risk of*
                  bleeding
   NSAIDs → *seizures*
   Beta blockers →↑ beta blocker effect
   H2 blockers →↓ [ofloxacin]
   Cyclophosphamide →↓ [ofloxacin]
   Oral hypoglycemics →↑ *hypoglycemia*
   Theophylline →↑ toxicity
   Cyclosporine →↑ nephrotoxicity
LS: Caffeine →↑ caffeine effects
   Phenytoin →↑ [phenytoin]
   Diazepam →↓ [diazepam]
   Foscarnet →↑ seizures
   Diuretic →↑ [ofloxacin]
FOOD: →↓ oral absorption
ALCOHOL: → NONE

Adverse Reactions

C: Nausea
   Insomnia
   Headache
   Pruritus vulvae
   Dizziness
   Vaginitis
   Diarrhea
   Vomiting
O: Abdominal cramps
   Chest pain
   Anorexia
   Dysgeusia
   Fatigue
   Flatulence
   Fever
   Rash
   Constipation

R: Asthenia
   Chills
   Malaise
   Extremity pain
   Epistaxis
   ↑ BUN/
     Creatinine
   ↑ Prothrombin
     time

Cat. C
③

I	II	III	
200–400 mg q12h	200–400 mg q24h	100–200 mg q24 h	NONE

Do not use in patients <18 years old!

Ofloxacin ophthalmic solution, 0.3%
(Ocuflox®)   [$22.78/5 ml]

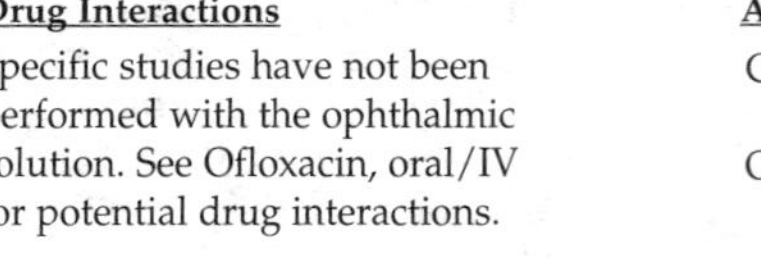

<u>Dosage Modifications</u>

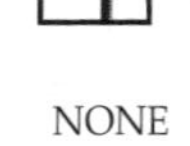 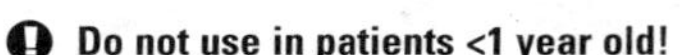

	I	II	III
Cat. C ②		NONE	NONE

Drug Interactions
Specific studies have not been performed with the ophthalmic solution. See Ofloxacin, oral/IV for potential drug interactions.

Adverse Reactions
C: Ocular discomfort
   Ocular burning
O: Stinging
   Redness
   Itching
R: Keratitis
   Periocular edema
   Facial edema
   Foreign body sensation
   Photophobia
   Blurred vision
   Tearing
   Dizziness

❶ **Do not use in patients <1 year old!**

Oxacillin
(Bactocill®, Prostaphlin®) [$6.61–10.48]

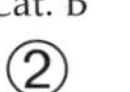

Cat. B
②

	I	II	III	
	500 mg q4–6h	250 mg q6–8h	250 mg q12–24h	NONE

Drug Interactions

VS: Oral anticoagulant →↑ risk of
      bleeding
    Cyclosporine →↑↓ [cyclosporine]
    Methotrexate →↑ [MTX]
    Tetracyclines 〉→↓ oxacillin
    Chloramphenicol 〉 effect
    Atenolol →↓ atenolol absorption
LS: Erythromycin →↓ effects of
    both drugs
    Aminoglycoside →↓ oxacillin effect
    Oral contraceptives →↓ contraceptive
    effect

FOOD: →↓ [oxacillin] (oral)
ALCOHOL: → NONE

Adverse Reactions

C: Nausea
   Vomiting
   Dysgeusia
   Diarrhea
   Steatorrhea
O: Leukopenia
   Thrombocytopenia
   Eosinophilia
   ↑ SGOT/SGPT (AST/ALT)
   ↑ BUN/↓ K^+
R: Anaphylaxis

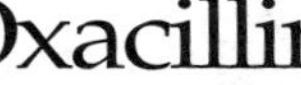 **Not for PCN-allergic patients!**

Oxamniquine
(Vansil®)   [$21.77]   [Ped-$10.88]

Dosage Modifications

	I	II	III
Cat. C ②		NONE	NONE

Drug Interactions

NONE
FOOD: → better tolerated
ALCOHOL: → NONE

Adverse Reactions

C: Nausea
   Vomiting
   Abdominal pain
   Anorexia
   Dizziness
   Drowsiness
   Headache
O: NONE
R: Epileptiform seizures

Paromomycin sulfate
(Humatin®)   [$14.49–20.29]

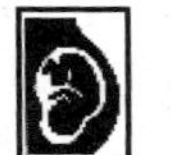 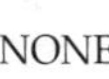 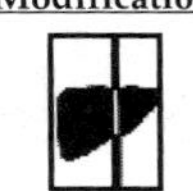

Drug Interactions

VS: Polypeptide →↑ risk of respiratory
antibiotics   depression and
                   nephrotoxicity
Succinyl choline →↑ respiratory
                   depression
Digoxin →↑↓ [digoxin]
LS: Oral anticoagulants →↑ risk of
                        bleeding
Methotrexate →↓ [MTX]
FOOD: →↑ absorption
ALCOHOL: → NONE

Adverse Reactions

C: Nausea
   Abdominal cramps
   Diarrhea
O: Tinnitus
   ↓ Hearing
   Dizziness
   ↑ SGOT/SGPT (AST/ALT)

Cat. C
③

I   II   III

Normal dose — 25–50% normal dose — 10–20% normal dose — NONE

Penicillin-G benzathine (IM) or Potassium (IV)

(Bicillin® C-R, Bicillin® L-A,
Permapen® [benzathine]) **[$25.36]**
(Pfizerpen® [potassium]) **[$3.44–10.09]**

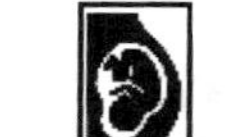 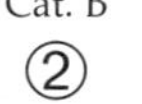 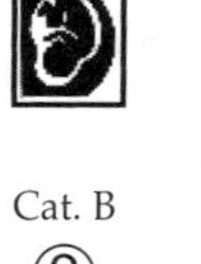

<u>Dosage Modifications</u>

	I	II	III
Cat. B		NONE	NONE
②			

Drug Interactions

VS: Oral anticoagulants →↑ risk of
    bleeding
Cyclosporine →↓↑ [cyclosporine]
Methotrexate →↑ [MTX]
Tetracyclines →↓ PCN effect
Probenecid →↑ [PCN]
Atenolol →↓ [atenolol]
LS: Erythromycin →↓ PCN effects
Oral contraceptives →↓ contraceptive
    effect

FOOD: → NONE
ALCOHOL: → NONE

Adverse Reactions

C: Nausea
Vomiting
Diarrhea
Dysgeusia
O: Anemia
Leukopenia
Thrombocytopenia
R: Hypersensitivity reactions
Neuropathy
Nephropathy
Leukopenia
Thrombocytopenia

❶ **Not for PCN-allergic patients!**

Penicillin-V (oral) [$0.54]

(Veltids®, Ledercillin® VK, V-Cillin® K, Beepen®-VK, Truxcillin® VK, Aoracillin® B, Pen-Vee® K, Pen®-V)   **[$0.60–0.92]**

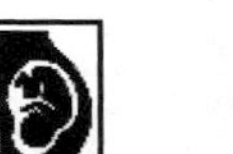

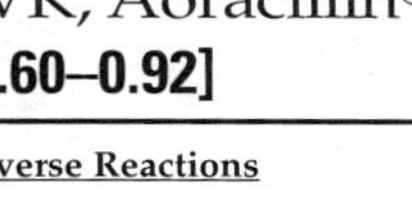

Drug Interactions	**Adverse Reactions**			
See Penicillin-G	C: Nausea	Cat. B	NONE	NONE
FOOD: →↓ [PCN]	Epigastric distress	②		
ALCOHOL: → NONE	Diarrhea			
	Black hairy tongue			
	O: Fever			
	Eosinophilia			
	R: Hemolytic anemia			
	Leukopenia			
	Thrombocytopenia			
	Neuropathy			
	Nephropathy			
	Hypersensitivity reactions			

❶ Not for PCN-allergic patients!

Pentamidine isethionate aerosol inhaler/IV

(Nebupent®, Pentam® 300)   **[$98.75]**
(Pentam® 300 IV)   **[$98.75]**

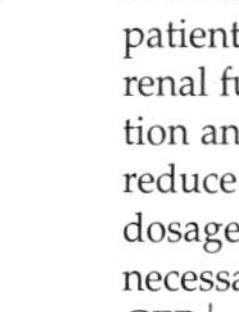
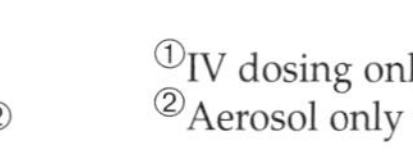

Drug Interactions	Adverse Reactions				
None Known	C: Leukopenia[1]	Anemia	Cat. C	Monitor patients' renal function and reduce dosage if necessary if GFR↓	NONE
FOOD: → NONE	Thrombocytopenia[1]	Neuralgia	②		
ALCOHOL: → NONE	↑ Creatinine[1]	Thrombocytopenia			
	Pain at injection site[1]	Phlebitis[1]			
	↑ LFTs[1]	Headache[2]			
	Nausea	Myalgia[2]			
	Anorexia	Edema[2]			
	Hypotension[1]	R: EKG abnormalities[1]			
	Hypoglycemia[1]	Diarrhea[1]			
	Fatigue	↑ Ca++[1]			
	Metallic taste	Tachycardia[2]			
	Shortness of breath[2]	Hypotension[2]			
	Dizziness[2]	Palpitations[2]			
	Rash[2]	Tremors			
	Cough[2]	Pruritus			
	Bronchospasm[2]	Melena[2]	[1]IV dosing only		
	O: Confusion/hallucinations	Gingivitis[2]	[2]Aerosol only		
		Colitis[2]			

❶ Do not use inhaler in pediatric patients!

Piperacillin Na
(Pipracil®)   [$69.00–92.00]

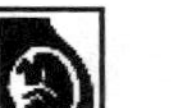 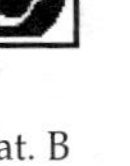

Drug Interactions

VS: Oral anticoagulants →↑ risk of
          bleeding
    Muscle relaxants →↑ respiratory
          depression
    Methotrexate →↑ [MTX]
    Tetracyclines →↓ piperacillin effect
    Oral contraceptives →↓ contraceptive
          effect

LS: Chloramphenicol →↓ piperacillin
          effect

FOOD: → NONE
ALCOHOL: → NONE

Adverse Reactions

C: Thrombophlebitis
   Local injection site inflammation
   Diarrhea
O: Vomiting
   ↑ SGOT/SGPT (AST/ALT)
   ↑ Bilirubin
   Headache
R: Hepatitis
   Bloody diarrhea
   Colitis
   Hypersensitivity reactions
   ↑ BUN/creatinine
   Leukopenia
   Thrombocytopenia
   ↑ K$^+$

Cat. B
②

I   12–16 gm/d given q4–6h
II 3–4 gm q8h
III 3–4 gm q12h
    NONE

❶ **Do not use in patients < 12 years old!**
❶ **Not for PCN-allergic patients!**

Piperacillin + Tazobactam
(Zosyn®)   [$61.24]

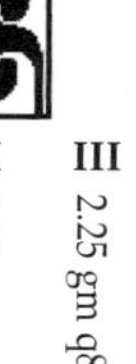

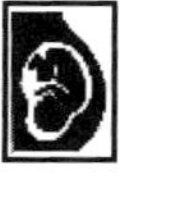

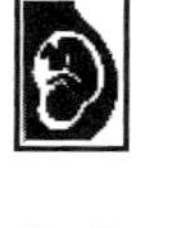

	I	II	III
Cat. B	3.375 gm q6h	2.25 gm q6h	2.25 gm q8h
②			NONE

Drug Interactions

See Piperacillin, plus:
VS: Aminoglycosides →↑
    aminoglycoside effect
    Tobramycin →↓ [tobramycin]
    Probenecid →↑ [zosyn]
FOOD: → NONE
ALCOHOL: → NONE

Adverse Reactions

C: Phlebitis
   Diarrhea
   Headache
   Constipation
   Nausea
   Insomnia
   Rash
   Vomiting
   Dyspepsia
   Pruritus
   Fever
   Agitation

O: Pain
   Moniliasis
R: Chest pain
   Edema
   Rhinitis
   Dyspnea
   ↑ SGOT/SGPT
    (AST/ALT)
   ↑ Prothrombin
    time
   ⊕ Coombs' Test

❶ Do not use in patients < 12 years old!
❶ Not for PCN-allergic patients!

Piperazine citrate [$0.27–0.38]

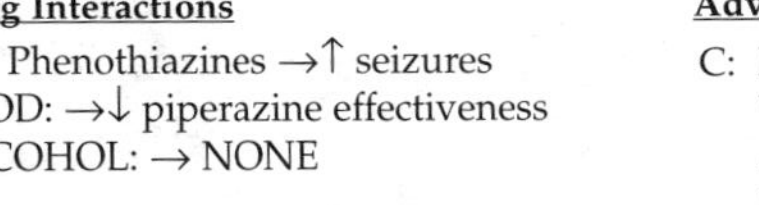

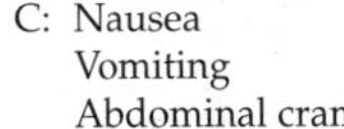

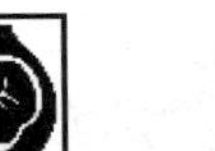

I   II   III

Drug Interactions

VS: Phenothiazines →↑ seizures
FOOD: →↓ piperazine effectiveness
ALCOHOL: → NONE

Adverse Reactions

C: Nausea
   Vomiting
   Abdominal cramps
   Diarrhea
O: Headache
   Vertigo
   Ataxia
   Tremors
   Chorea
   Muscular weakness
   Paresthesias
   Seizures
   EEG abnormalities
R: Hypersensitivity reactions

Cat.
③

Do not use in patients with renal or hepatic impairment.

❶ Do not use in pediatric patients!

Pneumococcal vaccine
(Pneumovax® 23, Pnu-Imune® 23)   [$12.36]

	I	II	III
Cat. C		NONE	NONE
②			

Drug Interactions

VS: Chemotherapy or radiation
therapy within 14 days
→↓ response to vaccine
FOOD: → NONE
ALCOHOL: → NONE

Adverse Reactions

C: Local injection site inflammation
and soreness
O: Fever
Malaise
Myalgia
Headache
Nausea
Vomiting
Asthenia
R: Rash
Urticaria
Arthritis
Serum sickness
Anaphylactoid reactions

❶ **Do not use in patients < 2 years old!**

Podofilox topical solution, 0.5%

(Condylox®)   **[$52.44/3.5 ml]**

I   II   III

Cat. C   NONE   NONE

②

Drug Interactions

NONE
FOOD: → NONE
ALCOHOL: → NONE

Adverse Reactions

C: Burning
Pain
Inflammation
Erosion
Itching
O: Dyspareunia
Insomnia
Tingling
Bleeding
Chafing
Malodor
Dizziness
Scarring
R: Hematuria
Vomiting
Ulceration

❶ **Do not use in pediatric patients!**

Podophyllin
(Podoben®, Pododerm®,
Podocon®-25)   **[$16.19–35.00/15ml]**

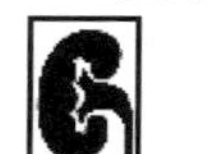 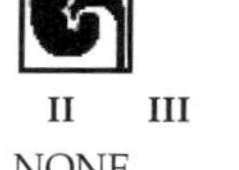 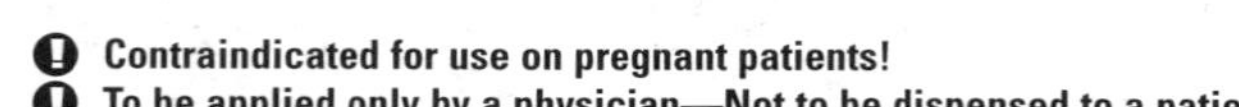

	I	II	III
Cat. C ③		NONE	NONE

Drug Interactions

VS: Steroids → DO NOT USE!
FOOD: → NONE
ALCOHOL: → NONE

Adverse Reactions

C: Local inflammation
O: Paresthesia
   Polyneuritis
R: Paralytic ileus
   Pyrexia
   Leukopenia
   Thrombocytopenia
   Coma

❶ **Contraindicated for use on pregnant patients!**
❶ **To be applied only by a physician—Not to be dispensed to a patient!**

Polio vaccine, inactivated
(Ipol®) [$19.05]

Drug Interactions

NONE
FOOD: → NONE
ALCOHOL: → NONE

Adverse Reactions

C: Local injection site inflammation
Fever
O: Sleepiness
Fussiness
Crying
↓ Appetite
Spitting up
R: Guillain-Barré syndrome

I   II   III

Cat. C   NONE   NONE
②

❗ **Do not use in patients with allergy to Neomycin, Streptomycin, or Polymyxin-B**

Polio vaccine, oral
(Orimune®) [$16.80]

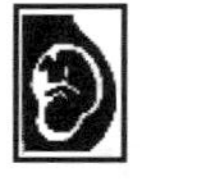

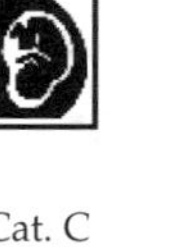

Drug Interactions	**Adverse Reactions**		I	II	III
NONE	C: Fever	Cat. C		NONE	NONE
FOOD: → NONE	Sleepiness	②			
ALCOHOL: → NONE	Fussiness				
	Crying				
	↓ Appetite				
	Spitting up				
	O: NONE				
	R: Paralytic poliomyelitis				

❶ **Avoid use in pregnant women!**
❶ **Do *not* use in patients with immune deficiency diseases or who are immunocompromised!**

Polymyxin + trimethoprim ophthalmic solution

(Polytrim®)　[$19.80/10 ml]

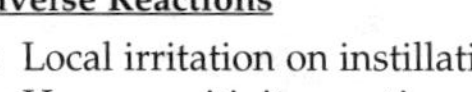

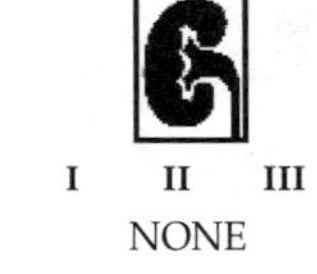

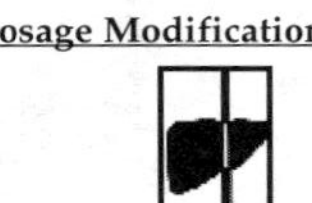

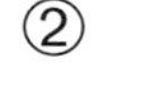

	I	II	III

Drug Interactions

NONE
FOOD: → NONE
ALCOHOL: → NONE

Adverse Reactions

C: Local irritation on instillation
O: Hypersensitivity reactions
R: Photosensitivity

Cat. C
②

NONE　　NONE

❗ **Do not use in patients < 2 months old!**

Praziquantel
(Biltricide®) [$75.09]

Drug Interactions

VS: Chloroquine →↓ [praziquantel]
Phenytoin
Carbamezepine ⟩ →↓ [praziquantel]
FOOD: →↑ tolerability of drug
ALCOHOL: → NONE

Adverse Reactions

C: Malaise
Headache
Abdominal discomfort
Dizziness
O: Fever
R: Urticaria

Cat. B
③

I II III

NONE   NONE

❶ Do not use in patients < 4 years old!

Primaquine phosphate [$0.86]

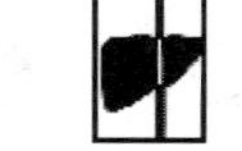

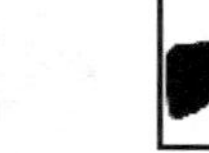
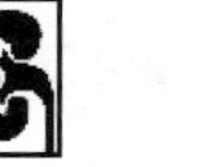

	I	II	III

Drug Interactions

VS: Quinacrine → ↑ toxicity
FOOD: → NONE
ALCOHOL: → NONE

Adverse Reactions

C: Nausea
Vomiting
Epigastric distress
Abdominal cramps
Hemolytic anemia (in G-6-PD
   deficient patients)
O: Leukopenia
R: Methemoglobinemia

Cat. C
③

I —
II — NONE
III — Monitor LFTs frequently—drug accumulates in the liver

Probenecid
(Benemid®, Col Benemid®)   [$0.34]

I   II   III

Cat. C   NONE   NONE

②

Drug Interactions

VS: Penicillins →↑ [PCN]
    Methotrexate →↑ [MTX]
    NSAIDs →↑ [NSAID]
    Benzodiazepine →↑ sedative effect
    Zidovudine →↑ [AZT]
    Cephalosporins →↑ [cephalosporin]
    Salicylates →↓ probenecid effect
LS: Hypoglycemic agents →↑ effects
    Acyclovir →↑ [acyclovir]
FOOD: → NONE
ALCOHOL: →↓ drug effect

Adverse Reactions

C: Nausea
   Vomiting
   Anorexia
   Sore gums
O: Precipitation of acute gouty arthritis
   ↑ SGOT/SGPT (AST/ALT)
   Anemia
   Leukopenia
   Dermatitis
R: Hepatitis
   Uric acid stones
   Nephrotic syndrome
   Alopecia

❶ Do not use in patients < 2 years old
❶ Do not use in patients with uric acid kidney stones

Propamidine isethionate, 0.1%
(Brolene®)

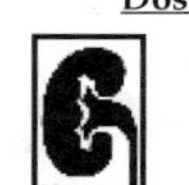 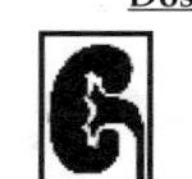

Dosage Modifications

I   II   III

Drug Interactions

Adverse Reactions

Drug information available from Bausch & Lomb Pharmaceuticals, (813) 975–7700.

Pyrantel pamoate
(Antiminth®, Pin-Rid®)   [$5.65]

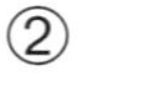

<u>Dosage Modifications</u>

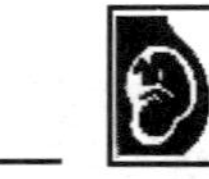

I   II   III

Cat. C   NONE   Contraindicated
②   in hepatic
         disease

Drug Interactions

VS: Piperazine → mutually antagonistic
LS: Theophylline →↑ [theophylline]
FOOD: → NONE
ALCOHOL: → NONE

Adverse Reactions

C: Headache
   Dizziness
O: Abdominal pain
   Diarrhea
R: Vomiting
   Rash

❶ **Avoid use in pregnant women!**
❶ **Do not use in children < 2 years old!**

Pyrazinamide [$4.04]

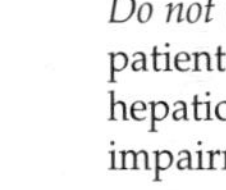

	I	II	III
Cat. C ②		NONE	*Do not use* in patients with hepatic impairment

Drug Interactions

VS: Cyclosporine →↓ [cyclosporine]
LS: Rifabutin →↓ [rifabutin]
    Rifampin →↓ [rifampin]
FOOD: → NONE
ALCOHOL: → NONE

Adverse Reactions

C: Hepatotoxicity
   Nausea
   Vomiting
   Anorexia
   Arthralgia
   Myalgia
O: Hypersensitivity reactions
R: Fever
   Porphyria
   Dysuria
   Thrombocytopenia
   Sideroblastic anemia
   Blood clotting disorders
   Acne
   Photosensitivity
   Interstitial nephritis

Pyrimethamine
(Daraprim®) [$0.82–1.23]

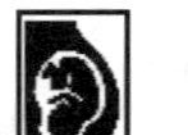 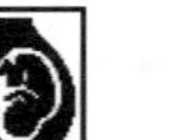 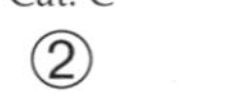

	I	II	III

Drug Interactions

VS: Folic acid →↓ pyrimethamine effect
Sulfonamides ⟩ →↑ bone marrow
TMP-SMX / suppression
LS: Lorazepam → hepatotoxicity
FOOD: → NONE
ALCOHOL: → NONE

Adverse Reactions

C: Anorexia
Vomiting
Atropic glossitis
Hypersensitivity reactions
O: Megaloblastic anemia
Leukopenia
Thrombocytopenia
Pancytopenia
Hematuria
Cardiac arrhythmias
R: Insomnia
Diarrhea
Headache
Light-headedness
Dermatitis
Fever
Malaise
Depression

Cat. C
②

I   II III

NONE   NONE

Pyrimethamine + Sulfadoxine
(Fansidar®)   [$6.74–10.11]

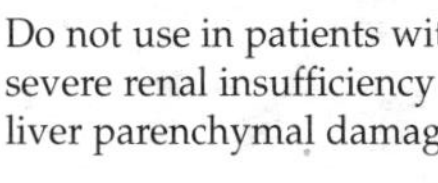

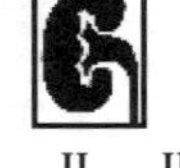 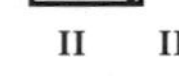

Drug Interactions

VS: Chloroquine →↑ toxicity

Sulfonamides ⟩ →↑ bone marrow
TMP-SMX ⟩ suppression

Anticoagulants →↑ risk of bleeding

MAO inhibitors →↑ toxicity

FOOD: → NONE

ALCOHOL: → NONE

Adverse Reactions

C: Nausea
Vomiting
Abdominal pain
Diarrhea
Anorexia

O: Pancreatitis
Stomatitis
Megaloblastic anemia
Severe allergic skin rash
Headache
Peripheral neuritis
Fever

R: *Stevens-Johnson syndrome*
Toxic epidermal necrolysis
Anaphylaxis

Cat. C

③

I   II   III

Do not use in patients with
severe renal insufficiency or
liver parenchymal damage

❶ **Do not use in patients < 2 months old!**

Quinacrine HCl [$0.97]

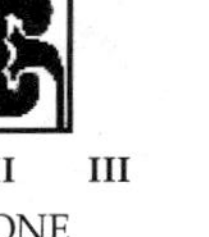

Drug Interactions

VS: Primaquine → ↑ toxicity
FOOD: → ↑ absorption
ALCOHOL: → disulfiram-like
      reaction

Adverse Reactions

C: Diarrhea
   Anorexia
   Nausea
   Abdominal cramps
   Vomiting
   Headache
   Dizziness
O: Yellowing of skin
R: Skin rash
   Fever
   Acute, toxic psychosis

Cat. X
③   NONE   NONE

Quinidine gluconate
(Quinaglute®)   [$1.12]

Drug Interactions

VS: Thiazide diuretics
Carbonic anhydrase
inhibitors   →↑ [quinidine]
Sodium bicarbonate

Amiodarone
Cimetidine   →↑ [quinidine]

Phenobarbital
Phenytoin   →↓ [quinidine]
Rifampin

Ketoconazole →↑ [quinidine]

Nifedipine
Verapamil   →↓ [quinidine]

Digoxin →↑ [digoxin]
Procainamide →↑ [procainamide]
Haloperidol →↑ [haloperidol]
Neuromuscular blockers
→↑ neuromuscular blockade

FOOD: →↑ [quinidine] (especially
alkaline foods: dairy
products, citrus juices,
nuts, some vegetables)

ALCOHOL: → NONE

Adverse Reactions

C: Diarrhea
Fever
Rash
Cardiac arrhythmias
Nausea/vomiting
Dizziness
Headache

O: Asthenia
Cinchonism
Depression
Mydriasis
Optic neuritis
Photosensitivity

R: Autoimmune syndromes
Hepatotoxicity
Urticaria
Hypotension
Ataxia

Cat. C
③

I   II   III

NONE   NONE

Quinine sulfate [$0.72]

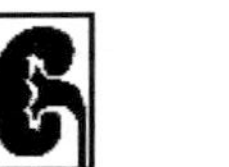

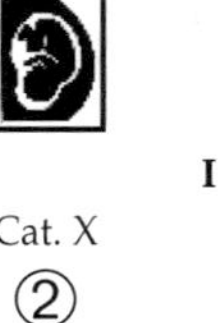

	I	II	III
Cat. X ②		NONE	NONE, but monitor LFTs while patient is taking drug

Drug Interactions

VS: Antacids →↓ quinine absorption
Oral anticoagulants →↑ risk of bleeding
Cometidine →↑ [quinine]
Digoxin→↑ [digoxin]
Mefloquine → risk of cardiac toxicity
Neuromuscular blockers → respiratory depression
Urinary alkalizers →↑ [quinine]
Terfenadine ⎫
Astemizole ⎭ → cardiac toxicity

LS: Rifabutin →↓ [quinine]

FOOD: →↓ GI irritation, but may ↑ absorption → toxicity

ALCOHOL: → NONE

Adverse Reactions

C: Cinchonism
Hemolytic anemia
Agranulocytosis
Hypoprothrom-binemia
Nausea
Vomiting
Abdominal pain
Diarrhea
Dysgeusia

O: Visual disturbances
Tinnitus
Vertigo
Headache
Fever
Restlessness
Confusion
Dizziness
↑ SGOT/SGPT (AST/ALT)

R: Hypersensitiv-ity reactions
Angina
Flushing
Asthma
Hemoglobinuria

Rabies immune globulin

(Imogam® rabies, Bayrab®, Hyperab®)

[$565.56 – 725.00/dose]

Drug Interactions

VS: Rabies vaccine →↓ immunity
from vaccine (if RIG
given repeatedly once
vaccine treatment is
initiated)
Live viral vaccine (M-M-R,
polio) →↓ response to
vaccine

FOOD: → NONE
ALCOHOL: → NONE

Adverse Reactions

C: Soreness at injection site
O: Fever
R: Angioneurotic edema
Skin rash
Nephrotic syndrome
Anaphylaxis

Cat. C
②

I   II   III

NONE   NONE

❗ **Use with caution in patients with IgA deficiency!**

Rabies vaccine
(Imovax®) **[$140.56/dose]**

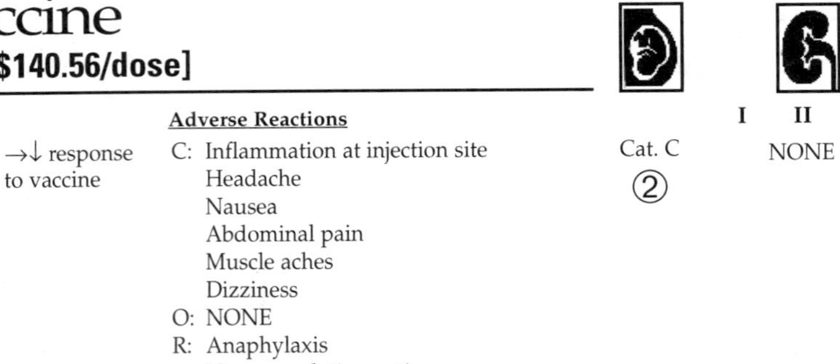

I II III

Cat. C	NONE	NONE
②		

Drug Interactions

VS: Corticosteroids
Immunosuppressive } →↓ response to vaccine
agents
FOOD: → NONE
ALCOHOL: → NONE

Adverse Reactions

C: Inflammation at injection site
Headache
Nausea
Abdominal pain
Muscle aches
Dizziness
O: NONE
R: Anaphylaxis
Neuroparalytic reactions

❗ **Use with caution in patients with immunosuppressive illnesses!**

Ranitidine-Bismuth citrate

(Tritec®)   [**$3.48** plus cost of clarithromycin]

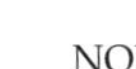

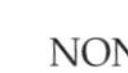

Drug Interactions

VS: Clarithromycin ⟩ ↑ [ranitidine]
　　　　　　　　　 ↑ [bismuth]

LS: Antacids →↓ [ranitidine]
FOOD: → NONE
ALCOHOL: → NONE

Adverse Reactions

C: Dysgeusia
　 Diarrhea
O: Nausea
　 Vomiting
　 Headache
　 Sleep disorder
　 Chest symptoms
　 Pruritus
　 Gynecological problems
R: Abdominal discomfort
　 ↑ SGOT/SGPT (AST/ALT)
　 Anaphylaxis
　 Tremors

I　**II**　**III**

I　Normal dose

II　Use with extreme caution!

III　Do not use if GFR < 25 ml/min!

NONE

❶ **Do not use in pediatric patients!**

Ribavirin inhaler
(Virazole®) [$1319.85]

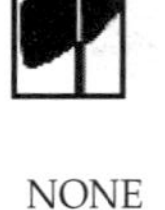

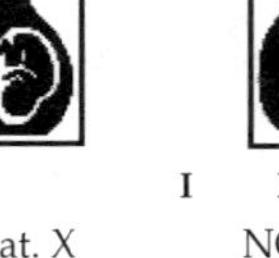 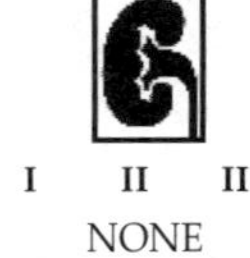 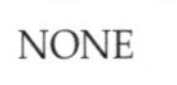

	Drug Interactions	Adverse Reactions		I	II	III

Drug Interactions

Clinical drug interaction
studies have not been
performed
FOOD: → NONE
ALCOHOL: → NONE

Adverse Reactions

C: *Sudden deterioration of respiratory
   function!*
   Cardiotoxicity!
   Anemia
O: Rash
   Conjunctivitis
R: Seizures
   Asthenia

Cat. X
③

I II III

NONE   NONE

❶ Do not use in adults! For pediatric use only.
❶ Use with caution in mechanically-ventilated patients!

Rifabutin
(Mycobutin®)   **[$7.48]**

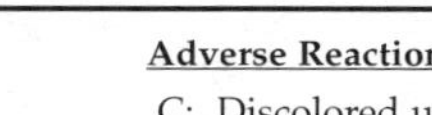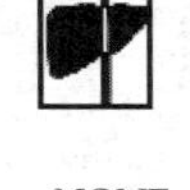

Drug Interactions

VS: Oral anticoagulants →
   ↓ anticoagulant effect
Corticosteriods →↓ steroid effect
Cyclosporine→↓ [cyclosporine]
Phenytoin →↓ [phenytoin]
Beta blockers →↓ anti-hypertensive
   effect
Zidovudine →↓ [AZT]
Azole antifungals →↓ [antifungal]
Quinine
Quinidine ⟩ →↓ [quinine/quinidine]
Indinavir →↓ [indinavir]
Oral contraceptives →↓ contraceptive
   effect

FOOD: →↓ absorption (especially
   high-fat foods)

ALCOHOL: → NONE

Adverse Reactions

C: Discolored urine/saliva
   Rash
   Neutropenia
   Leukopenia
   ↑ SGOT/SGPT (AST/ALT)
O: Anorexia
   Diarrhea
   Dyspepsia
   Eructation
   Flatulence
   Dysgeusia
   Nausea
R: Uveitis

Cat. B

I	II	III
	NONE	NONE

Rifampin (oral) ($3.89)
(Rifadin®) [$4.22]; (Rifadin® IV) [$79.38]

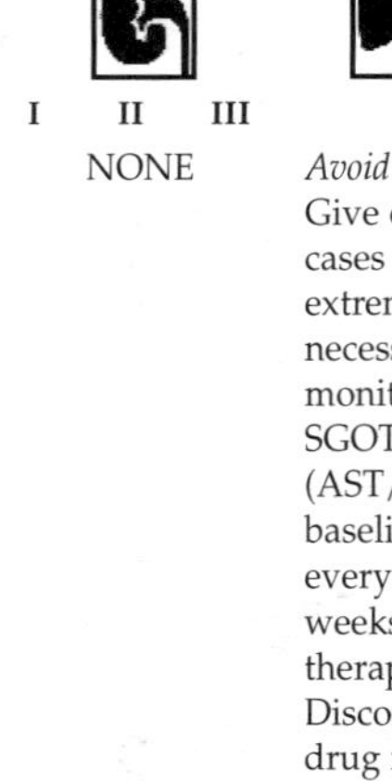

Dosage Modifications

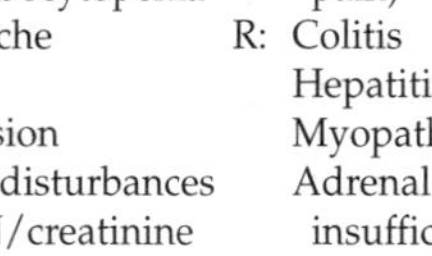	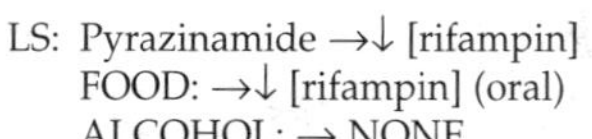	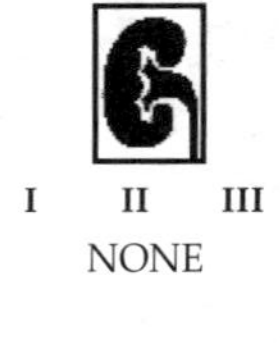

Drug Interactions

Adverse Reactions

VS: Oral anticoagulants →
  ↓ anticoagulant effect
Corticosteroids →↓ steroid effect
Cyclosporine →↓ [cyclosporine]
Calcium channel blockers →
  →↓ [CCB]
Ritonavir →↓ [ritonavir]
Oral hypoglycemic →↓ hypoglycemic
  effect
Phenytoin →↓ [phenytoin]
Digoxin →↓ [digoxin]
Isoniazid→↑ hepatotoxicity
Zidovudine →↓ [AZT]
Azole antifungal→↓ [azole] &↓ [rifampin]
Quinine/Quinidine →↓ [quinine/quinidine]
Theophylline →↓ [theophylline]
Oral contraceptives →↓ contraceptive
  effect

Indinavir →↓ [indinavir]

C: Liver dysfunction
Jaundice
Leukopenia
Hemolytic anemia
Thrombocytopenia
O: Headache
Fever
Confusion
Visual disturbances
↑ BUN/creatinine
Flushing
Itching

GI distress
  (nausea/
  vomiting/
  epigastric
  pain)
R: Colitis
Hepatitis
Myopathy
Adrenal
  insufficiency
Hypersensi-
  tivity
  reactions

LS: Pyrazinamide →↓ [rifampin]
  FOOD: →↓ [rifampin] (oral)
  ALCOHOL: → NONE

Cat. C
②

NONE

Avoid use.
Give only in
cases of
extreme
necessity, and
monitor
SGOT/SGPT
(AST/ALT) at
baseline and
every 2–4
weeks during
therapy.
Discontinue
drug if signs
of hepatocel-
lular damage
occur.

Rifampin + Isoniazid
(Rifamate®)   [$4.86]

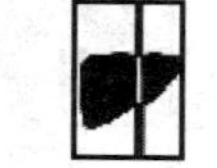

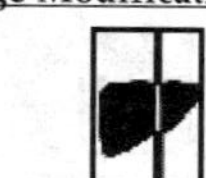

I   II   III

Drug Interactions

Adverse Reactions

See listings for Isoniazid and Rifampin. Rifamate is simply a combination capsule of the two drugs.

Rifampin + Isoniazid + Pyrazinamide
(Rifater®)   [$10.80]

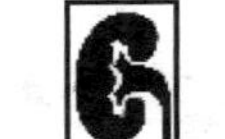 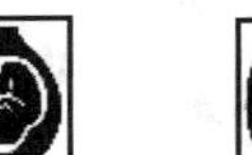 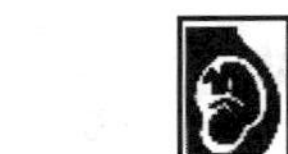

Dosage Modifications

I   II   III

Drug Interactions

Adverse Reactions

See listings for Isoniazid, Rifampin, & Pyrazinamide. Rifater is simply a combination tablet containing the three drugs.

❶ **Avoid this combination in patients < 15 years old!**

Rimantadine
(Flumadine®) [$3.00]

Drug Interactions

LS: Cimetidine →↑ [rimantadine]
    Acetaminophen →↓ [rimantadine]
FOOD: → NONE
ALCOHOL: → NONE

Adverse Reactions

C: Nausea
    Vomiting
    Anorexia
O: Insomnia
    Dizziness
    Headache
    Nervousness
    Dry mouth
    Abdominal pain
    Asthenia
R: Dyspepsia
    Constipation
    Stomatitis
    Ataxia

Dosage Modifications

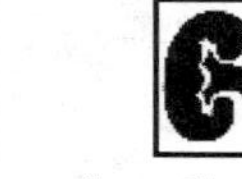

Cat. C
③

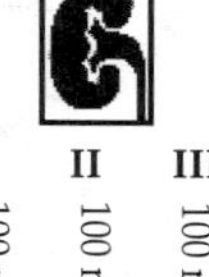

I	II	III	
100 mg BID	100 mg qd	100 mg qd	100 mg qd

All patients with hepatic or renal insufficiency should be monitored for adverse effects, with further dose adjustments made as necessary

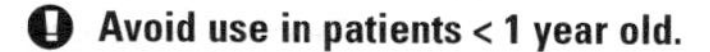 **Avoid use in patients < 1 year old.**

Ritonavir
(Norvir®) [$22.26]

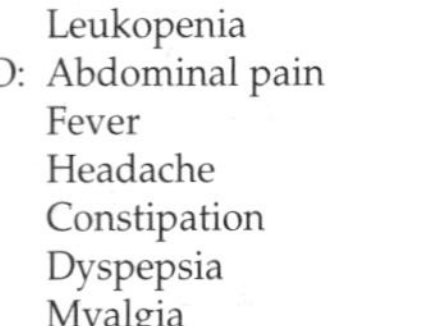
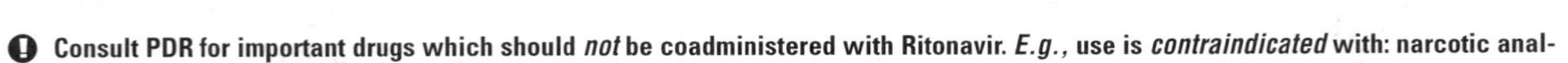

	I	II	III
Cat. B 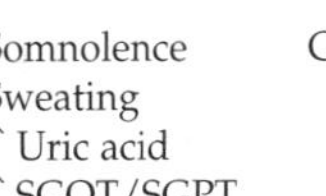	NONE		*Use with extreme caution.* Clinical and laboratory monitoring of hepatic function must be performed frequently. May start patients at 300 mg BID and dose titrate by 100 mg BID increments.

Drug Interactions

VS: Encainide →↑↑ [encainide]
Bepridil →↑↑ [bepridil]
Amiodarone →↑↑ [amiodarone]
Propoxyphene →↑↑ [propoxyphene]
Meperidine →↑↑ [meperidine]
Terfenadine ⎫
Astemizole ⎭ → cardiotoxicity
Rifabutin →↓ [ritonavir]
Clozapine→↑↑ [clozapine]
Flecainide →↑↑ [flecainide]
Propafenone →↑↑ [propafenone]
Quinidine →↑↑ [quinidine]
Cisapride →↑↑ [cisapride]
LS: Benzodiazepines → severe sedation
Piroxicam →↑ [piroxicam]
FOOD: →↑ absorption
ALCOHOL: → NONE

Adverse Reactions

C: Diarrhea
Nausea/vomiting
Dysgeusia
Asthenia
↑ GGT
↑ Triglycerides
↑ CPK
Anemia
Leukopenia
O: Abdominal pain
Fever
Headache
Constipation
Dyspepsia
Myalgia
Paresthesias
Dizziness

Somnolence
Sweating
↑ Uric acid
↑ SGOT/SGPT (AST/ALT)
R: Malaise
Flatulence
Thought disturbances
Pharyngitis
↑ Glucose
↑ Creatinine
↑ K^+/Ca^{++}
↑ LDH

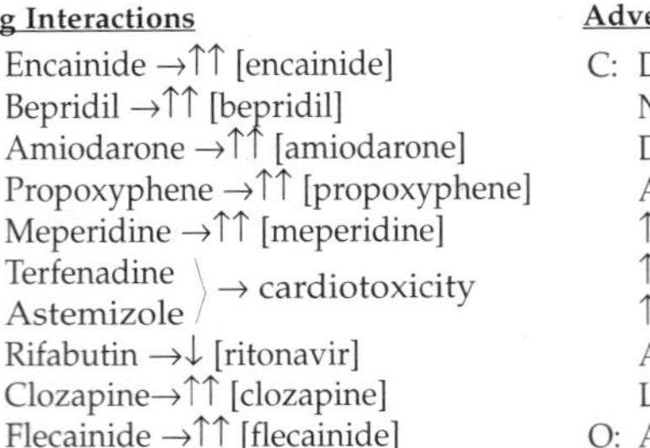
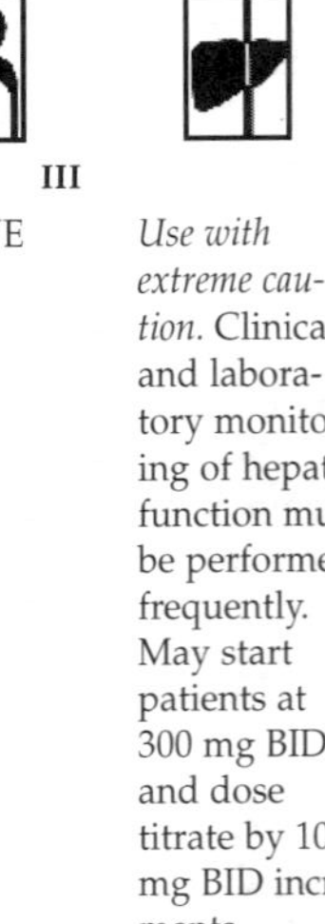

❶ Consult PDR for important drugs which should *not* be coadministered with Ritonavir. *E.g.*, use is *contraindicated* with: narcotic analgesics, piroxicam, antiarrhythmics, certain anti-depressants, anti-emetics, nonsedating antihistamines, Rifabutin, & calcium channel blockers!

Saquinavir mesylate
(Invirase®, Fortovase®)   [$19.07–19.12]

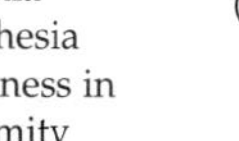 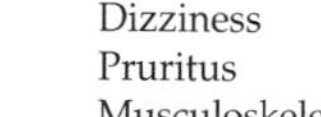 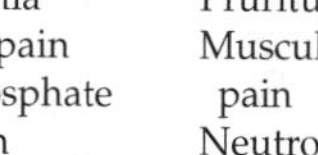

Drug Interactions

VS: Ritonavir →↑↑ [saquinavir]
LS: Ketoconazole →↑ [saquinavir]
Rifampin ⟩ →↓ [saquinavir]
Rifabutin
Phenobarbital
Phenytoin ⟩ may ↓
Dexamethasone → [saquinavir]
Carbamazepine
FOOD: →↑ absorption
ALCOHOL: → NONE

Adverse Reactions

C: Diarrhea
   Nausea
   Cheilitis
   Headache
   Peripheral neuropathy
   Rash
   Hypoglycemia
O: Abdominal pain
   ↑ K^+ / ↓ Phosphate
   Constipation
   Eructation
   Discolored feces
   Gastritis
   Melena
   ↑ SGOT / SGPT
   (AST / ALT)

R: Hepatitis
   Asthenia
   Paresthesia
   Numbness in
   extremity
   Dizziness
   Pruritus
   Musculoskeletal
   pain
   Neutropenia
   Thrombocyto-
   penia

	I	II	III
Cat. B ②		NONE	*Use with extreme caution and frequent clinical and laboratory monitoring*

 Do not use in patients < 16 years old!
 Consult PDR for use of drugs which, if coadministered with saquinavir, may result in serious toxicity!

Silver nitrate solution/ ointment, 1% [$18.75/30 ml; $30.00/30 gm]

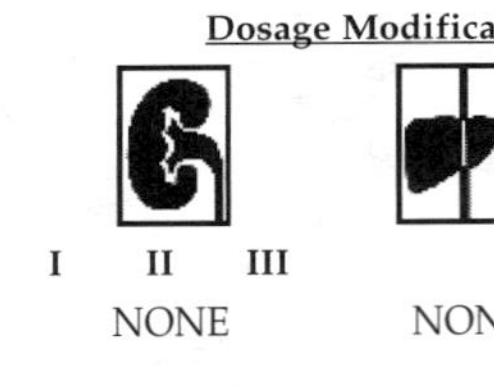

Drug Interactions

VS: Sulfonamides → incompatibility
FOOD: → NONE
ALCOHOL: → NONE

Adverse Reactions

C: Chemical conjunctivitis
   Skin discoloration

	I	II	III
Cat. C 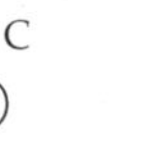		NONE	NONE

Stavudine (d4T)
(Zerit ®)   **[$8.46]**

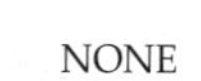 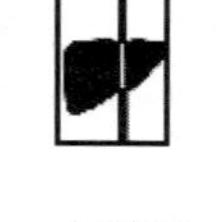 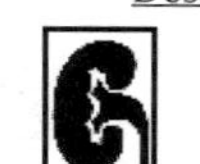

Drug Interactions

VS: Zidovudine → antagonism with stavudine—do not use concurrently

FOOD: →↓ [stavudine] (especially high fat foods)

ALCOHOL: → NONE

Adverse Reactions

C: Peripheral neuropathy
↑ SGOT/SGPT (AST/ALT)
Headache
Chills
Fever
Diarrhea
Nausea/vomiting
Anorexia
Dyspepsia
Constipation
Myalgia
Insomnia
Allergic reaction
↑ Amylase

O: Ulcerative colitis
Aphthous stomatitis
Pancreatitis
Neutropenia
Thrombo-cytopenia
↑ Bilirubin

Cat. C
③

	I	II	III	
	40 mg q12h	20 mg q12h	20 mg q24h	NONE

Streptomycin sulfate [$0.58]

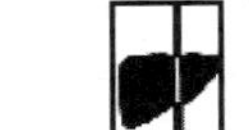 Cat. D 

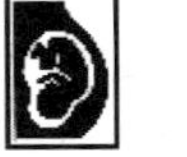 I II III

Drug Interactions

VS: Diuretics →↑ ototoxicity
Muscle relaxants →↑ respiratory
depression
NSAIDs →↑ [streptomycin] &
↓ GFR
Digoxin →↓ [digoxin]
Cephalosporins→↑ nephrotoxicity
Amphotericin B →↑ nephrotoxicity
LS: Penicillins →↓ PCN effect
FOOD: → NONE
ALCOHOL: → NONE

Adverse Reactions

C: Vestibular
ototoxicity
Facial paresthesia
Rash
Fever
Urticaria
Angioneurotic edema
Eosinophilia
O: Cochlear ototoxicity
Exfoliative dermatitis
Anaphylaxis
Azotemia
Leukopenia
Thrombocytopenia

Hemolytic
anemia
Muscle
weakness
Amblyopia
R: Nephrotoxicity

I Normal dose
II 25–50% normal dose
III 10–20% normal dose
NONE

❶ **Consult PDR for list of important drugs that should *not* be coadministered with streptomycin!**

Sulfacetamide sodium ophthalmic solution/cream, 10%

(AK-Sulf®, Bleph®-10, Cetamide®, Sulf®-10)

[$3.15/5 ml or $3.39/3.5 gm]

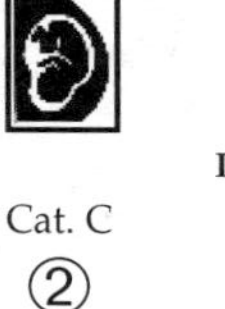

Drug Interactions

VS: Silver-containing ophthalmic preparations → incompatibility
Local ophthalmic anesthetics →↓ sulfacetamide effect

FOOD: → NONE
ALCOHOL: → NONE

Adverse Reactions

C: Local irritation
O: Secondary corneal infections (viral, fungal)
   Allergic reactions
R: Stevens-Johnson syndrome
   Toxic epidermal necrolysis
   Hepatic necrosis
   Agranulocytosis

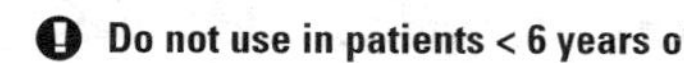 **Do not use in patients < 6 years old.**

Sulfacetamide + prednisone ophthalmic solution
(Blephamide®, Blephamide® S.O.P.) [$18.04/5 ml]

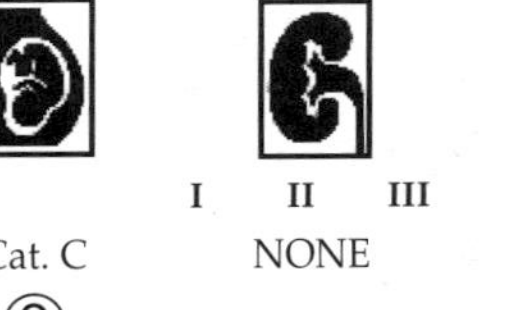

<u>**Dosage Modifications**</u>

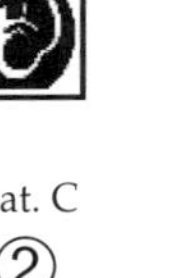

	I	II	III
Cat. C 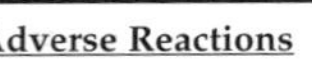		NONE	NONE

<u>Drug Interactions</u>

See sulfacetamide sodium

<u>Adverse Reactions</u>

C: Local irritation
O: Secondary corneal infections
  ↑ Intraocular pressure
  Glaucoma
  Cataract formation
R: Optic nerve damage
  Stevens-Johnson syndrome
  Toxic epidermal necrolysis
  Hepatitic necrosis
  Agranulocytosis
  Fungal invasion
  Corneal ulceration
  Acute anterior uveitis

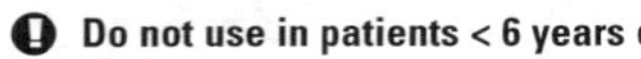 **Do not use in patients < 6 years old.**

Sulfadiazine topical cream, 1%
(Silvadene®, SSD®, Thermazene®)   [$4.25/20 gm]

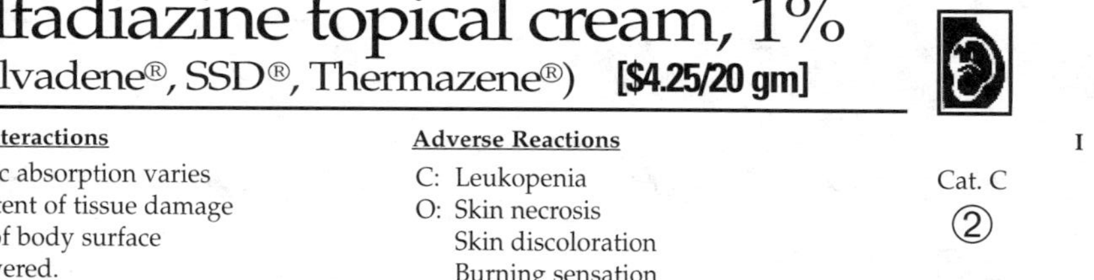

Dosage Modifications

	I	II	III
Cat. C		NONE	NONE
②			

Drug Interactions

Systemic absorption varies
with extent of tissue damage
and % of body surface
area covered.
FOOD: → NONE
ALCOHOL: → NONE

Adverse Reactions

C: Leukopenia
O: Skin necrosis
 Skin discoloration
 Burning sensation
 Rashes
R: Interstitial nephritis
 Erythema multiforme

Suramin
(Fourneau® 309, Bayer® 205)

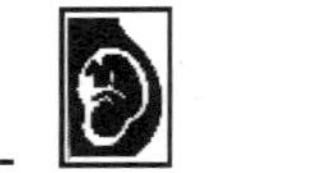

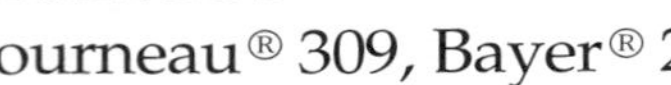

I   II   III

Drug Interactions

Adverse Reactions

Drug information is available from the Centers for Disease Control & Prevention, Center for Infectious Diseases, by calling (404) 639-3670 (8 AM–4:30 PM EST, M–F) or (404) 639-2888 (for emergencies).

Terbinafine topical cream, 1%

(Lamisil®)   [$27.12/15 gm]

	I	II	III
Cat. B		NONE	NONE
②			

Drug Interactions

NONE
FOOD: → NONE
ALCOHOL: → NONE

Adverse Reactions

C: Irritation
O: Burning
   Tingling
R: Itching
   Dryness

❶ **Nursing mothers should avoid application of Terbinafine topical cream to the breast!**
❶ **Do not use in patients < 12 years old!**

Terconazole vaginal cream / suppositories
(Terazol® 3, Terazol® 7) **[$8.34]**

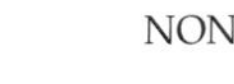

Dosage Modifications

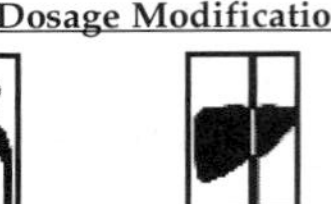  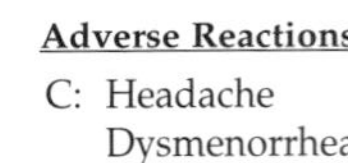

Drug Interactions

NONE
FOOD: → NONE
ALCOHOL: → NONE

Adverse Reactions

C: Headache
   Dysmenorrhea
O: Genital burning
   Genital itching
   Abdominal pain
R: Fever

	I	II	III
Cat. C ②		NONE	NONE

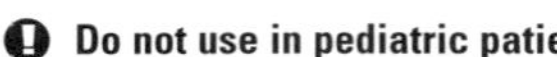 **Do not use in pediatric patients!**

Tetanus immune globulin
(Baytet®)   [$62.00/dose]

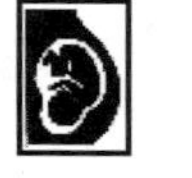

	I	II	III
Cat. C		NONE	NONE
②			

Drug Interactions

VS: Live viral vaccine
   (M-M-R, polio) →
      ↓ vaccine response
   (Defer such vaccinations
   for ≥ 3 months)
FOOD: → NONE
ALCOHOL: → NONE

Adverse Reactions

C: Soreness at injection site
   Fever
O: NONE
R: Angioneurotic edema
   Nephrotic syndrome
   Anaphylactic shock

❗ **Do not use in patients < 7 years old!**

Tetanus toxoid [$3.23/dose]

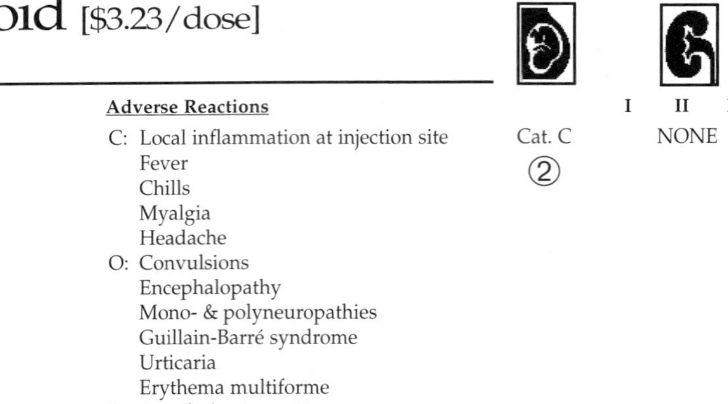

Drug Interactions

VS: Immunosuppressive
     drugs or
     corticosteroids →
          ↓ antibody response
FOOD: → NONE
ALCOHOL: → NONE

Adverse Reactions

C: Local inflammation at injection site
   Fever
   Chills
   Myalgia
   Headache
O: Convulsions
   Encephalopathy
   Mono- & polyneuropathies
   Guillain-Barré syndrome
   Urticaria
   Erythema multiforme
R: Anaphylactic reaction

❗ **Do not use in patients with allergy to Thimerosal!**

Tetanus + diphtheria toxoids
(Td®)   [$3.04/dose]

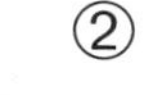

	I	II	III
Cat. C ②		NONE	NONE

Drug Interactions

VS: Immunosuppressive
agents or corticosteroids →
↓ antibody response
FOOD: → NONE
ALCOHOL: → NONE

Adverse Reactions

C: Local inflammation at injection site
Fever
Chills
Myalgias
Headaches
O: Convulsions
Encephalopathy
Mono- & polyneuropathies
Guillain-Barré syndrome
Urticaria
Erythema multiforme
R: Anaphylactic reaction

❶ **Do not use in patients < 7 years of age!**

Tetracycline [$0.15]

(Brodspec®, Sumycin®, Tetracap®, Panmycin®, Achromycin®, Wesmycin®, ALA-TET®)   [$0.12–0.60]

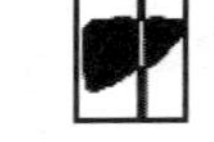

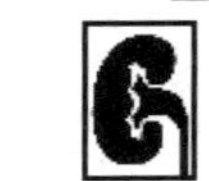

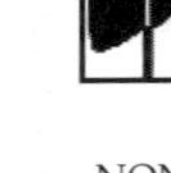

Dosage Modifications

I	II	III	
500 mg QID	250 mg QID	250 mg BID	NONE

Cat. D ③

Drug Interactions

VS: Antacids →↓ TCN absorption
Digoxin →↑ [digoxin]
Anticoagulants →↑ risk of
       bleeding
Vitamins →↓ TCN absorption
Iron →↓ TCN absorption
Penicillins →↓ PCN effect
Oral contraceptives
    ↓ contraceptive effect
Insulin →↑ hypoglycemic
    effects
Bismuth →↓ TCN absorption
LS: Diuretics →↑ BUN
Theophylline ↑ toxicity
Lithium →↑ toxicity
FOOD: →↓ TCN absorption
ALCOHOL: →↑ TCN clearance

Adverse Reactions

C: Nausea
Vomiting
Diarrhea
Glossitis
Stomatitis
Anorexia
O: ↑ BUN
Rashes
Hemolytic anemia
Thrombocytopenia
Dizziness
Tinnitus
Visual disturbances
Pseudotumor cerebri
Photosensitivity

R: ↑ SGOT/SGPT
(AST/ALT)
Esophagitis
Colitis
Balanitis
Anaphylaxis
Eosinophilia
Myasthenic
  syndrome

❶ **Do not use in patients < 8 years old!**

Thiabendazole
(Mintezol®) [$3.13]

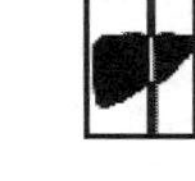

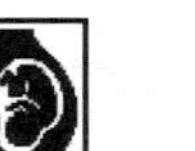

	I	II	III
Cat. C		NONE	NONE
②			

Drug Interactions

VS: Theophylline →
    ↑ [theophylline]
FOOD: → NONE
ALCOHOL: → NONE

Adverse Reactions

C: Anorexia
   Vomiting
   Diarrhea
   Epigastric distress
   Dizziness
   Drowsiness
   Headache
   Numbness
   Confusion
   Floating sensation
   Hematuria
   Cholestasis
   Jaundice
O: Erythema multiforme
   Drying of mucous membrane
   Fever
R: ↑ SGOT/SGPT (AST/ALT)
   Hepatic failure
   Leukopenia

Ticarcillin
(Ticar®)   [$23.22–46.44]

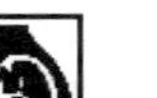 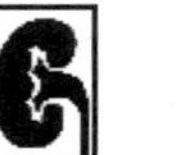

Dosage Modifications

Drug Interactions

VS: Oral anticoagulants →↑ risk of
　　　　　　　　　bleeding
　　Cyclosporine →↑↓ [cyclosporine]
　　Methotrexate →↑ [MTX]
　　Tetracyclines →↓ ticarcillin effect
　　Oral contraceptives →
　　　　　　↓ contraceptive effect
　　Chloramphenicol →↓ ticarcillin
　　　　　　　　　effect

FOOD: → NONE
ALCOHOL: → NONE

Adverse Reactions

C: Nausea
　　Vomiting
　　Diarrhea
O: Anemia
　　Thrombocytopenia
　　Neutropenia
　　Eosinophilia
　　↑ SGOT/SGPT (AST/ALT)
　　Phlebitis
R: Seizures
　　Pseudomembranous colitis

Cat. C
②

	I	II	III	
	3 gm q4h	2 gm q4–8h	2 gm q12h	NONE, unless there is concomitant renal insufficiency, then 1 gm q12h or 2gm q24h

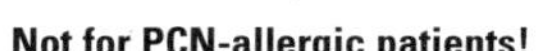 **Not for PCN-allergic patients!**

Ticarcillin + clavulanate
(Timentin®) [$67.70]

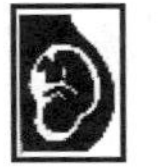

Drug Interactions

See Ticarcillin

Adverse Reactions

See Ticarcillin, plus:
C: False ⊕ Coombs' Test

Cat. B
②

I	II	III	
2–3.1 gm q4h	2 gm q8h	2 gm q12h	NONE, unless there is concomitant renal insufficiency, then 2gm q24h.

❶ **Do not use in patients < 12 years old!**
❶ **Not for PCN-allergic patients!**

Tioconazole vaginal cream, 6.5%
(Vagistat®)   [$24.20/4.6 gm]

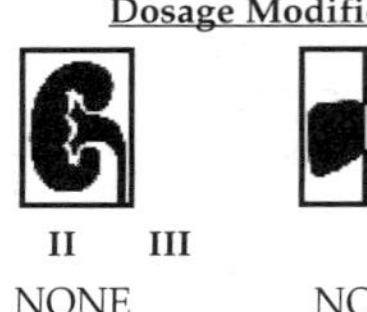
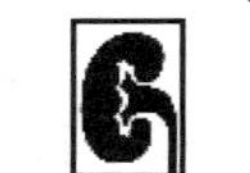
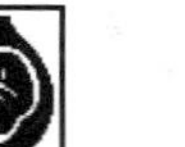

	I	II	III
Cat. C ③		NONE	NONE

Drug Interactions

NONE
FOOD: → NONE
ALCOHOL: → NONE

Adverse Reactions

C: Burning
   Itching
O: Irritation
   Discharge
   Vulvar swelling
   Vaginal pain
   Dysuria
   Dyspareunia
   Dryness of vagina
   Vaginitis
   Headache
   Abdominal pain
R: Rash
   Vulvovaginal disorder

Tobramycin
(Nebcin®) [$19.12–31.90]

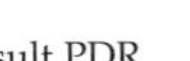 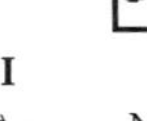 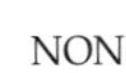

Drug Interactions

VS: Bumetanide → ototoxicity
Methoxyflurane → nephrotoxicity
Muscle relaxants → respiratory
depression
Diuretics → ototoxicity
Torsemide → ototoxicity
Vancomycin → nephrotoxicity
NSAIDs →↑ [tobramycin]
Dogoxin→↑↓ [digoxin]
Cephalosporins →↑ nephrotoxicity
Amphotericin B →↑ nephrotoxicity
Cyclosporine →↑ nephrotoxicity
LS: Anticoagulants →↑ risk of bleeding
FOOD: → NONE
ALCOHOL: → NONE

Adverse Reactions

C: Eighth nerve neurotoxicity
↑ BUN/creatinine
Oliguria
Proteinuria
O: Anemia
Granulocytopenia
Thrombocytopenia
Rash
Fever
Nausea
Diarrhea
R: Exfoliative dermatitis
↑ SGOT/SGPT (AST/ALT)
Disorientation
Mental confusion

Cat. D
③

I II III
Normal dose 20–60% normal dose 10–15% normal dose NONE

Consult PDR
for reduced
dosage nomo-
gram

Tobramycin ophthalmic solution/cream, 1%

(Tobrasol®, Tobrex®)   [$7.45–21.25/5 ml]

Dosage Modifications

	I	II	III
Cat. B		NONE	NONE
②			

Drug Interactions

NONE
FOOD: → NONE
ALCOHOL: → NONE

Adverse Reactions

C: Lid itching
   Lid swelling
   Conjunctival erythema

❶ **Avoid use in pediatric patients!**

Tobramycin + dexamethasone ophthalmic ointment/solution

(TobraDex®)   [$24.38/3.5 gm; $12.50/2.5 ml]

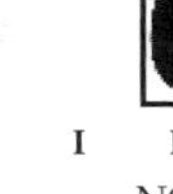

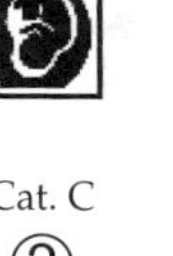

	I	II	III
Cat. C ②		NONE	NONE

Drug Interactions

NONE
FOOD: → NONE
ALCOHOL: → NONE

Adverse Reactions

C: Hypersensitivity
Lid itching
Lid swelling
Conjunctival erythema

O: ↑ Intraocular pressure
Glaucoma
Secondary infections (viral/fungal)

R: Optic nerve damage
Posterior subcapsular cataract
Delayed wound healing

❶ Do not use in pediatric patients!
❶ Do not use for viral infections of the eye!

Tolnaftate topical cream/solution, 1%
(Various OTC Products)   **[$1.38–4.95/15 gm]**

Dosage Modifications

Drug Interactions

NONE
FOOD: → NONE
ALCOHOL: → NONE

Adverse Reactions

C: Mild irritation
O: Sensitization

Cat. B
②

	I	II	III
	NONE	NONE	NONE

Tretinoin cream/gel

[$21.00–25.00/20 gm]
   (Renova®, Retin-A®)   **[$48.00–53.40/40 gm]**
   (Retin-A® Micro)   **[$32.90–20 gm]**

I   II   III

Cat. C   NONE   NONE

③

Drug Interactions

VS: Medicated/abrasive
       soaps
    Drying cosmetics   → drying
    Alcohol-containing   Excessive of skin
       astringents
    Topicals containing sulfur,
    resorcinol or salicylic acid
    should *not* be used with
    Tretinoin

FOOD: → NONE
ALCOHOL: → NONE

❶ **Avoid use in pregnant patients!**

Adverse Reactions

C: Erythema
   Skin edema
   Blistering
   Crusting
O: Hyper- or hypo-pigmentation
   Photosensitivity
R: Liver disorders

Trifluridine ophthalmic solution, 1%
(Viroptic®) [$53.13/7.5 ml]

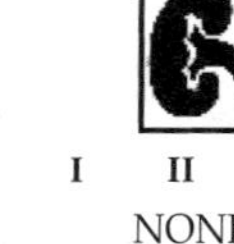

Dosage Modifications

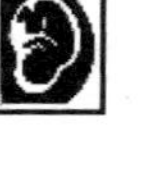 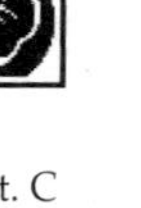 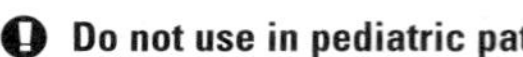

	I	II	III
Cat. C		NONE	NONE
②			

Drug Interactions

NONE
FOOD: → NONE
ALCOHOL: → NONE

Adverse Reactions

C: Burning
   Stinging
   Palpebral edema
O: Superficial punctate keratopathy
   Epithelial keratopathy
R: Hypersensitivity
   Stromal edema
   Keratitis sicca
   Hyperemia
   ↑ Intraocular pressure

❶ **Do not use in pediatric patients!**

Trimethoprim [$0.32]
(Proloprim®) **[$1.66]**

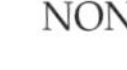  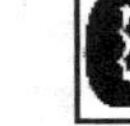

Drug Interactions

VS: Phenytoin →↑ [phenytoin]
Dapsone →↑ [trimethoprim] &
↑ [dapsone]
Amantadine →↑ [amantadine] &
↑ [trimethoprim]
Cyclosporine →↓ [cyclosporine]
Procainamide →↑ [procainamide]
LS: Digoxin →↑ [digoxin]
Zidovudine →↑ [AZT]
FOOD: → NONE
ALCOHOL: → NONE

Adverse Reactions

C: Rash
Pruritus
O: Epigastric disorders
Nausea
Vomiting
Glossitis
↑ SGOT/SGPT
(AST/ALT)
Fever
↑ BUN/creatinine
Thrombocytopenia
Leukopenia
$\uparrow K^+ / \downarrow Na^+$
R: Cholestatic jaundice
Exfoliative dermatitis

Erythema mul-
tiforme
Stevens-
Johnson
syndrome
Lyell
syndrome
Anaphylaxis
Aseptic
meningitis

Cat. C
②

I — 100 mg q12h
II — 50 mg q12h
III — DO NOT USE
NONE

❗ **Avoid use as a single agent in patients < 12 years old!**

Trimethoprim + Sulfamethoxazole

(Septra®, Septra® DS/Bactrim®,
Bactrim® DS)   [$2.52/2.50] (Septra® IV/
Bactrim® IV)   [$34.87–69.74/$70.09–140.18]

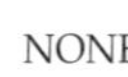 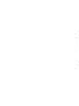 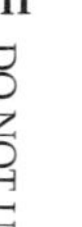

<u>Dosage Modifications</u>

	I	II	III	
Cat. C ③	Normal dose	50% normal dose	DO NOT USE	NONE

Drug Interactions

VS: Anticoagulants →↑ risk of
     bleeding
   Diuretics →↑ incidence of
   (esp. thiazides) thrombocytopenia
     (esp. in elderly)
   Phenytoin →↑ [phenytoin]
   Methotrexate →↑ [MTX]
LS: See Trimethoprim
FOOD: → NONE
ALCOHOL: → NONE

Adverse Reactions

C: Nausea
   Vomiting
   Anorexia
   Rash
   Urticaria
O: Agranulocytosis
   Aplastic anemia
   Thrombocytopenia
   Leukopenia
   ↓ Prothrombin time
   Eosinophilia
   ↓ Iron/folate
   ↑ BUN/creatinine

R: Stevens-Johnson
     syndrome
   Toxic epidermal
     necrolysis
   Erythema
     multiforme
   Renal failure
   Interstitial
     nephritis

❶ Do *not* use in pregnant patients!
❶ Do not use in patients < 2 months old!

Trimetrexate glucuronate
(Neutrexin®) [$121.68 + cost of leucovorin]

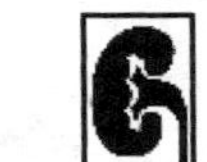
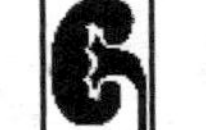

I   II   III

Drug Interactions

VS: Erythromycin ⎫
    Rifampin   ⎬ ↓↑ [trimetrexate]
    Rifabutin   ⎪ and
    Ketoconazole⎬ ↑↓ [interacting
    Fluconazole ⎭   index drug]
    Cimetidine →↑ [trimetrexate]
    Acetaminophen → altered
        trimetrexate metabolites
FOOD: → NONE
ALCOHOL: → NONE

Adverse Reactions

C: Neutropenia
   Thrombocytopenia
   Anemia
   ↑ SGOT/SGPT
     (AST/ALT)
   Fever
   Rash
   Pruritis
   Nausea/Vomiting
   ↑ Alkaline phosphatase
   ↓ Na⁺
O: Confusion
   Fatigue
   ↑ Bilirubin
   ↓ Ca⁺⁺

R: ↑ Creatinine
   Neurologic
   toxicity

Cat. D
③

Interrupt treatment if serum creatinine levels ↑ to >2.5 mg/dL. Drug may be restarted when lab values return to baseline.

Interrupt treatment if SGOT/SGPT or alkaline phosphatase levels ↑ to >5× upper limit of normal. Drug may be restarted when lab values return to baseline.

❶ **MUST be given with Leucovorin concomitantly!**
❶ **Avoid in patients < 18 years old!**
❶ **See PDR for dose modifications for hematologic toxicity!**

Typhoid vaccine, live oral
(Vivotif Berna®)   **[$32.95/series]**

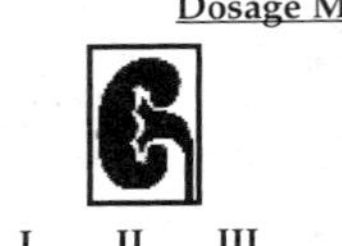

Dosage Modifications

	I	II	III
Cat. C		NONE	NONE
②			

Drug Interactions

VS: Sulfonamides
Antibiotics
(See PDR for specific agents) } →↓ immune response to vaccine

FOOD: → NONE
ALCOHOL: → NONE

Adverse Reactions

C: Abdominal pain
Nausea
Headache
Fever
Diarrhea
Vomiting
O: Skin rash
R: Anaphylactic shock

❶ **Do not use in patients < 6 years old!**

Typhoid Vi Polysaccharide vaccine, intramuscular
(Typhim® Vi) [$35.69]

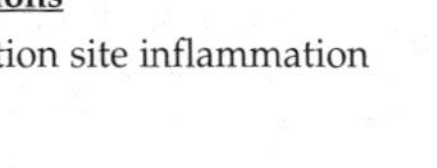

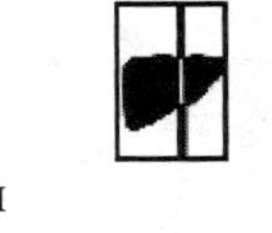 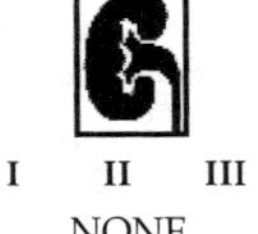

	I	II	III

Drug Interactions

NONE
FOOD: → NONE
ALCOHOL: → NONE

Adverse Reactions

C: Local injection site inflammation
   Headache
   Malaise
   Nausea
O: Myalgia
   Diarrhea
   Fever
R: Allergic reactions

Cat. C
②

NONE   NONE

❶ **Do not use in patients < 2 years old!**

Valacyclovir
(Valtrex®)   [$16.92]

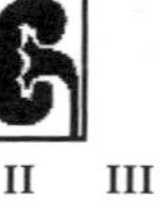

Drug Interactions

VS: Probenecid ⎱ →↑ rate of valocyclovir
Cimetidine ⎰ to acyclovir conversion
& ↑ [acyclovir]

FOOD: → NONE
ALCOHOL: → NONE

Adverse Reactions

C: Nausea
Headache
Vomiting
Diarrhea
O: Constipation
Asthenia
Dizziness
Abdominal pain
Anorexia
R: TTP
Hemolytic uremia syndrome
Facial edema
Thrombocytopenia
Erythema multiforme

Cat. B
②

	I	II	III
	1 gm q8–12h	1 gm q12–24h	500 mg q24h

NONE

❗ **Do not use in pediatric patients!**

Vancomycin IV [$47.50]
(Vancoled®, Vancocin®, Lyphocin®) [$23.04–40.70]

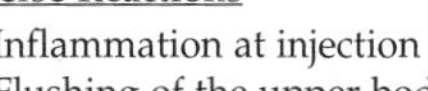

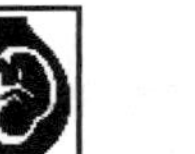
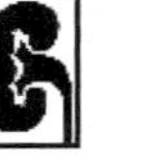

Drug Interactions

VS: Succinylcholine →↑ neuromuscular
    blockade
    Muscle relaxants → prolonged
    respiratory
    depression

Aminoglycosides
Amphotericin B
Bacitracin
Polymyxin B
Colistin
Viomycin
Cisplatin
} →↑ nephrotoxicity

Anesthetic agents → erythema and
    histamine-like
    flushing

LS: Methotrexate →↓ [MTX]
    Indomethacin →↑ [vancomycin]
FOOD: → NONE
ALCOHOL: → NONE

Adverse Reactions

C: Inflammation at injection site
O: Flushing of the upper body
R: Anaphylactoid reactions
   Renal failure
   Interstitial nephritis
   Pseudomembranous colitis
   Ototoxicity
   Neutropenia
   Thrombocytopenia
   Drug fever
   Nausea
   Chills
   Stevens-Johnson syndrome
   Vasculitis

Cat. C
②

	I	II	III
	1 gm q24h	500–750 mg q24h	150 mg q24h

NONE

❶ **Should not be given as rapid bolus—infuse *slowly!***

Varicella-Zoster Virus immune globulin [$448.20]

	I	II	III
Cat. C		NONE	NONE
②			

Drug Interactions

NONE
FOOD: → NONE
ALCOHOL: → NONE

Adverse Reactions

C: Injection site inflammation
O: Fever
   Asthenia
   Myalgia
R: Anaphylaxis

❶ Not recommended for pregnant women.

Varicella-Zoster Virus vaccine
(Varivax®)   [$51.76]

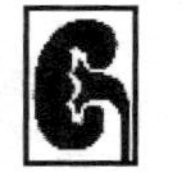 

Drug Interactions	Adverse Reactions			

Drug Interactions

VS: Blood transfusion ⎫
Plasma transfusion ⎬ → interference with vaccine for 2–5 months
Immune globulin (including VZIG) ⎭
Salicylates →↑ incidence of Reye's syndrome

FOOD: → NONE
ALCOHOL: → NONE

Adverse Reactions

C: Injection site inflammation
Fever
Varicella-like rash
O: Headache
Fatigue
Cough
Myalgia
Nausea
Malaise
R: Anaphylaxis
Thrombocytopenia
Guillain-Barré syndrome
Stevens-Johnson syndrome
Reye's syndrome

Cat. C ②   NONE   NONE

❗ **Do not use in pregnant patients!**
❗ **Do not use in patients < 12 months old!**

Vidarabine ophthalmic ointment, 3%

(Vira-A®)   **[$20.77/3.5 gm]**

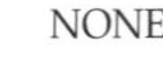

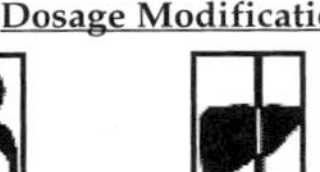 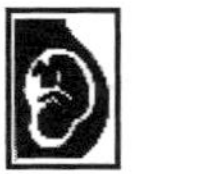 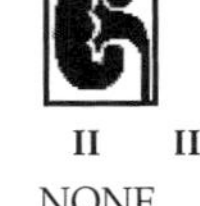

Dosage Modifications

I   II   III

Drug Interactions

NONE
FOOD: → NONE
ALCOHOL: → NONE

Adverse Reactions

C: Lacrimation
    Foreign body sensation
    Temporary visual haze
O: Burning
    Irritation
    Pain
    Photophobia
R: Superficial punctate keratitis
    Punctal occlusion
    Hypersensitivity reaction

Cat. C

③

NONE   NONE

Yellow Fever vaccine
(YF-VAX®)   [$52.06]

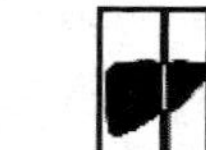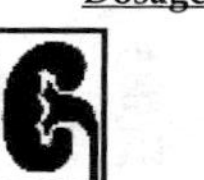

I   II   III

Drug Interactions

Adverse Reactions

In the U.S., Yellow Fever vaccine is supplied only to authorized designated vaccination centers. Information regarding the vaccine and the nearest center may be obtained from the Centers for Disease Control & Prevention (404-639-3670), or your local or state health department.

Zalcitabine (ddC)
(Hivid®) [$6.90]

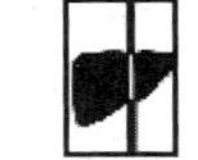

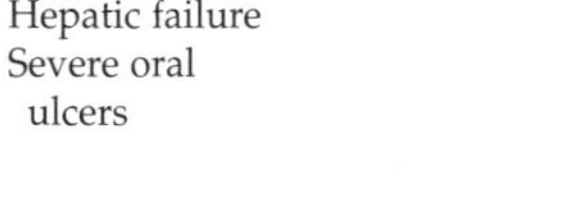

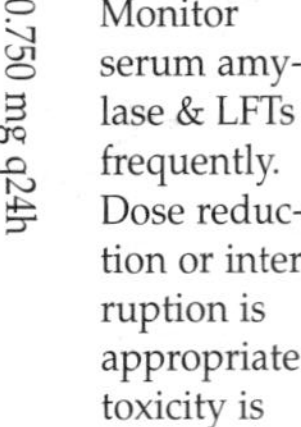

Drug Interactions

VS: Probenecid →↑ [ddC]
Cimetidine →↑ [ddC]
Maalox →↓ [ddC]
LS: Metoclopramide →↓ [ddC]
FOOD: →↓ absorption
ALCOHOL: →↑ risk of
pancreatitis

Adverse Reactions

C: Peripheral neuropathy
Leukopenia/
neutropenia
↑ Amylase
Abnormal hepatic
function
(↑ SGOT/SGPT)
Anemia
O: Fatigue
Headache
Fever
Abdominal pain
Stomatitis/glossitis
Nausea/vomiting
Diarrhea

Rash
Pruritus/
urticaria
Eosinophilia
Thrombocyto-
penia
R: Pancreatitis
Lactic acidosis
Hepatomegaly
with steatosis
Hepatic failure
Severe oral
ulcers

Cat. C
③

I 0.750 mg q8h
II 0.750 mg q12h
III 0.750 mg q24h

Monitor
serum amy-
lase & LFTs
frequently.
Dose reduc-
tion or inter-
ruption is
appropriate if
toxicity is
noted.

❶ **Do not use in patients < 13 years old!**

Zidovudine (AZT)

(Retrovir®) [$9.56]; (Retrovir® IV) [$34.46]

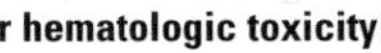
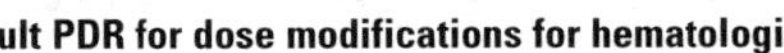

I II III

Drug Interactions

VS: Ganciclovir
Interferon-alpha
Dapsone
Flucytosine
Vincristine
Vinblastine
Adriamycin } ↑ hematologic toxicity
Probenecid →↑ [AZT]
Fluconazole →↑ [AZT]
Atovaquone →↑ [AZT]
Valproic Acid →↑ [AZT]
LS: Lamivudine →↑ [AZT]
Acyclovir →↑ lethargy
Clarithromycin →↓ [AZT]
FOOD: →↓ absorption
ALCOHOL: → NONE

Adverse Reactions

C: Nausea
Abdominal pain
Diarrhea
Vomiting
Dyspepsia
Granulocytopenia
Anemia
Headache
Asthenia
Fever
Anorexia
Myalgia
Rash
Constipation
O: Diaphoresis
Malaise

Dyspepsia
Dizziness
Insomnia/
somnolence
Paresthesia
Dyspnea
Dysgeusia
R: Bone marrow
suppression
Myopathy
Lactic acidosis
Severe hepa-
tomegaly with
steatosis
Pancreatitis
Anaphylaxis

Cat. C
③

600 mg po qd
or 6 mg/kg iv qd

100 mg po q 6–8h
or 1 mg/kg iv q 6–8h

Monitor LFTs
frequently.
Reduce dose
or
discontinue
drug for
severe
toxicity.

❶ Consult PDR for dose modifications for hematologic toxicity!

Zidovudine + lamivudine
(Combivir®)   [$17.24]

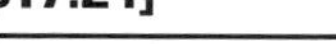 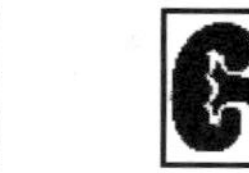 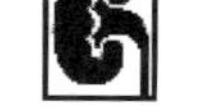 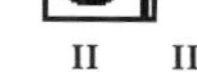

Drug Interactions   **Adverse Reactions**

See listings for Zidovudine and Lamivudine; each Combivir tablet contains 300 mg of Zidovudine and 150 mg of Lamivudine.

Index